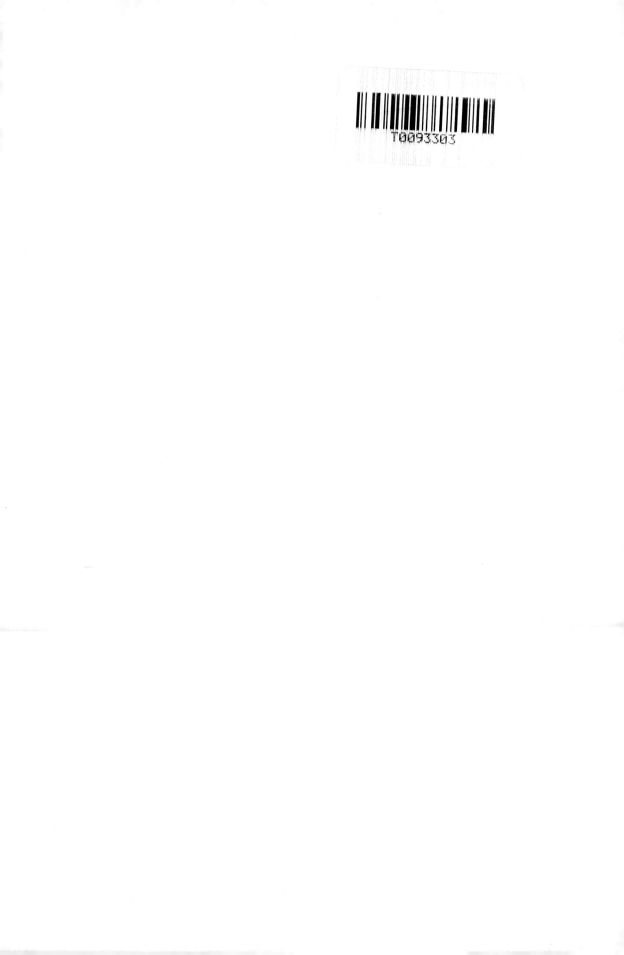
T0093303

Complementary and Alternative Medicines in Prostate Cancer

A Comprehensive Approach

Traditional Herbal Medicines for Modern Times

Each volume in this series provides academia, health sciences, and the herbal medicines industry with in-depth coverage of the herbal remedies for infectious diseases, certain medical conditions, or the plant medicines of a particular country.

Series Editor: Dr. Roland Hardman

Traditional Herbal Medicines for Modern Times

Complementary and Alternative Medicines in Prostate Cancer
A Comprehensive Approach

edited by
K. B. Harikumar

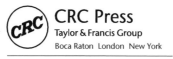

CRC Press
Taylor & Francis Group
Boca Raton London New York

CRC Press is an imprint of the
Taylor & Francis Group, an **informa** business

CRC Press
Taylor & Francis Group
6000 Broken Sound Parkway NW, Suite 300
Boca Raton, FL 33487-2742

First issued in paperback 2021

© 2017 by Taylor & Francis Group, LLC
CRC Press is an imprint of Taylor & Francis Group, an Informa business

No claim to original U.S. Government works

ISBN 13: 978-1-03-209732-9 (pbk)
ISBN 13: 978-1-4987-2987-1 (hbk)

This book contains information obtained from authentic and highly regarded sources. Reasonable efforts have been made to publish reliable data and information, but the author and publisher cannot assume responsibility for the validity of all materials or the consequences of their use. The authors and publishers have attempted to trace the copyright holders of all material reproduced in this publication and apologize to copyright holders if permission to publish in this form has not been obtained. If any copyright material has not been acknowledged please write and let us know so we may rectify in any future reprint.

Except as permitted under U.S. Copyright Law, no part of this book may be reprinted, reproduced, transmitted, or utilized in any form by any electronic, mechanical, or other means, now known or hereafter invented, including photocopying, microfilming, and recording, or in any information storage or retrieval system, without written permission from the publishers.

For permission to photocopy or use material electronically from this work, please access www.copyright.com (http://www.copyright.com/) or contact the Copyright Clearance Center, Inc. (CCC), 222 Rosewood Drive, Danvers, MA 01923, 978-750-8400. CCC is a not-for-profit organization that provides licenses and registration for a variety of users. For organizations that have been granted a photocopy license by the CCC, a separate system of payment has been arranged.

Trademark Notice: Product or corporate names may be trademarks or registered trademarks, and are used only for identification and explanation without intent to infringe.

Publisher's Note
The publisher has gone to great lengths to ensure the quality of this reprint but points out that some imperfections in the original copies may be apparent.

Library of Congress Cataloging-in-Publication Data

Names: Harikumar, K. B., editor.
Title: Complementary and alternative medicines in prostate cancer : a comprehensive approach / [edited by] K.B. Harikumar.
Other titles: Traditional herbal medicines for modern times.
Description: Boca Raton, FL : CRC Press, Taylor & Francis Group, 2017. | Series: Traditional herbal medicines for modern times
Identifiers: LCCN 2016027060| ISBN 9781498729871 (hardback : alk. paper) | ISBN 9781498729888 (e-book)
Subjects: LCSH: Prostate--Cancer--Alternative treatment. | Alternative medicine. | Materia medica, Vegetable.
Classification: LCC RC280.P7 C638 2017 | DDC 616.99/463--dc23
LC record available at https://lccn.loc.gov/2016027060

Visit the Taylor & Francis Web site at
http://www.taylorandfrancis.com

and the CRC Press Web site at
http://www.crcpress.com

Contents

Series Preface

Global warming and global travel are contributing factors in the spread of infectious diseases such as malaria, tuberculosis, hepatitis B and HIV. These are not well controlled by the present drug regimes. Antibiotics are also failing because of bacterial resistance. Formerly less well-known tropical diseases are reaching new shores.

A whole range of illnesses, such as cancer, occur worldwide. Advances in molecular biology, including methods of *in vitro* testing for a required medical activity, give new opportunities to draw judiciously on the use and research of traditional herbal remedies from around the world. The re-examining of the herbal medicines must be done in a multidisciplinary manner.

There have been 51 volumes published since the start of the book series *Medicinal and Aromatic Plants – Industrial Profiles* in 1997. The series continues.

The same Series Editor, Dr Roland Hardman, is also covering a second series entitled *Traditional Herbal Medicines for Modern Times*. Each volume of this series reports on the latest developments and discusses key topics relevant to interdisciplinary health sciences, research by ethnobiologists, taxonomists, conservationists, agronomists, chemists, pharmacologists, clinicians and toxicologists. The series is relevant to all these scientists and enables them to guide business, government agencies and commerce in the complexities of these matters. The background of the subject is outlined next.

Over many centuries, the safety and limitations of herbal medicines have been established by their empirical use by the 'healers' who also took a holistic approach. The healers are aware of the infrequent adverse effects and often know how to correct contraindications when they occur. Consequently, and ideally, the preclinical and clinical studies of a herbal medicine need to be carried out with the full cooperation of the traditional healer. The plant's composition of the medicine, the stage of the development of the plant material, when it is to be collected from the wild or from its cultivation, its postharvest treatment, the preparation of the medicine, the dosage and frequency and much other essential information is required. Consideration of the intellectual property rights and appropriate models of benefit sharing, may also be necessary.

Wherever the medicine is being prepared, the first requirement is a well-documented reference collection of dried plant material. Such collections are encouraged by organizations including the World Health Organization and the United Nations Industrial Development Organization. The Royal Botanic Gardens at Kew (United Kingdom) is now increasing its collection of traditional Chinese dried plant material relevant to its purchase and use by those who sell or prescribe traditional Chinese medicine in the United Kingdom.

In any country, the control of the quality of raw plant material, of its efficacy and of its safety in use, is essential. The work requires sophisticated laboratory equipment and highly trained personnel. This kind of 'control' cannot be applied to the locally produced herbal medicines in the rural areas of many countries, on which millions of people depend. Local traditional knowledge of the healers has to suffice.

Conservation and protection of plant habitats are required and breeding for biological diversity is important. Gene systems are being studied for medicinal exploitation. There can never be too many seed conservation 'banks' to conserve genetic diversity. Unfortunately, such banks are usually dominated by agricultural and horticultural crops, with little space for medicinal plants. Developments, such as random amplified polymorphic DNA, enable the genetic variability of a species to be checked. This can be helpful in deciding whether specimens of close genetic similarity warrant storage.

From ancient times, a great deal of information concerning diagnosis and the use of traditional herbal medicines has been documented in the scripts of China, India and elsewhere. Today, modern formulations of these medicines exist in the form of powders, granules, capsules and tablets. They are prepared in various institutions, such as government hospitals in China and Korea and by companies such as the Tsumura Company of Japan, with good quality control. Similarly, products are produced by many other companies in India, the United States and elsewhere with a varying degree of quality control. In the United States, the Dietary Supplement and Health Education Act of 1994 *recognized* the class of physiotherapeutic agents derived from medicinal and aromatic plants. Furthermore, under public pressure, the US Congress set up an Office of Alternative Medicine. In 1994, this office assisted in the filing of several Investigational New Drug applications (IND) required for clinical trials of some Chinese herbal preparations. The significance of these applications was that each Chinese preparation involved several plants and yet was handled with a single IND. A demonstration of the contribution to efficacy, of *each* ingredient of *each* plant, was not required. This was a major step forward towards more sensible regulations with regard to phytomedicines.

The subject of Western herbal medicines is now being taught again to medical students in Germany and Canada. Throughout Europe, the United States, Australia and other countries, pharmacy and health-related schools are increasingly offering training in phytotherapy. Traditional Chinese medicine clinics are now common outside of China. An Ayurvedic hospital now exists in London, with a BSc. Honours degree course in Ayurvedic Medicine being available: Professor Shrikala Warrier, Registrar/Dean, MAYUR, Ayurvedic University of Europe, 81 Wimpole Street, London, WIG 9RF, email sw@unifiedherbal.com. This is a joint venture with a university in Manipal, India.

The term *integrated medicine*, which selectively combines traditional herbal medicine with 'modern medicine', is now being used. In Germany, there is now a hospital in which traditional Chinese medicine is integrated with Western medicine. Such co-medication has become common in China, Japan, India and North America by those educated in both systems. Benefits claimed include improved efficacy, reduction in toxicity and the period of medication, as well as a reduction in the cost of the treatment. New terms, such as *adjunct therapy, supportive therapy* and *supplementary medicine* now appear as a consequence of such co-medication. Either medicine may be described as an adjunct to the other, depending on the communicator's view. Great caution is necessary when traditional herbal medicines are used by doctors not trained in their use and likewise when modern medicines are used by traditional herbal doctors. Possible dangers from drug interactions need to be stressed.

Roland Hardman, BPharm, BSc (Chemistry), PhD (London), FRPharmS
Head of Pharmacognosy (retired), School of Pharmacy and Pharmacology
University of Bath, United Kingdom

Preface

Recent global cancer statistics clearly indicate that prostate cancer is the second most frequently diagnosed cancer (at 15% of all male cancers) and globally the sixth leading cause of cancer death in males. There has been tremendous development in various treatment strategies for prostate cancer in the last few decades. However, evidence suggests that along with conventional therapies a large number of patients still rely on various types of Complementary and Alternative Medicine (CAM). The National Cancer Institute definition of CAM states, "Complementary and alternative medicine is a form of treatment used in addition to (complementary) or instead of (alternative) standard treatments."

Medicinal plants constitute the major portion of various CAM-based treatment modalities. Several studies have been reported to show the potential benefits of medicinal plants and their isolated products in prostate cancer. The preclinical data is highly promising, but sufficient clinical data is still needed. Many patients also follow a variety of other systems such as Ayurveda, homeopathy, Siddha, acupuncture, yoga, and naturopathy approaches.

In this book we have summarized the available information on various preclinical and clinical trials involving CAM in prostate cancer. The book provides up-to-date references for academics, clinical practitioners, research scholars, as well as the general public.

I would like to express my sincere gratitude to Dr. Roland Hardman, series editor, for giving me an opportunity to edit this book and for his continuous support and valuable suggestions and for his own chapter.

I would like to acknowledge all the contributors for their valuable effort and time. Special thanks are due to my wife Kanni Das and my laboratory members Sabira Mohammed and Manendra Babu for proofreading the manuscript. My sincere thanks to John Sulzycki and Jill Jurgensen and her successor Jennifer Blaise of CRC Press for their unfailing help.

K.B. Harikumar

About the Editor

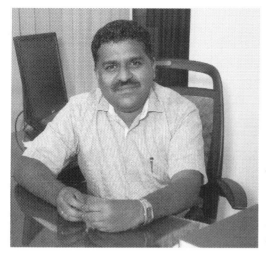

K.B. Harikumar, PhD, earned his bachelor's and master's degrees from Nagpur University in India. His doctoral research was conducted under the direction of Dr. Ramadasan Kuttan at Amala Cancer Research Centre, affiliated with Mahatma Gandhi University at Kottayam in India. Subsequently he conducted his post-doctoral research at the Department of Experimental Therapeutics, University of Texas MD Anderson Cancer Center (Houston, Texas) and the Department of Biochemistry and Molecular Biology, Virginia Commonwealth University (Richmond, Virginia). He is currently a faculty member in the cancer research program at the Rajiv Gandhi Centre for Biotechnology (an autonomous institution of the Department of Biotechnology, Government of India) in Thiruvananthapuram, India. He has over 40 peer-reviewed publications and several book chapters to his credit. His major research focuses are the role of bioactive lipid signaling in inflammation and cancer, and cancer chemoprevention.

Contributors

Hakima Amri
Department of Biochemistry and Cellular and
  Molecular Biology
Georgetown University
Washington DC, USA

T. Anandan
Central Council for Research in Siddha
Ministry of AYUSH, Government of India
Chennai, India

Frank Arfuso
Curtin Health Innovation Research Institute
Curtin University
Perth, Western Australia

Apoorva Arora
Amity Institute of Biotechnology
Amity University Uttar Pradesh
Noida, India

Sourav Bhattacharya
Department of Pathology
St. Louis University
St. Louis, Missouri, USA

V. Gayathri Devi
Regional Research Institute for Siddha
Ministry of AYUSH, Government of India
Thiruvananthapuram, India

Krishna Vanaja Donkena
Department of Urology
Mayo Clinic
Rochester, Minnesota, USA

Dallas Donohoe
Department of Nutrition
Laboratory for Cancer Research
University of Tennessee
Knoxville, Tennessee, USA

Christopher Funes
Department of Biochemistry and Cellular and
  Molecular Biology
Georgetown University
Washington, DC, USA

Manuela Martins-Green
Department of Cell Biology and Neuroscience
University of California
Riverside, California, USA

Sanjay Gupta
Department of Chemistry
Case Western Reserve University
Cleveland, Ohio, USA

K.B. Harikumar
Cancer Research Program
Rajiv Gandhi Centre for Biotechnology
Thiruvananthapuram, Kerala State, India

Roland Hardman
School of Pharmacy and Pharmacology
University of Bath
Bath, UK

S. Syed Hissar
National Institute for Research in Tuberculosis
  (NIRT)
Indian Council of Medical Research (ICMR)
Chetpet, Chennai, India

E-Chu Huang
Department of Nutrition
Laboratory for Cancer Research
University of Tennessee
Knoxville, Tennessee, USA

Omran Karmach
Department of Cell Biology and Neuroscience
University of California
Riverside, California, USA

Nikta Rezakahn Khajeh
Department of Urology
University of California
Irvine, California, USA

Cyrus Khoyilar
Department of Urology
University of California
Irvine, California, USA

Vaishali Kuchewar
Mahatma Gandhi Ayurved College
    Hospital and Research Centre
Wardha, Maharashtra, India

Alan Prem Kumar
Department of Pharmacology
Yong Loo Lin School of Medicine
National University of Singapore
Singapore

A. Rajendra Kumar
Siddha Regional Research Institute
Ministry of AYUSH, Government of India
Kuyavarpalayam, Puducherry, India

Manendra Babu L.
Cancer Research Program
Rajiv Gandhi Centre for Biotechnology
Thiruvananthapuram, Kerala State, India

Amber MacDonald
Department of Nutrition
Laboratory for Cancer Research
University of Tennessee
Knoxville, Tennessee, USA

Jeniece Montellano
Department of Chemistry
Case Western Reserve University
Cleveland, Ohio, USA

Revathy Nadhan
Cancer Research Program
Rajiv Gandhi Centre for Biotechnology
Thiruvananthapuram, Kerala State, India

Sudhir Rawal
Rajiv Gandhi Cancer Institute
    and Research Centre
Rohini, New Delhi, India

Ratna B. Ray
Department of Pathology
St. Louis University
St. Louis, Missouri, USA

R.S. Reshma
Cancer Research Program
Rajiv Gandhi Centre for Biotechnology
Thiruvananthapuram, Kerala State, India

S. Selvarajan
Regional Research Institute for Siddha
Ministry of AYUSH, Government of India
Thiruvananthapuram, India

Gautam Sethi
Department of Pharmacology
Yong Loo Lin School of Medicine
National University of Singapore
Singapore

Girish Sharma
Amity Center for Cancer Epidemiology and
    Cancer Research
Amity Institute of Biotechnology
Amity University Uttar Pradesh
Noida, India

Eswar Shankar
Department of Urology
Case Western Reserve University
Cleveland, Ohio, USA

Muthu K. Shanmugam
Department of Pharmacology
Yong Loo Lin School of Medicine
National University of Singapore
Singapore

Priya Srinivas
Cancer Research Program
Rajiv Gandhi Centre for Biotechnology
Thiruvananthapuram, Kerala State, India

Muthuirulappan Srinivasan
Department of Biochemistry
Jaya College of Arts & Science
Thiruninravur, Chennai, India

Athira Thampy
Pranavam Clinic, Mudavanmugal
Thiruvananthapuram, Kerala State, India

Robert Thomas
Cranfield University
Bedford, UK

Yadu Vijayan
Cancer Research Program
Rajiv Gandhi Centre for Biotechnology
Thiruvananthapuram, Kerala State, India

Arman Walia
Department of Urology
University of California
Irvine, California, USA

Jay Whelan
Department of Nutrition
Laboratory for Cancer Research
University of Tennessee
Knoxville, Tennessee, USA

Michael Wu
Department of Urology
University of California
Irvine, California, USA

Charles Y.F. Young
Department of Urology
Mayo Clinic
Rochester, Minnesota, USA

Yi Zhao
Department of Nutrition
Laboratory for Cancer Research
University of Tennessee
Knoxville, Tennessee, USA

Xiaolin Zi
Department of Urology
University of California
Irvine, California, USA

CHAPTER 1

Prostate Cancer: An Introduction

Manendra Babu L., Yadu Vijayan, and K.B. Harikumar

CONTENTS

1.1   INTRODUCTION

Prostate cancer (PC) is the leading malignancy among men around the world. Although it is the second most incident cancer, it stands only at the sixth position in death rate. This huge difference between incidence and mortality is due to the slow and constant rate of headway of the disease resulting in a long latent preclinical stage. Almost 80% of men in their eighties have a high chance of developing PC, and around 50% of men in their late fifties have prostatic intraepithelial neoplasia, which greatly increases the risk of PC. Prostate cancer also shows great dependency on the effect of race and genetic and epigenetic changes. Black men have a higher chance of developing PC, and native Japanese have the lowest (Altekruse et al., 2010; Bunker et al., 2002). People migrating from Southeast Asia to the west have a higher risk of PC, indicating the effect of epidemiological and environmental factors in PC (Peto, 2001). Most men affected with PC have an apathetic form of disease which does not require treatment. Only 10–20% of those affected with the more aggressive form of the disease may develop metastasis, ultimately resulting in death. The inability to distinguish between the two forms of PC has resulted in undertreatment or overtreatment in many cases (Delpierre et al., 2013; Lee et al., 2013; Moyer, 2012).

1.2   THE PROSTATE GLAND

The prostate gland is the compound exocrine gland associated with the human male reproductive system. On average the size of a walnut, the prosate is positioned at the bottom of the urinary bladder. It is incompletely surrounded by a thin capsule anteriorly supported by pubovesical ligament and inferiorly by urogenital diaphragm. During puberty the size of the prostate gland expands counter to the level of serum testosterone. The prostate gland is made of three kinds of cells: the gland cells, which secrete the fluid portion of semen; the muscle cells, which regulate urine flow and ejaculation; and the fibrous cells, which support the gland. The glandular cells of the prostate comprise the luminal cells, basal cells, and neuroendocrine cells. The urethra, which allows the passage of urine, passes through the prostate gland. The prostate gland also has a very important role in making the semen alkaline, and increases the life span of sperm (Kim and Kim, 2013).

1.3   THE ORIGIN AND EVOLUTION OF PROSTATE CANCER

One of the most interesting questions in cancer biology is whether the oncogenic transformation of different cell types in a single tissue gives rise to the same or different cancers. In the context of PC, the answer is yes. The tumors developed from different cell lineages act as different entities regardless of whether their origin is from the same tissue or organ. Subclones originate as a result of the rivalry for various niches, and this follows the Darwinian theory of evolution. The rejuvenative capacity of the prostate organ is integral, as it perpetuates adult stem cells in luminal and basal layers. The luminal cells express high androgen receptor levels, whereas basal cells express markers like CK5, CK14 and p63 (Shen and Abate-Shen, 2010). The phenotype of the tumor is also dependent on the cell of origin. These are elucidated by lineage tracing experiments. In the cell-of-origin model, the heterogeneous tumors originating from different cell types show varied phenotypic and genotypic changes such as expression patterns, mutational status, prognostic markers, and differential response to treatment (Visvader, 2011). In PC, both luminal cells and basal cells have the potential to give rise to tumors with different phenotypic changes. In 2013, Wang et al. used genetic lineage marking to show the stemness property attained by each cell population and proved that both luminal and basal cells have the capacity to give rise to tumors but the aggression of the tumor will be elevated if it has a luminal origin. This is why certain patients develop aggressive tumors when compared to the indolent disease, which requires minimal treatment (Wang et al., 2013).

Almost 90% of cancer deaths are due to metastasis (Gupta and Massagué, 2006). The primary heterogeneous tumor usually evolves into the metastatic state by dissemination, but the principles superintending this process are less known. It was previously thought that cells that metastasize emanate from a single clone, but there is a great deal of evidence from mouse experiments that shows multiple clones at the same metastatic site (McFadden et al., 2014). Next-generation sequencing results from various primary and metastatic PC patients divulge some interesting facts. In 2015, Gundem et al. showed that the polyclonal seeding of metastasis occurs in many cases, and they were able to locate a set of mutations which are common in all the polyclonal metastatic sites representing the origin of those set from the founder cell. Most of the metastatic clones will be transformed into castration-resistant PC, which shows resistance to androgen deprivation therapy. They found that in the same patient, castration will be achieved by distinct independent mechanisms between different subclones. Some achieve it by amplification of the *MYC* gene, and a few by mutation in *AR* gene, and also by bypassing the *AR* pathway. Sequencing of multiple metastatic sites showed that they are different from the primary tumor, and a close similarity was observed between the metastatic regions from the same tissue, which raises questions about geological proximity or tissue-specific seeding. It has also been shown that multiple subclones from a primary tumor can give rise to multiple metastatic sites. Almost all the patients showed a similar clone with definite metastatic potential and the largest cluster of mutations. Most of the subclones are different but they maintain the genetic print of the ancestor and compete for supremacy across the entire system (Gundem et al., 2015).

1.4   RISK FACTORS

Familial factors are related to the risk of PC more than diet and other potential confounders. It has been observed that in affected family members risk increased as the number of affected family members increased, and was inversely related to age (Lesko et al., 1996). In breast cancer, it has been shown that mutations, especially in the susceptible genes *BRCA1/2*, are amalgamated with a more aggressive PC phenotype with a higher risk of nodal intimacy and distant metastasis (Castro et al., 2013). The presence of a germline BRCA2 mutation is a prognostic marker associated with deprived survival outcome. Thus BRCA mutations should be rated for analyzing the disease status of these patients (Bunker et al., 2002). Even though family history was found to be a significant risk factor for PC, its molecular mechanism is poorly understood. It has been shown through linkage studies that chromosome site 17q21-22 is a possible location of a PC vulnerability gene. A study by Ewing et al. scrutinized families by linkage analysis, and from 94 unrelated patients with PC, more than 200 gene variants in the 17q21-22 region were found by germline DNA sequencing. A significantly higher risk of hereditary PC is found to be linked with the novel *HOXB13* G84E variant, but the mechanism by which this mutation contributes to PC development is largely unknown. In prostate and other cancers HOXB13 is implicated both as a tumor suppressor and as an oncogene. The breast cancer susceptibility genes have not shown a possible role in hereditary PC, even though they were associated with elevations in the risk of PC. The *HOXB13* G84E mutation was also associated with increased risk of hereditary PC, and although this mutation is only found in a small portion of men it may have strong implications for PC risk factor assessment (Ewing et al., 2012). The prostatic intraepithelial neoplasia (PIN) which comes under the category of high grade does not depend on the PSA levels, which are usually used as an explorative marker for PC in African men who migrated to America. They are prone to PC with high incidence and mortality rates (Chornokur et al., 2013). In a small pilot study, it was observed that increase in relative telomere length after 5 years of follow-up in men with biopsy-proven low-risk PC was found to be coupled with comprehensive lifestyle involvement (Ornish et al., 2013). Insulin-like growth factor-I (IGF-I) is a mitogen and an anti-apoptotic signal for prostate epithelial cells (Cohen et al., 1994; Cohen et al., 1991; Rajah et al., 1997). Plasma IGF-I has been identified as a compelling predictor of PC risk (Chan et al., 1998). Enzalutamide and abiraterone are new treatment modalities for the management of castration-resistant PC which are directed at the androgen receptor (Scher et al., 2012; Ryan et al., 2013; Cunha et al., 1987). The androgen-receptor isoform encoded by splice variant 7, which is the target of enzalutamide and abiraterone, remains constitutively active as a transcription factor despite the fact that it lacks the ligand-binding domain. In men with advanced stage PC the resistance to enzalutamide and abiraterone could be due to the presence of androgen-receptor coded by the splice variant 7 messenger RNA (AR-V7) in the circulating tumor cells (Antonarakis et al., 2014). Sex steroids, mostly androgens, are found to have an important role in the pathogenesis of PC. Within normal endogenous ranges, high levels of circulating testosterone and low levels of sex hormone–binding globulin (SHBG) are related to a higher risk of PC. Low levels of circulating estradiol could also signify as an additional risk factor (Gann et al., 1996).

1.5 TUMOR MICROENVIRONMENT

In tumor development and progression, the interaction between cancer cells and microenvironment is vital. The role of micro-RNAs (miRs) on tumor microenvironments has not been vastly studied. In a study by Musumeci et al., the downregulation of miR-15 and miR-16 in fibroblasts bordering the prostate tumors was observed in most of the patients analyzed. Reduced post-transcriptional repression of Fgf-2 and its receptor Fgfr1 is responsible for such downregulation in cancer-associated fibroblasts (CAFs) promoting tumor growth and progression. It acts on both the stromal cells and the tumor cells to augment cancer cell survival, proliferation and migration. In fact, *in vitro* and *in vivo* tumor-supportive potential of stromal cells was impaired significantly by reconstituting miR-15 and miR-16. New avenues in treatment modalities can be opened by involving a reconstitution of miR-15 and miR-16 in highly developed PC (Musumeci et al., 2011).

During early PC development, reactive stroma initiates and coevolves with cancer progression, and the key markers are established for a reactive stroma. It has a key role in prostate tumorigenesis and progression. Even if the stem/progenitor cells of origin and their mechanism of regulation of recruitment are largely not identified, some key regulatory factors are recognized. These include transforming growth factor β, interleukin-8, fibroblast growth factors, connective tissue growth factor, wingless homologs-Wnts, and stromal cell-derived factor-1. New therapeutic strategies can focus on coevolution of reactive stroma and reactive stroma–carcinoma interactions that can control cancer development and metastasis. Similarly, uncoupling of reactive stroma to inhibit cancer progression can be used as a combined strategy with the current treatment regime (Berger et al., 2011).

Acquired resistance to anticancer drugs is another distressing problem found in malignant tumors. Cellular phenotypes, like susceptibilities to toxic insults, are influenced mainly by the machinery of tissue microenvironments. The Wnt family member, wingless-type MMTV integration site family member 16B (WNT16B), has been recognized among a spectrum of secreted proteins derived from the tumor microenvironment by analyzing genotoxic stress-induced transcriptional regulation by cancer therapeutics. WNT16B expression is regulated by the activation of the canonical Wnt signaling in tumor cells by a nuclear factor of κ light polypeptide gene enhancer in B cells 1 (NF-κB) following DNA damage and subsequent paracrine signaling. In the prostate tumor microenvironment, the expression of WNT16B attenuated the effects of cytotoxic chemotherapy *in vivo*, promoting tumor cell survival and disease development. This indicates that genotoxic therapies set in a cyclic manner can greatly contribute in overcoming treatment resistance by tumor microenvironment (Sun et al., 2012).

Tumor and stromal communications are indispensable during oncogenesis. The influence of reactive stromal fibroblasts – myofibroblast or CAFs and the molecular events driving the growth and invasion of PC – has been poorly understood. Cancer-activated or cancer-associated fibroblasts can be distinguished from normal fibroblasts (NSFs) by increased numbers of fibroblasts with a myofibroblastic phenotype (Ostman and Augsten, 2009). Incitement of stromal fibroblasts leading to cancer progression has a prognostic importance in PC (Ao et al., 2007; Yanagisawa et al., 2007). It has been shown that stromal cell–derived factor 1 (SDF-1 or CXCL12) and its receptors (CXCR4 and RDC1/CXCR7) play a crucial role in PC metastasis (Sun et al., 2005; Wang et al., 2008). The ATP-generating glycolytic enzyme, phosphoglycerate kinase-1 (PGK1) involves the glycolytic pathway and has direct implications in CXCL12–CXCR4 signaling. In a study by Wang et al., a strong upregulation of PGK1 was observed in prostate tumors by laser capture microdissection and cDNA microarray analysis. Normal fibroblasts overexpressing the PGK1 showed increased expression of smooth muscle α-actin and vimentin, and also elevated levels of CXCL12 similar to myofibroblasts. An elevated proliferative index was also shown by these cells. The overexpression of MMP-2 and MMP-3 along with the activation of AKT and ERK pathways highlight its contribution to tumor cell invasion *in vitro*. Tumor cell growth in PC cells was enhanced by co-implantation of PGK1 overexpressing fibroblasts *in vivo*. Together these implicate a pivotal role for microenvironment interactions and the expression of PGK1 in cancer development (Wang et al., 2010).

1.6 DISEASE PROGRESSION AND PSA LEVELS

During the initial stages of developing PC, the levels of PSA increase gradually and the tumor will be indolent and clinically localized to prostate (Figure 1.1). Surgical resection helps in saving the patient. After a few months of monitoring, if the PSA levels again rise, the chance of recurrence can be predicted. At this stage the clinician suggests androgen deprivation therapy. The PC cells depend on certain androgen hormones like testosterone for their growth, and diminishing the androgen signaling will lead to senescence. Testicles are the major androgen-synthesizing organ, and surgical resection will deprive the PC cells. Other methods are to use certain antagonists which can impede the synthesis of testosterone. Luteinizing hormone releasing hormone (LHRH) which is secreted by the brain stimulates testicles to produce testosterone through luteinizing hormone. Blocking LHRH leads to androgen deprivation, which replicates testicle removal clinically. Few

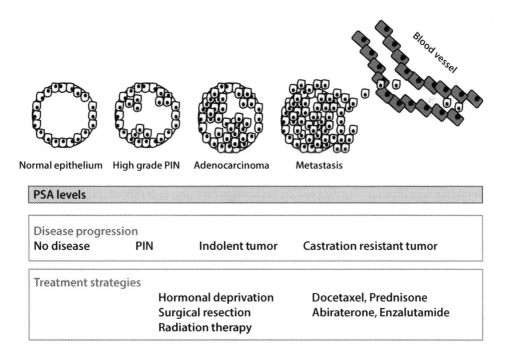

Figure 1.1 Development of prostate cancer from the normal epithelium. First, a high-grade prostate intraepithelial neoplasia develops which increases the chance of development of prostate cancer leading to indolent tumor and castration-resistant tumor. The PSA levels rise during the transformation from PIN to tumor. Certain treatment strategies are also highlighted during the disease progression.

drugs will directly target androgen receptor because of their higher efficiency of binding with androgen receptor than testosterone (Nouri et al., 2015). The patient responds well at first and the reduction in PSA levels can be seen, but gradually he will become resistant because the cancer cells evolve faster. The cancer cells become sensitive to hormonal deprivation by adapting various strategies, such as mutations in the androgen receptor. The PSA levels shoot up and the disease progresses to castration-resistant PC. Almost 15% of cancer patients enter into this stage and the levels of PSA in the serum increases. Docetaxel is the recommended drug during this stage, but only 48 to 50% of patients respond as indicated by the decrease in PSA levels. The rest are affected by the toxicity of the drug and a few cases acquired resistance to it, leading to incurable and more aggressive cancer (Prensner et al., 2012, Zhao et al., 2009).

1.7   SIGNALING PATHWAYS REGULATE CERTAIN HALLMARKS OF PC

1.7.1   Sustained Proliferative Signaling

Cytokine signaling plays a crucial role in PC progression. Protein inhibitors of activated signal transducers and activators of transcription (PIAS1) play a prime role in regulating cytokine signaling. It impedes the transcription factor STAT1 from binding to DNA, which results in downregulation of STAT1-regulated genes, mainly cytokines. It can also result in sumoylation of STAT1, resulting in the inhibition of IFN-γ mediated transactivation. The upregulation of PIAS1 protein leads to increased cell proliferation and downregulation results in increased p21 expression and cell cycle arrest at G0/G1 phase. It has been shown that PIAS1 expression is regulated by androgenic hormones and it also acts as a coactivator for androgenic receptor, which plays a central role in PC development (Hoefer et al., 2012). Next generation sequencing has brought an era of big data which has increased the complexity of existing signaling pathways and has also paved the way for finding new pathways. Along with the coding transcripts, other important molecules like antisense transcripts, miRNAs, and long noncoding RNAs and their biological significance were also identified. The C-terminal binding protein 1 (CTBP1) acts as a co-repressor for androgen receptor, and its androgen-responsive antisense transcript CTBP1-AS upregulates and localizes to nucleus in PC. Functional studies have shown that it promotes both androgen-dependent and castration-resistant tumor growth. It also procures PSF, an RNA-binding transcriptional repressor which inhibits CTBP1 and other tumor suppressor genes, resulting in cell cycle progression (Takayama et al., 2013). miRNAs are 21–24 nucleotide length short RNAs which regulate various cell functions, predominantly in pathological conditions. One of the most important miRNAs upregulated in PC is miR-153, and it has been shown to upregulate the expression of cyclinD1 and downregulate p21 expression. It carries out its function by directing the phosphorylation of FOXO1 and AKT and it directly targets 3′-UTR region of PTEN mRNA. Similarly it has another function by acting as an onco-miR which regulates PC development and progression (Wu et al., 2013).

1.7.2   Invasion and Metastasis

PC initiation and progression involves many alterations in genetic and epigenetic levels which involve various mutations in TP53, EGFR and KRAS, loss of functional PTEN, and other genomic rearrangements (Berger et al., 2011). These genome level changes are mediated by certain epigenetic factors by altered expression of histone demethylase LSD1, histone methyltransferases such as MMSET and EZH2, and histone deacetylases. Downregulation of MMSET showed reduced cell proliferation, migration, and colony formation ability, and its overexpression showed the opposite.

The MMSET binds on TWIST1 locus, leading to an increase in H3K36me2 resulting in upregulated TWIST1, which acts as one of the core EMT promoting genes, and similarly many epigenetic factors regulate various EMT markers for promoting metastasis (Ezponda et al., 2013). Certain genes have differential organ-specific functions that play different roles in the progression of diseases that are specific to different organs. For example, differentiation related gene-1 suppressed tumor growth in bladder cancer, whereas it no effect on colon cancer but showed reduction in liver metastasis. In PC, it suppressed tumor metastasis with no effect on primary tumor growth, but the molecular mechanism is still undiscovered (Bandyopadhyay et al., 2003). The most common mutation or alteration found in PC is within *PTEN*. Almost 30% of primary tumors and 63% of metastatic tumors have *PTEN* mutations or express truncated proteins. Its phosphatase activity is involved in termination of PI3K/AKT pathways, and thus loss of PTEN leads to accumulation of PIP3 and activation of AKT, which in turn results in activation of key signaling molecules like BAD, which plays a role in cell survival and metabolism. The homozygous deletion of PTEN in mouse models resulted in early metastatic tumor development which exactly mimicked the human model, but a single PTEN deletion did not lead to metastasis (Wang et al., 2003). In humans, many other alterations along with PTEN can lead to aggressive tumor development and metastasis. Microarray analysis of patient samples revealed the activation of the RAS/MAPK pathway in both primary and metastatic lesions. The activation of RAS cannot induce tumors and metastasis alone, but when it is combined with loss of PTEN results in 100% penetrance towards metastasis. Thus, targeting PI3K/AKT pathway and PTEN/RAS/MAPK helps in reducing the tumor burden (Mulholland et al., 2012).

In normal prostate tissue, the expression of fibroblast growth factor receptor 1 (FGFR1) is confined to stroma with no expression in epithelial cells, whereas in cancer cells, its expression goes up. The ligand for FGFR1 is FGF2 which is overexpressed in tumor stroma. This gives a clue that stromal cells are supporting the activation of FGFR1 in the cancer cells. The targeted deletion of FGFR1 results in small-sized tumors with 0% metastasis and prolonged survival in mice. Leaky expression resulted in poorly differentiated phenotypes, suggesting a permissive role of ectopic FGFR1 signaling in tumor progression mainly in metastasis (Yang et al., 2013). G protein–coupled receptors occupy a distinct position in the developmental stages of cancer. The signaling is mediated by their interaction with the associated G proteins, leading to several downstream-signaling pathways. Among various G proteins, GNA12/GNA13 is the most important in the context of cancer. GNA13 expression is high in PC and is involved in SDF-1 induced invasion and metastasis, but the correlation is gone astray between the protein and transcript levels. This happens due to the loss of miRNA-182 and miRNA-200a, which can transcriptionally regulate the expression of GNA13 (Rasheed et al., 2013).

1.7.3 Angiogenesis

Angiogenesis is the capillary sprouting of new blood vessels from the preexisting ones, which helps in fueling solid tumors with the adequate and required nutrient supply (Van Moorselaar and Voest, 2002). PC cells have the ability to produce certain angiogenic-inducing factors such as fibroblast growth factor 2, vascular endothelial growth factor, cyclooxygenase-2, transforming growth factor-B, and metalloproteases such as MMP2 and 9 (Wood et al., 1997). VEGF, an important angiogenic factor, was shown to be overexpressed in most PC patients, and its expression correlated with tumor grade and clinical outcome (Ling et al., 2005). In the prostate, the epithelial homeostasis occurs by perpetuating TGF-β through its three receptors. In PC, the loss of TGF-β1 receptors leads to high-grade tumors and the tumors will become insensitive to TGF-B, leading to more aggressive tumors (Kim et al., 1998). Cycloxygenase-2 is an important enzyme which catalyzes the conversion of arachidonic acid to prostaglandins and other eicosanoids and is regulated by various cytokines. COX-2 inhibition leads to reduced tumor growth and angiogenesis (Van Moorselaar and Voest,

2002) but the COX-2 inhibitors failed in the market because of their side effects. Jain et al. showed that targeting prostaglandin E2, which is a metabolite of COX-2, can reduce tumor angiogenesis by targeting epidermal growth factor receptor through EP-2 and EP-4 mediated pathways. Targeting PEG2 also halts the activation of activating transcription factor 4, which leads to reduced expression of vascular endothelial growth factor and urokinase-type plasminogen activator, which are imperative for invasion and angiogenesis (Jain et al., 2008).

1.7.4　Metabolic Reprogramming in PC

The postulation by Warburg on the new and emerging hallmarks of cancer has brought in metabolic reprogramming as one of the crucial and indispensable characters of cancer. In the field of cancer biology, metabolic reprogramming was dominated by the glycolytic pathway and fluorodeoxyglucose positron emission tomography (FDG-PET) is an emerging technique which detects cancer by metabolic imaging (Yeh et al., 1996). Cancer cells devour a large amount of glucose as an energy source and by labeling this glucose, it enters the cell in high amounts mimicking the usual glucose import mechanism. The glucose will be metabolized to lactate through glycolysis by the cancer cell, and the rate of glycolysis is 200 times higher than a normal cell. This lactate will be then rapidly effluxed out by monocarboxylate transporters, which are always overexpressed in cancer cells. In the advanced stages, PC shows a high glycolytic phenotype, which correlates with a poor prognosis (Pertega-Gomes et al., 2015). Recently, tricarboxylic acid cycle (TCA) and oxidative phosphorylation (OXPHOS) were also shown to be involved. In PC, androgen receptor, which is mainly involved in cancer progression, plays a critical role in metabolic switching. This is done by activating 5′-AMP activated protein kinase, which acts as a master metabolic sensor. AMPK governs the cellular energetics by modulating the usage of sugars, fats and proteins as fuel. The activated AMPK potentiates PGC-1alpha, leading to high mitochondrial function and increased β-oxidation, generating surplus amounts of ATP. This mechanism is somewhat contradictory to the already established glycogen-dominant models, but the blockage of mitochondrial biogenesis leads to cancer cell death, which highlights the authenticity of this model (Tennakoon et al., 2014). The metabolic reprogramming of tumor stromal cells also influences PC growth. In tumor biology, cancer-associated fibroblasts occupy a distinct status in the microenvironment. In PC, p62 levels were reduced in the stromal cells, resulting in the inactivation of mTORC1 leading to metabolic reprogramming through c-Myc inactivation. This reprogramming leads to elevated IL6 production by the stromal cells, which further increases the proliferative and invasive capabilities of malignant epithelial cells and creates a proinflammatory environment around the tumor (Valencia et al., 2014).

1.7.5　Inflammation

Chronic inflammation is one of the insults faced by the cells through their own host machinery. It is known for its promotion in initiation and progression of various malignancies by inducing both epigenetic and genetic factors. Many epidemiological studies have highlighted this risk factor, which causes inflammation-induced cancer. In PC, almost 20% of patients suffering with chronic inflammation develop tumors which arise due to various reasons (De Marzo et al., 2007). There is always a bias due to unawareness of prostatitis, which does not show many symptoms, and ideally many people with PC would have a history of prostatitis. The chronic inflammation causes accumulation of proinflammatory cytokines and various growth factors, which leads to uncontrolled proliferation leading to a higher chance of oncogenic mutations. Many reports have shown that the tumor milieu of the prostate consists of CD4+, CD25+ and CD8+ FoxP3+ regulatory T cells, which play a vital role in immune suppression (Stallone et al., 2014).

Inflammation-induced tumors usually show high immune cell infiltrations. COX-2, an important molecule in inflammation, is already known for its contribution towards inducing tumor growth, angiogenesis, and metastasis. In PC, COX-2 upregulation is observed in epithelial cells when they are surrounded by the immune cells. This gives an additional Bcl2 support to these COX-2 positive cells, resulting in evading apoptosis (Wang et al., 2004). The mechanistic insights of the initiation of PC through inflammation have been poorly understood. In 2013, Kwon et al. showed that various urogenital infections caused by the *Escherichia coli* strain CP9 induce an inflammatory environment in the prostate leading to initiation of intra-epithelial neoplasia. They showed that the acute prostatitis caused by bacterial infections leads to tissue damage which progresses to reprogramming of basal cells to luminal cells (Kwon et al., 2014).

1.7.6 Genomic instability

Whole-generation sequencing has emerged as a powerful tool for finding genomic alterations. It involves translocations, rearrangements, deletions, and mutations in the genome. Sequencing of around 57 PC genomes showed a punctuated evolution with regard to somatic alterations and their accumulation during oncogenic transformation. The evolution of oncogenicity is mainly by chromoplexy, a complex DNA rearrangement process observed mainly in cancer cells. Certain events have been recorded through chromoplexy, such as deletion of NKX3-1 or FOXP-1 and the fusion between TMPRSS2 and ERG, leading to disruption of normal differentiation of prostate epithelial cells. Following these insults are TP53 and CDKN1B mutations, which give survival support and genomic instability. Lastly, attaining loss of the PTEN gene, which is a gating event, will lead to a more aggressive form of tumor. Altogether, this shows that PC attains genomic instability through sequential events. The chromoplexy occurs even in the subclones and they start to attain new genomic alterations after they get separated from the primary tumor, and the extent of aggressiveness actually depends on accumulation of these alterations (Baca et al., 2013).

Mutations are among the most important features of cancer progression, and Kras is an important example. Recently, a study by Geng et al. showed that almost 15% of PC patients have speckle-type poxvirus and zinc finger domain protein (SPOP). The wild-type SPOP binds with SRC-3, which is known to be overexpressed in most of the cancer. This interaction leads to cullin-3 dependent ubiquitination and proteolysis, assigning its function as tumor suppressor. In PC, p160 SRCs play a central role in regulating the transcriptional activity of the androgen receptor, leading to increased cell proliferation, metastasis, and invasiveness. The team found out that the SPOP-mutated type was unable to bind with SRC-3, which is a key pleiotropic master regulator of transcription factor activity necessary for cancer cell proliferation, metabolism, survival, and even metastasis. Certain mutations like F102C and W131G in *SPOP* may lead to gain of function oncogenic effect by increasing the protein turnover of SRC-3 (Geng et al., 2013).

Double strand breaks and rearrangements are most commonly seen in many cancers, but the molecular mechanisms are unpinned. The most common rearrangement leading to fusion protein occurring in nearly 50% of PC is TMPRSS2-ERG. TMPRSS2 is an androgen-regulated gene and ERG is an ETS transcription factor gene fusion that leads to an oncogenic fusion protein. The initiation of androgen signaling leads to co-recruitment of androgen receptor and TOP2B, an enzyme which catalyzes the double strand breaks that can resolve topological constraints to the TMPRSS2 and ERG genomic loci, resulting in rearrangement, and this progresses to more aggressive PC (Haffner et al., 2010).

1.8 BIOMARKERS

The management of PC involves detection and follow-up by certain biomarkers. In the 1930s, prosthetic acid phosphatase (PAP) was detected in the serum of PC patients, and it was the gold standard until PSA came into the picture after about 50 years. PSA rapidly replaced PAP, as it is a secretory protein, encoded by prostate specific gene, kallikrein 3, a serein protease family. The immature PSA will undergo two proteolytic cleavages, leading to an active form which is secreted into the serum. PSA levels will be very low under normal conditions but very high in PC. The US Food and Drug Administration (FDA) approved PSA as a biomarker for assessing the status of PC in 1986. A major disadvantage of using PSA as the biomarker is that the levels of PSA can become elevated due to conditions such as prostatitis, benign prostate hyperplasia, urinary tract infection, and so forth, and the high rate of using PSA has resulted in overdiagnosis. The biomarkers after the era of PSA were called next-generation biomarkers, and some of the most prominent are PC antigen 3(PCA3), TMPRSS2-ERG and alpha-methylacyl-coenzyme A racemase. None of these can compete with PSA, which is the gold standard for PC detection (Nouri et al., 2015).

1.9 RECURRENCE OF PC

Prostate cancer in its initial stages is responsive to androgen deprivation therapy, which is accomplished by surgical or medical castration, lowering levels of testosterone needed in the development and growth of PC. Even after androgen deprivation therapy, recurrence of PC occurs and can progress to terminal stage cancer. The majority of recurrent PCs have been found to have high expression of TIF2 and SRC1. This high expression of TIF2 and SRC1 in recurrent PC increases the response to other steroid hormones like adrenal androgens, through androgen receptor (AR), thus providing a mechanism for AR-mediated recurrence of PC (Gregory et al., 2001). Micro RNAs have been found to exert either tumor suppressor or tumor promoting activity. A study was conducted by Hudson et.al about the importance of MicroRNA-106b-25 in early disease recurrence. The MicroRNA-106b-25 cluster encodes microRNAs miR-106b, miR-93 and miR-25 which are upregulated in primary human prostate tumor. This miR cluster, located at 7q23.1, is involved in many epithelial cancers and is also similar in function to the miR-17-92 cluster, but only the MicroRNA-106b-25 cluster is deregulated in PC. It was discovered that MicroRNA-106b-25 cluster cooperates with its host gene MCM7 by targeting the tumor suppressor gene PTEN. The expression of the MicroRNA-106b-25 cluster was high in both primary prostate tumors and metastasized PCs, and patients with high median expression of miR-106b were at high risk of recurrence of PC. The MiR-25 homolog miR-32 was found to be associated with high recurrence of PC. Additional comparison showed that miR-375 but not miR 101 was associated with early recurrence. It was found that CASP7 is the novel target of the MicroRNA-106b-25 cluster. Tumors with high miR-106b and low expression of their target CASP7 were shown to have a high possibility of recurrence (Hudson et al., 2013).

1.10 TREATMENT STRATEGIES

Various epidemiological studies have revealed that intake of cruciferous vegetables may reduce the risk of many malignancies, including PC (Ambrosone et al., 2004). These vegetables are rich in phenethyl isothiocyanate, which has shown an antitumor effect in many of the cancer cell lines. It inhibits the growth of PC-3, a PC cell line which is orthotopically injected in mice (Xiao et al., 2006). The induction of cell death is through different pathways, including G2/M phase cell cycle arrest, selective degradation of cellular tubulins, ROS generation, and lowering the expression of androgen signaling. It reduces the tumor burden *in vivo* by targeting AKT, which is involved in angiogenesis. It blocks the complex 3 of mitochondria, leading to high ROS generation, Bax activation, loss of mitochondrial membrane permeability, caspase 3 activation, and finally leads to cell death (Xiao et al., 2010).

Certain novel strategies have arrived on the market, as most of the drugs started failing in clinical scenarios due to the rapid evolution of tumor cells. The new-generation oligomers with phosphorodiamidate morpholino backbone come with the additional advantage of RNase H tolerance with neutral chemistry. London et al. showed that intratumoral administration of this novel PMO antisense MMP9 molecule in DU145 xenograft revealed a high apoptotic cell population and reduced angiogenesis, with lowered tumor burden (London et al., 2003). Targeting metabolic activities of a cancer cell ideally reduces the tumor burden. Most cancers show a glycogenic phenotype with shutting down of the mitochondrial oxidative phosphorylation event. 2-Deoxyglucose acts as an inhibitor of glycolysis by inhibiting hexokinase, leading to depletion of intracellular ATP and induction of autophagy (DiPaola et al., 2008). Metformin, an antidiabetic, showed its anticancer potential against many cancers by inhibiting the energy-sensitive mTOR signaling pathway, regulating the cell metabolism. Combination of these two drugs showed a synergistic effect on PC cell lines but when used alone, 2DG induced autophagy and metformin induced G0-G1 phase arrest in the cell cycle. But after the combination, the apoptosis proceeded through G2-M phase arrest and AMP kinase pathway (Sahra et al., 2010).

Castration-resistant PC is an incurable advanced state with a 90% incidence towards bone metastasis. Most of the deaths in PC come under this category. Recently two large phase III clinical trials showed that cabazitaxel and sipuleucel-T were effective combatants, and FDA approved the usage of sipuleucel-T (Delpierre et al., 2013). Most CRPC patients receive chemotherapy, but eventually they attain resistance, while the use of abiraterone, a known inhibitor of androgen biosynthesis, improved the overall survival of patients who received chemotherapy (De Bono et al., 2011). Few patients cross this stage and enter into hormone refractory PC, which attains resistance to androgen therapy and is detected by a rise in PSA levels even after hormone treatment. The overexpression of Notch and hedgehog signaling pathways were observed in a subset of the population during this stage, and it shows resistance to docetaxel. Targeting these pathways and blocking them depleted this population through inhibition of Bcl-2 and AKT cell survival molecules, resulting in improved response to docetaxel (Domingo-Domenech et al., 2012).

MALAT1, a long noncoding RNA known for its high expression in many of the solid tumors, showed a positive effect in reducing PC. The knockdown of MALAT1 resulted in reduced cell growth, migration and increased apoptosis rate. The androgen-dependent expression of MALAT1 emphasized its role in PC, as androgen signaling and PC are inseparable (Figure 1.2). Silencing of MALAT1 results in inhibition of growth and metastasis *in vivo* (Ren et al., 2013). Androgen plays an important role in prostate development which acts through androgen receptors (Cunha et al., 1987; Yeh et al., 2002). It is also shown that androgen receptor signaling is crucial and plays an important role in all stages of PC development (Chiin Lim and Attard, 2013). There are many important signaling pathways which are AR dependent; for example, PSA and certain genes linked to cell survival (Heinlein and Chang, 2004). After disease development, in a certain subset of the population, a new function will be assigned to AR signaling, due to the ETS rearrangements, like control over invasion and metastasis. In order to tackle this, androgen deprivation therapy (ADP), which is achieved by removal of the testes surgically, is done. The other way to block is via blocking the hypothalamic stimulus for production of testosterone through testicular cells. This will be achieved by gonadotrophin releasing analogues. Although ADT showed initial success and patient responses were positive, it later led to the reactivation of AR signaling, and an increase in PSA levels was also observed, leading to a lethal castration-resistant form of PC (Rodrigues et al., 2014).

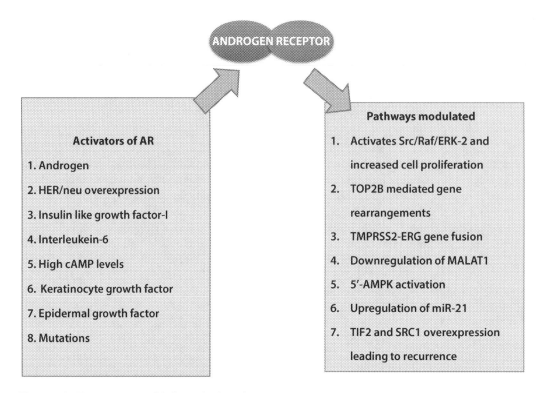

Figure 1.2 Factors responsible for activation of androgen receptor and the pathways modulated in prostate cancer leading to malignancy.

1.11 CONCLUSION

Much progress has been made in recent years in understanding the initiation and progression of PC. High grade PIN, biomarkers, and the various risk factors help us to predict disease outcome. In-depth knowledge is lacking in the tumor microenvironment, and this is emerging as one of the important supportive factors for malignancy maintenance, projecting it as a crucial strategy for targeting. New biomarkers which should be more sensitive and cost-effective than PSA should hit the market soon. The lethal castration-resistant tumor should be addressed with more focus on the signaling pathways which will sensitize the tumor against various available drugs.

ACKNOWLEDGEMENTS

The authors express their gratitude to the University Grants Commission, Government of India, New Delhi for the research fellowship to MBL, the Council for Scientific and Industrial Research, Government of India, New Delhi for supporting YV and the Department of Biotechnology, Government of India, New Delhi – Ramalingaswami Fellowship to KBH.

REFERENCES

Altekruse, S.F. Kosary, C.L. Krapcho, M. et al. 2010. SEER cancer statistics review, 1975–2007. Bethesda, MD: *National Cancer Institute* 7.

Ambrosone, C.B. McCann, S.E. Freudenheim, J.L. et al. 2004. Breast cancer risk in premenopausal women is inversely associated with consumption of broccoli, a source of isothiocyanates, but is not modified by GST genotype. *J Nutr* 134(5), 1134–1138.

Antonarakis, E.S. Lu, C. Wang, H. et al. 2014. AR-V7 and resistance to enzalutamide and abiraterone in prostate cancer. *N Engl J Med* 371(11), 1028–1038.

Ao, M. Franco, O.E. Park, D. et al. 2007. Cross-talk between paracrine-acting cytokine and chemokine pathways promotes malignancy in benign human prostatic epithelium. *Cancer Res* 67(9), 4244–4253.

Baca, S.C. Prandi, D. Lawrence, M.S. et al. 2013. Punctuated evolution of prostate cancer genomes. *Cell* 153(3), 666–677.

Bandyopadhyay, S. Pai, S.K. Gross, S.C. et al. 2003. The Drg-1 gene suppresses tumor metastasis in prostate cancer. *Cancer Res* 63(8), 1731–1736.

Berger, M.F. Lawrence, M.S. Demichelis, F. et al. 2011. The genomic complexity of primary human prostate cancer. *Nature* 470(7333), 214–220.

Bunker, C.H. Patrick, A.L. Konety, B.R. et al. 2002. High prevalence of screening-detected prostate cancer among Afro-Caribbeans: The Tobago Prostate Cancer Survey. *Cancer Epidemiol Biomarkers Prev* 11(8), 726–729.

Castro, E. Goh, C. Olmos, D. et al. 2013. Germline BRCA mutations are associated with higher risk of nodal involvement, distant metastasis, and poor survival outcomes in prostate cancer. *J Clin Oncol* 31(14), 1748–1757.

Chan, J.M. Stampfer, M.J. Giovannucci, E. et al. 1998. Plasma insulin-like growth factor-I and prostate cancer risk: a prospective study. *Science* 279(5350), 563–566.

Chiin Lim, A. Attard, G. 2013. Improved therapeutic targeting of the androgen receptor: rational drug design improves survival in castration-resistant prostate cancer. *Curr Drug Targets* 14(4), 408–419.

Chornokur, G. Han, G. Tanner, R. et al. 2013. High grade prostate intraepithelial neoplasia (PIN) is a PSA-independent risk factor for prostate cancer in African American men: results from a pilot study. *Cancer Lett* 331(2), 154–157.

Cohen, P. Peehl, D.M. Lamson, G. et al. 1991. Insulin-like growth factors (IGFs), IGF receptors, and IGF-binding proteins in primary cultures of prostate epithelial cells. *J Clin Endocrinol Metab* 73(2), 401–407.

Cohen, P. Peehl, D.M. Rosenfeld, R.G. 1994. The IGF axis in the prostate. *Horm Metab Res* 26(2), 81–84.

Cunha, G.R. Donjacour, A.A. Cooke, P.S. et al. 1987. The endocrinology and developmental biology of the prostate. *Endocr Rev* 8(3), 338–362.

De Bono, J.S. Logothetis, C.J. Molina, A. et al. 2011. Abiraterone and increased survival in metastatic prostate cancer. *N Engl J Med* 364(21), 1995–2005.

De Marzo, A.M. Platz, E.A. Sutcliffe, S. et al. 2007. Inflammation in prostate carcinogenesis. *Nat Rev Cancer* 7(4), 256–269.

Delpierre, C. Lamy, S. Kelly-Irving, M. et al. 2013. Life expectancy estimates as a key factor in over-treatment: the case of prostate cancer. *Cancer epidemiology* 37(4), 462–468.

DiPaola, R.S. Dvorzhinski, D. Thalasila, A. et al. 2008. Therapeutic starvation and autophagy in prostate cancer: a new paradigm for targeting metabolism in cancer therapy. *The Prostate* 68(16), 1743–1752.

Domingo-Domenech, J. Vidal, S.J. Rodriguez-Bravo, V. et al. 2012. Suppression of acquired docetaxel resistance in prostate cancer through depletion of notch-and hedgehog-dependent tumor-initiating cells. *Cancer Cell* 22(3), 373–388.

Ewing, C.M. Ray, A.M. Lange, E.M. et al. 2012. Germline mutations in HOXB13 and prostate-cancer risk. *N Engl J Med* 366(2), 141–149.

Ezponda, T. Popovic, R. Shah, M.Y. et al. 2013. The histone methyltransferase MMSET/WHSC1 activates TWIST1 to promote an epithelial–mesenchymal transition and invasive properties of prostate cancer. *Oncogene* 32(23), 2882–2890.

Gann, P.H. Hennekens, C.H. Ma, J. et al. 1996. Prospective study of sex hormone levels and risk of prostate cancer. *J. Natl. Cancer Inst* 88(16), 1118–1126.

Geng, C. He, B. Xu, L. et al. 2013. Prostate cancer-associated mutations in speckle-type POZ protein (SPOP) regulate steroid receptor coactivator 3 protein turnover. *Proc Natl Acad Sci U S A* 110(17), 6997–7002.

Gregory, C.W. He, B. Johnson, R.T. et al. 2001. A mechanism for androgen receptor-mediated prostate cancer recurrence after androgen deprivation therapy. *Cancer Res* 61(11), 4315–4319.

Gundem, G. Van Loo, P. Kremeyer, B. et al. 2015. The evolutionary history of lethal metastatic prostate cancer. *Nature* 520(7547), 353–357.

Gupta, G.P. Massagué, J. 2006. Cancer metastasis: building a framework. *Cell* 127(4), 679–695.

Haffner, M.C. Aryee, M.J. Toubaji, A. et al. 2010. Androgen-induced TOP2B-mediated double-strand breaks and prostate cancer gene rearrangements. *Nat Genet* 42(8), 668–675.

Heinlein, C.A. Chang, C. 2004. Androgen receptor in prostate cancer. *Endocr Rev* 25(2), 276–308.

Hoefer, J. Schäfer, G. Klocker, H. et al. 2012. PIAS1 is increased in human prostate cancer and enhances proliferation through inhibition of p21. *Am J Pathol* 180(5), 2097–2107.

Hudson, R.S. Yi, M. Esposito, D. et al. 2013. MicroRNA-106b-25 cluster expression is associated with early disease recurrence and targets caspase-7 and focal adhesion in human prostate cancer. *Oncogene* 32(35), 4139–4147.

Jain, S. Chakraborty, G. Raja, R. et al. 2008. Prostaglandin E2 regulates tumor angiogenesis in prostate cancer. *Cancer Res* 68(19), 7750–7759.

Kim, B. Kim, P.A.C.K. 2013. Embryology, anatomy, and congenital anomalies of the prostate and seminal vesicles. In *Abdominal Imaging*, Hamm, B. Ros, P.R. (Eds.) Berlin Heidelberg: Springer, pp. 1797–1812.

Kim, I.Y. Ahn, H.J. Lang, S. et al. 1998. Loss of expression of transforming growth factor-beta receptors is associated with poor prognosis in prostate cancer patients. *Clin Cancer Res* 4(7), 1625–1630.

Kwon, O.J. Zhang, L. Ittmann, M.M. et al. 2014. Prostatic inflammation enhances basal-to-luminal differentiation and accelerates initiation of prostate cancer with a basal cell origin. *Proc Natl Acad Sci U S A* 111(5), E592–E600.

Lee, Y.J. Park, J.E. Jeon, B.R. et al. 2013. Is prostate-specific antigen effective for population screening of prostate cancer? A systematic review. *Ann Lab Med* 33(4), 233–241.

Lesko, S.M. Rosenberg, L. Shapiro, S. 1996. Family history and prostate cancer risk. *Am J Epidemiol* 144(11), 1041–1047.

Ling, M.T. Lau, T.C. Zhou, C. et al. 2005. Overexpression of Id-1 in prostate cancer cells promotes angiogenesis through the activation of vascular endothelial growth factor (VEGF). *Carcinogenesis* 26(10), 1668–1676.

London, C.A. Sekhon, H.S. Arora, V. et al. 2003. A novel antisense inhibitor of MMP-9 attenuates angiogenesis, human prostate cancer cell invasion and tumorigenicity. *Cancer Gene Ther* 10(11), 823–832.

McFadden, D.G. Papagiannakopoulos, T. Taylor-Weiner, A. et al. 2014. Genetic and clonal dissection of murine small cell lung carcinoma progression by genome sequencing. *Cell* 156(6), 1298–1311.

Moyer, V.A. 2012. Screening for prostate cancer: US Preventive Services Task Force recommendation statement. *Ann Intern Med* 157(2), 120–134.

Mulholland, D.J. Kobayashi, N. Ruscetti, M. et al. 2012. Pten loss and RAS/MAPK activation cooperate to promote EMT and metastasis initiated from prostate cancer stem/progenitor cells. *Cancer Res* 72(7), 1878–1889.

Musumeci, M. Coppola, V. Addario, A. et al. 2011. Control of tumor and microenvironment cross-talk by miR-15a and miR-16 in prostate cancer. *Oncogene* 30(41), 4231–4242.

Nouri, M. Ratther, E. Stylianou, N. et al. 2015. Androgen-targeted therapy-induced epithelial mesenchymal plasticity and neuroendocrine transdifferentiation in prostate cancer: an opportunity for intervention. *Front Oncol* 4, 1–19.

Ornish, D. Lin, J. Chan, J.M. et al. 2013. Effect of comprehensive lifestyle changes on telomerase activity and telomere length in men with biopsy-proven low-risk prostate cancer: 5-year follow-up of a descriptive pilot study. *Lancet Oncol* 14(11), 1112–1120.

Ostman, A. Augsten, M. 2009. Cancer-associated fibroblasts and tumor growth – bystanders turning into key players. *Curr Opin Genet Dev* 19(1), 67–73.

Pertega-Gomes, N. Felisbino, S. Massie, C.E. et al. 2015. A glycolytic phenotype is associated with prostate cancer progression and aggressiveness: a role for monocarboxylate transporters as metabolic targets for therapy. *J Pathol* 236(4), 517–530.

Peto, J. 2001. Cancer epidemiology in the last century and the next decade. *Nature* 411(6835), 390–395.

Prensner, J.R. Rubin, M.A. Wei, J.T. et al. 2012. Beyond PSA: the next generation of prostate cancer biomarkers. *Sci Transl Med* 4(127), 127rv3–127rv3.

Rajah, R. Valentinis, B. Cohen, P. 1997. Insulin-like growth factor (IGF)-binding protein-3 induces apoptosis and mediates the effects of transforming growth factor-β1 on programmed cell death through a p53-and IGF-independent mechanism. *J Biol Chem* 272(18), 12181–12188.

Rasheed, S.A.K. Teo, C.R. Beillard, E.J. et al. 2013. MicroRNA-182 and microRNA-200a control G-protein subunit α-13 (GNA13) expression and cell invasion synergistically in prostate cancer cells. *J Biol Chem* 288(11), 7986–7995.

Ren, S. Liu, Y. Xu, W. et al. 2013. Long noncoding RNA MALAT-1 is a new potential therapeutic target for castration resistant prostate cancer. *J Urol* 190(6), 2278–2287.

Rodrigues, D.N. Butler, L.M. Estelles, D.L. et al. 2014. Molecular pathology and prostate cancer therapeutics: from biology to bedside. *J Pathol* 232(2), 178–184.

Ryan, C.J. Smith, M.R. De Bono, J.S. et al. 2013. Abiraterone in metastatic prostate cancer without previous chemotherapy. *N Engl J Med* 368(2), 138–148.

Sahra, I.B. Laurent, K. Giuliano, S. et al. 2010. Targeting cancer cell metabolism: the combination of metformin and 2-deoxyglucose induces p53-dependent apoptosis in prostate cancer cells. *Cancer Res* 70(6), 2465–2475.

Scher, H.I. Fizazi, K. Saad, F. et al. 2012. Increased survival with enzalutamide in prostate cancer after chemotherapy. *N Engl J Med* 367(13), 1187–1197.

Shen, M.M. Abate-Shen, C. 2010. Molecular genetics of prostate cancer: new prospects for old challenges. *Genes Dev* 24(18), 1967–2000.

Stallone, G. Cormio, L. Netti, G.S. et al. 2014. Pentraxin 3: a novel biomarker for predicting progression from prostatic inflammation to prostate cancer. *Cancer Res* 74(16), 4230–4238.

Sun, Y. Campisi, J. Higano, C. et al. 2012. Treatment-induced damage to the tumor microenvironment promotes prostate cancer therapy resistance through WNT16B. *Nat Med* 18(9), 1359–1368.

Sun, Y.X. Schneider, A. Jung, Y. et al. 2005. Skeletal localization and neutralization of the SDF-1 (CXCL12)/CXCR4 axis blocks prostate cancer metastasis and growth in osseous sites in vivo. *J Bone Miner Res* 20(2), 318–329.

Takayama, K.I. Horie-Inoue, K. Katayama, S. et al. 2013. Androgen-responsive long noncoding RNA CTBP1-AS promotes prostate cancer. *EMBO J* 32(12), 1665–1680.

Tennakoon, J.B. Shi, Y. Han, J.J. et al. 2014. Androgens regulate prostate cancer cell growth via an AMPK-PGC-1α-mediated metabolic switch. *Oncogene* 33(45), 5251–5261.

Valencia, T. Kim, J.Y. Abu-Baker, S. et al. 2014. Metabolic reprogramming of stromal fibroblasts through p62-mTORC1 signaling promotes inflammation and tumorigenesis. *Cancer Cell* 26(1), 121–135.

Van Moorselaar, R.J.A. Voest, E.E. 2002. Angiogenesis in prostate cancer: its role in disease progression and possible therapeutic approaches. *Mol Cell Endocrinol* 197(1), 239–250.

Visvader, J.E. 2011. Cells of origin in cancer. *Nature* 469(7330), 314–322.

Wang, J. Shiozawa, Y. Wang, J. et al. 2008. The role of CXCR7/RDC1 as a chemokine receptor for CXCL12/SDF-1 in prostate cancer. *J Biol Chem* 283(7), 4283–4294.

Wang, J. Ying, G. Wang, J. et al. 2010. Characterization of phosphoglycerate kinase-1 expression of stromal cells derived from tumor microenvironment in prostate cancer progression. *Cancer Res* 70(2), 471–480.

Wang, S. Gao, J. Lei, Q. et al. 2003. Prostate-specific deletion of the murine Pten tumor suppressor gene leads to metastatic prostate cancer. *Cancer Cell* 4(3), 209–221.

Wang, W. Bergh, A. Damber, J.E. 2004. Chronic inflammation in benign prostate hyperplasia is associated with focal upregulation of cyclooxygenase-2, Bcl-2, and cell proliferation in the glandular epithelium. *The Prostate* 61(1), 60–72.

Wang, Z.A. Mitrofanova, A. Bergren, S.K. et al. 2013. Lineage analysis of basal epithelial cells reveals their unexpected plasticity and supports a cell-of-origin model for prostate cancer heterogeneity. *Nature Cell Biol* 15(3), 274–283.

Wood, M. Fudge, K. Mohler, J.L. et al. 1997. In situ hybridization studies of metalloproteinases 2 and 9 and TIMP-1 and TIMP-2 expression in human prostate cancer. *Clin Exp Metastasis* 15(3), 246–258.

Wu, Z. He, B. He, J. et al. 2013. Upregulation of miR-153 promotes cell proliferation via downregulation of the PTEN tumor suppressor gene in human prostate cancer. *The Prostate* 73(6), 596–604.

Xiao, D. Lew, K.L. Zeng, Y. et al. 2006. Phenethyl isothiocyanate-induced apoptosis in PC-3 human prostate cancer cells is mediated by reactive oxygen species-dependent disruption of the mitochondrial membrane potential. *Carcinogenesis* 27(11), 2223–2234.

Xiao, D. Powolny, A.A. Moura, M.B. et al. 2010. Phenethyl isothiocyanate inhibits oxidative phosphorylation to trigger reactive oxygen species-mediated death of human prostate cancer cells. *J Biol Chem* 285(34), 26558–26569.

Yanagisawa, N. Li, R. Rowley, D. et al. 2007. Stromogenic prostatic carcinoma pattern (carcinomas with reactive stromal grade 3) in needle biopsies predicts biochemical recurrence-free survival in patients after radical prostatectomy. *Hum Pathol* 38(11), 1611–1620.

Yang, F. Zhang, Y. Ressler, S.J. et al. 2013. FGFR1 is essential for prostate cancer progression and metastasis. *Cancer Res* 73(12), 3716–3724.

Yeh, S.D. Imbriaco, M. Larson, S.M. et al. 1996. Detection of bony metastases of androgen-independent prostate cancer by PET-FDG. *Nucl Med Biol* 23(6), 693–697.

Yeh, S. Tsai, M.Y. Xu, Q. et al. 2002. Generation and characterization of androgen receptor knockout (ARKO) mice: an in vivo model for the study of androgen functions in selective tissues. *Proc Natl Acad Sci U S A* 99(21), 13498–13503.

Zhao, L. Lee, B. Y, Brown, D. et al. 2009. Identification of candidate biomarkers of therapeutic response to docetaxel by proteomic profiling. *Cancer Res* 69(19), 7696–7703.

CHAPTER 2

Global Epidemiology of Prostate Cancer

Girish Sharma, Apoorva Arora, and Sudhir Rawal

CONTENTS

2.1 INTRODUCTION

Second to cardiovascular diseases, cancer is becoming one of the leading causes of death worldwide. In 2012, global estimates of new cancer cases were 14.1 million, while 8.2 million deaths occurred due to cancer. Lung and breast cancers are the most frequently occurring cancers in the world, causing enormous mortality in men and women, respectively. However, in more developed countries prostate cancer in men and lung cancer in women are the leading causes of cancer death. In the developing countries, men are most commonly diagnosed with lung, bronchus and tracheal cancers, while in women breast cancer is the most prevalent. Whereas the less developed countries have a larger share in the world population, i.e. 82%, they only account for 57% of the estimated new cancer cases in the world. The burden of cancer is expected to grow worldwide, and especially in the economically weaker countries due to the adoption of lifestyle behaviors that are associated with increased risk of cancer. These include smoking, poor diet, lack of physical activity, and reproductive changes (Torre et al., 2015).

Prostate cancer, the most common cancer among men in developed countries, primarily affects elderly men. Additionally, black men have a greater risk of developing prostate cancer than Caucasian, Hispanic, and Asian men. The tumor forms in the prostate gland and slowly spreads to the other parts of the body. Ninety percent of prostate cancers are acinar adenocarcinomas that start from the glands in the prostate. Others are ductal adenocarcinoma, transitional cell (urothelial) cancer, squamous cell cancer, carcinoid, small cell cancer, sarcomas, and sarcomatoid cancer (Falconer, 2013). Usually no proper symptoms are produced during the early stages of prostate cancer. However, sometimes mild symptoms similar to those of benign prostatic hyperplasia are seen. These include frequent urination (especially at night), painful urination and difficulty in starting and maintaining a steady flow of urine, sense of not being able to empty the bladder, and blood in urine or semen (Sharma et al., 2014). Rarely, symptoms such as hip, pelvis, back, and other bony area pain occur when the prostate cancer has metastasized to the surrounding bones. This is known as metastatic prostate cancer (Falconer, 2013).

The high rate of incidence and mortality due to prostate cancer in men in the developed countries deems it necessary to study the epidemiology of prostate cancer. These numbers and figures related to prostate cancer are the best way of assessing the situation of the cancer burden globally and show how the world is coping with prostate cancer and what can be predicted for the future (Sharma et al., 2014).

2.2　THE EPIDEMIOLOGY OF PROSTATE CANCER

2.2.1　Sources of Data

The data presented here have been taken from GLOBOCAN, the Surveillance, Epidemiology and End Results (SEER) program of the National Cancer Institute (NCI) of the United States, as well as research papers related to prostate cancer. The GLOBOCAN 2012 project of the International Agency for Research on Cancer (IARC), World Health Organization (WHO) is a database that provides estimates of incidence, mortality and 5-year prevalence of all major types of cancers. These data have been collected from population-based cancer registries (PBCRs) in 184 countries. The SEER program provides statistical data for cancer collected from the PBCRs in the United States.

2.2.2　Incidence

Prostate cancer is the second most frequently diagnosed cancer in men, accounting for 15% of all the cancer cases (Ferlay et al., 2013). In 2012, 1.1 million new cases of prostate cancer were documented. In the developed countries, having only 17% of the world's male population, it is the most frequently diagnosed cancer in men (Torre et al., 2015). Among the worldwide new prostate cancer cases, 70% (759,000) occur in developed countries. It is most prevalent in Australia and New Zealand, having 111.6 new cases per 100,000, followed closely by North America, which had an incidence of 97.2 per 100,000 in 2012. Incidence of prostate cancer is also quite high in northern Europe (Ferlay et al., 2013). Figure 2.1 (A) in the color insert shows the worldwide incidence of prostate cancer.

As opposed to more developed regions that had 742,000 new cases in 2012, less developed regions had only 353,000 new cases (Ferlay et al., 2013). In fact, in developing countries, prostate cancer is the fourth most prevalent cancer among men. This variation in incidence in developed versus developing countries could be attributed to the use of different methods of prostate-specific antigen (PSA) testing for diagnosis. As the use of PSA testing is becoming more widespread in developed countries like Australia/New Zealand, the United States, and in Europe, the incidence of prostate cancer is also increasing. There was a rapid rise in incidence in the developed countries after the 1990s when PSA testing was introduced (Torre et al., 2015). The test detects even the latent, slow growing, asymptomatic cancers, thereby inflating the observed cancer incidence in developed countries. Therefore, in developing countries where PSA testing is not being used as widely, the incidence of prostate cancer is apparently low (Baade et al., 2013). The incidence rate is increasing even in countries including Japan, Thailand, and the United Kingdom, where PSA testing began later or is not as common (Torre et al., 2015). Among the less developed countries, incidence rates are high in the Caribbean (79.8 new cases per 100,000), South Africa (61.8 new cases per 100,000), and South America (60.1 per 100,000). In Eastern and South-Central Asia, the incidence is quite low (10.5 and 4.5 new cases per 100,000 respectively) (Ferlay et al., 2013).

In the United States, the highest incidence rate of prostate cancer from 2006 to 2010 was in California, which had 23,010 cases per 100,000 during that period. It was also high in Florida (16,590 per 100,000), Texas (15,900 per 100,000), and New York (15,440 per 100,000). The lowest incidences were in North Dakota (460 per 100,000), Wyoming (490 per 100,000), and the District of Columbia (510 per 100,000) (Siegel et al. 2014). Among the registries in India, the Kamrup Urban District (2009–2011) and Delhi (2008–2009) had the highest incidence at 11.1 and 10.1 per 100,000, respectively. The lowest rate was in Barshi (both rural and expanded), at 1.9 during 2009, and at Wardha, which had an incidence rate of 2.0 per 100,000 during 2010–2011 (Jain et al., 2010).

2.2.3 Mortality

Prostate cancer is the fifth leading cause of death across the world (Torre et al., 2015). In 2012, there were 307,000 deaths (6.6% of total deaths in men) worldwide due to prostate cancer. Figure 2.1 (B) in the color insert shows the mortality due to prostate cancer all over the world. Mortality is highest in the Caribbean, where the mortality rate is 29.8 per 100,000, followed by southern, middle, and western Africa, having mortality rates of 24.4, 24.2 and 21.2, respectively per 100,000 (Ferlay et al., 2013). The lowest mortality rate was reported in South-Central Asia, where 2.9 deaths occur per 100,000. The mortality rate in Asia was consistent with the low incidence of prostate cancer in this continent. In regions with the highest incidence, such as Australia/New Zealand, the United States, and northern and western Europe, the number of deaths was relatively low, with mortality rates of 12.9, 9.8, 14.5, and 10.7, respectively. The death rates have actually decreased in these regions. The main reason for this decline is early detection and improved treatment facilities (Torre et al., 2015). The disparity in the incidence of prostate cancer in developed and developing countries is not seen for mortality, as PSA screening has more effect on incidence and less on mortality. Higher mortality is seen in black populations as compared to Caucasians and Asians (Ferlay et al., 2013). Figures 2.1 and 2.2 show a comparison of prostate cancer incidence and mortality across the world.

In America, the highest prostate-specific mortality was in California (3,380 per 100,000), concordant with the high incidence rate in this state. In Florida, Texas, and New York, where the incidence was also quite high, mortality rates were respectively 2,170, 1,660, and 1,760 per 100,000. Deaths due to prostate cancer were surprisingly high in Illinois (1,190 per 100,000), Pennsylvania (1,370 per 100,000), and Ohio (1,200 per 100,000), where the incidence was lower compared to California (8,820; 10,930, and 8,690 per 100,000 respectively) (Siegel et al., 2014).

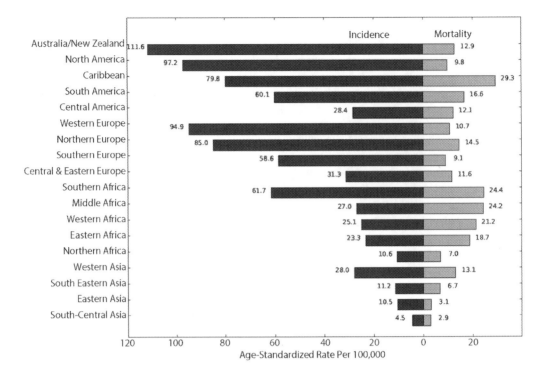

Figure 2.2   Prostate cancer incidence (left) and mortality (right) in specific countries and regions across the world. Age-adjusted rate (per 100,000). (Torre et al. 2015.)

2.2.4   Five-Year Prevalence

The 5-year prevalence of prostate cancer across the world documented for 2012 was 3,858,000. The developed countries showed a higher prevalence than developing countries until 2012. The 5-year prevalence in more developed countries was 2,871,000, while in less developed regions it was 987,000. In Southeast Asia, where the incidence and mortality rates are also quite low, the 5-year prevalence from 2008 to 2012 was 123,000 cases. The east Mediterranean region showed the lowest 5-year prevalence at 47,000 cases in the 2008–2012 period, second to which was India, where the 5-year prevalence was 64,000 cases (Bray et al., 2012).

2.2.5   Projected New Cases

The trend for prostate cancer incidence and mortality is an upward curve. The number of cases is increasing globally. The estimated number of new cases across the world in 2015 is 220,800, forming 13.3% of the total cancer cases. It has been projected that there would be 27,540 deaths, i.e. 4.7% of all cancer deaths, in 2015 (SEER 2015).

2.3   RISK FACTORS ASSOCIATED WITH PROSTATE CANCER

Identifying the risk factors associated with any disease allows understanding of the mechanism of pathology of the disease. Risk factors can be broadly divided into two categories, modifiable and non-modifiable. Non-modifiable risk factors include gene mutations, single nucleotide polymorphisms

(SNPs), age, and race, while modifiable risk factors are lifestyle and environmental risk factors (Cuzick et al., 2014). Age, race/ethnicity, and family history are the most well-established risk factors associated with development of prostate cancer (Center et al., 2012). Other factors like SNPs in specific genes and lifestyle factors (such as smoking, drinking, etc.) are being explored for their association with this morbid disease. Certain mutations have been identified to be strongly associated with the risk of developing prostate cancer. Dietary habits and sedentary lifestyle have also been found to contribute to the risk of developing prostate cancer. All these risk factors are discussed in the following sections.

2.3.1 Age

The risk of developing prostate cancer is directly proportional to age. More than 80% of all cancers are diagnosed in men over 65 years of age. It is expected that in Asian countries, where the incidence of prostate cancer is the lowest in the world, life expectancy is going to increase markedly in the near future. As a result of this, the burden of prostate cancer is expected to increase in these regions (Baade et al., 2013).

Prostate cancer incidence shows a sharp increase for ages beyond 55 years. Figures 2.3 (A) and (B) show incidence of and mortality due to prostate cancer in different age groups in the United States. However, as PSA testing became more common and people became more aware, median age at diagnosis dropped from 72 in 1986 to 66 in 2011. Furthermore, it was found that prostate cancers that developed at a younger age behaved more aggressively. It is noteworthy to mention young age prostate cancer, which is defined as prostate cancer detected in men less than 55 years of age. For younger men (<50 years of age), a low grade and low stage tumor that is detected early has a better prognosis than in older men with the same grade and stage of tumor (Hussein et al. 2015). The chances of recurrence are significantly low, and long-term disease-free survival is also higher if aggressive therapy is implemented (Smith et al., 2000).

2.3.2 Race/Ethnicity

Incidence and mortality rates of prostate cancer are markedly higher in African-American and Jamaican men of African origin compared to white men. The incidence rate in black men in the United States was 1.6 times higher and mortality rate was 2.3 times higher than in white men.

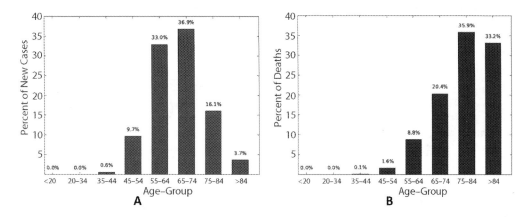

Figure 2.3 (A) Percentage of new cases of prostate cancer by age in the United States in 2012. (B) Percentage of deaths due to prostate cancer by age in the United States in 2012. Prostate cancer is diagnosed most frequently in the 65–74 age group, and the maximum number of deaths occurs in the 75–84 age group. (SEER cancer statistics for 2008–2012.)

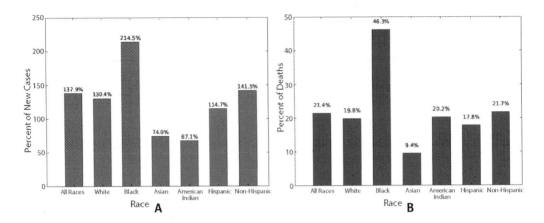

Figure 2.4   (A) Incidence of prostate cancer in 2012 in the United States among different races. (B) Mortality due to prostate cancer in 2012 in the United States among different races. Age-adjusted rate (per 100,000). Prostate cancer is most frequent in the black population and least frequent in Asians. (SEER Cancer Statistics for 2008–2012.)

African-American men in the United States were also reported to present their prostate cancer 2–3 years earlier than Caucasian men and have higher Gleason scores (Center et al., 2012; Hussein et al., 2015). Incidence and mortality rates are also high in the Caribbean and southern Africa (Torre et al., 2015). Figure 2.4 (A) shows the incidence of prostate cancer across different races, and Figure 2.4 (B) shows race-wise mortality associated with prostate cancer.

The reasons for this increased susceptibility in black men are not yet understood completely, although it has been suggested that it is due to inherent genetic factors. More specifically, increased susceptibility has been attributed to allelic variants found in black men at 8q24 and 17q21 loci, among others, but this remains to be confirmed (Center et al., 2012). While the incidence rates are relatively lower in western Africa, the occurrence of prostate cancer among African-American men originating from the same regions but residing in United States is higher than that of US whites, indicating a strong influence of the environment on the disease (Hebert et al., 1998) (Figure 2.1 in color insert). Another study reported that the higher risk of developing prostate cancer in African-American men could be due to increased expression of fatty acid synthase and inflammatory cytokines like IL-6, IL-8 and IL-1β (Powell et al., 2014). After blacks, prevalence of prostate cancer is highest in Caucasians, followed by Hispanics and then Asians (Baade et al. 2013; Cuzick et al., 2014).

2.3.3 Familial and Genetic Factors

The relative risk of developing prostate cancer is higher among men with an affected first-degree relative. In fact, family history is the strongest risk factor for development of prostate cancer among all the racial and ethnic groups. Of all the men affected with prostate cancer, about 10–15% have a positive family history. Moreover, the risk of developing prostate cancer is significantly higher for men less than 65 years of age than those greater than 65 years of age, having a positive family history of prostate cancer, as well as in men who have more than one first-degree relative with prostate cancer. Many studies also report a higher risk if the affected family member is the brother than if it is the father, which points to the possibility that the genetic component is X-linked or recessive (Schaid, 2004). Clinically, the only difference between hereditary and non-hereditary forms of prostate cancer is the early age (~6–7 years) at diagnosis in the case of hereditary prostate cancer (Schaid, 2004).

2.3.3.1 Gene Mutations

As mentioned earlier, there seems to be a strong correlation between risk of developing prostate cancer and allelic variants found in black men at loci 8q24 and 17q21 (Center et al., 2012).

Other studies have reported an association between *BRCA1* and *BRCA2* mutations and risk of prostate cancer in men. These mutations are also known to increase the risk of developing breast cancer in women several-fold. *BRCA1* is a gene at locus 17q21. It encodes a protein involved in the regulation of cell cycle progression. A study conducted on Ashkenazi Jews found that the prostate cancer risk was double in carriers of mutations 185delAG and 5382insC in *BRCA1* compared to non-carriers. However, the frequency of occurrence of these mutations is quite low (~2%), so they are not considered significant risk factors overall. *BRCA2* lies on locus 13q12 and can lead to about a 5- to 7-fold increase in relative risk, especially at a young age (≤ 65 years) and is also associated with more aggressive cancers (Schaid, 2004; Cuzick et al., 2014). However, *BRCA2* mutations are also seldom found in men having a positive family history of prostate cancer. Due to the low frequency of occurrence of *BRCA1* and *BRCA2* mutations in the population, they explain a very small percentage of hereditary prostate cancers (Schaid, 2004). The *HOXB13* G84E mutation also increases the relative risk of prostate cancer by three to four times, though it is also rare and occurs in 1.3–1.4% of the general population (Cuzick et al., 2014).

Among the other genes, missense and non-sense mutations in *MSR1* gene (which codes for macrophage scavenger receptor 1) have been postulated to be linked to the susceptibility of prostate cancer, although the exact contribution of these mutations in the risk of developing this cancer remains to be proven (Schaid, 2004).

Genetic polymorphisms in genes involved in metabolism of testosterone were thought be associated with prostate cancer, especially in the androgen receptor gene (*AR*), the steroid 5-α-reductase type II (*SRD5A2*) gene, the cytochrome P450C17α (*CYP17*) gene and two genes of the *HSD3B* family. But of these five genes, strong conclusive evidence has only been found for the *AR* gene. Longer variants of microsatellite repeats *CAG* and *CGN* in exon 1 of the *AR* gene provide a protective effect against prostate cancer, while shorter variants increase the risk (Schaid, 2004).

2.3.4 Dietary and Lifestyle-Related Risk Factors

Several studies point to the influence of diet and lifestyle on the risk of developing prostate cancer. For example, African-Americans from western Africa who reside in United States have a higher risk of developing prostate cancer and also show higher incidence than native western Africans (Hebert et al., 1998). Asians living in the United States also have a higher incidence than Asians living in their native countries (Baade et al., 2013). These migrant studies indicate that there is strong correlation between prostate cancer mortality and affluence.

Positive association of animal fat (total and saturated), milk, and dairy products (dairy protein) and energy from alcohol and sugar with prostate cancer have been shown by a substantial number of studies (Hebert et al., 1998; Schaid, 2004). Other dietary components that have shown a positive association include red meat (Schaid, 2004) and coffee (Cuzick et al., 2014). As the mechanism of pathology of prostate cancer is not yet understood, several hypotheses have been put forth to justify the link between dietary components and prostate cancer risk. For example, meat could be contributing to the increased risk by any one of the following three reasons (Schaid, 2004):

1. Meat is cooked at high temperatures at which certain carcinogens (heterocyclic aromatic amines and polycyclic aromatic hydrocarbons) form in it.
2. Red meat is a rich source of zinc, an essential element for the synthesis of testosterone. As the levels of zinc elevate, levels of testosterone also increase, in turn increasing the risk of prostate cancer.
3. Diets rich in meat are generally deficient in anti-carcinogenic components found in plant foods.

Animal fats may raise the sex hormone levels, thereby increasing the risk of adult cancers at sites sensitive to serum hormone levels, such as breast and prostate, a mechanism that was proposed by Hutchison about 20 years ago (Hebert et al., 1998).

Food components that are negatively associated, i.e. they do not contribute to the risk of prostate cancer, include cabbage, cereals, vegetables, soybeans, and fish (Hebert et al., 1998).

Foods that have been seen to confer protection from prostate cancer include cereals, nuts, oilseeds (including soybean), fish, and vegetables such as tomatoes and legumes (Hebert et al., 1998; Schaid, 2004). Fish seems to protect from cancers at many sites, including the prostate, because it is rich in ω-3 fatty acids (Hebert et al., 1998). Tomatoes are rich in the antioxidant carotenoid lycopene, which is why they have a protective effect against cancer. Other antioxidants like vitamin E and selenium may also reduce the risk (Schaid, 2004). Certain soybean components (isoflavonoids and lignans) also have antioxidant activity. They have also shown to increase the production of sex hormone–binding globulin (SHBG) in the liver, consequently keeping the serum levels of testosterone at bay and reducing hormonal activity. Yet another mechanism by which these soybean components protect against cancer may be their effect on hormone-sensitive target cells as opposed to that of biologic steroids, even though both have similar metabolisms. These phytoestrogens bind competitively to hormone receptors in target cells. This binding, though weak, can displace the harmful stimulatory action of the endogenously produced steroid hormones. Soybeans also have phytic acid, plant sterols, and protease inhibitors that protect through other mechanisms (Hebert et al., 1998).

Studies have also shown that vitamin D protects against prostate cancer, while calcium increases its risk. Consistent findings of various studies have shown that a metabolite of vitamin D – 1,25-dihydroxy vitamin D_3 (1,25 D) – inhibits the growth and development of prostate cancer cells. Dairy calcium suppresses the circulating 1,25-D levels, thus contributing to higher risk of prostate cancer (Schaid, 2004).

Sedentary lifestyle and lack of physical activity as well as high body mass index (BMI) have been correlated to the risk of prostate cancer. Increase in BMI leads to an increase in advanced prostate cancer; however, it reduces the tissue-confined disease (Cuzick et al., 2014). A sedentary lifestyle may be responsible for prostate cancer, as it has been shown to increase serum PSA concentration, according to one study (Cuzick et al., 2014). According to the World Cancer Research Fund (WCRF) and American Institute of Cancer Research (AICR), if exposures of poor diet, physical inactivity and obesity were eliminated, 16% of the world's prostate cancers could be prevented, even when other risk factors remain unchanged (Baade et al., 2013).

In fact, regions in the world that show the least incidence, i.e. Asian countries, especially Japan, have diets rich in the components that protect against cancer, such as soybeans, lentils, and fish. Soybeans are consumed as tofu, tempeh, miso, and soymilk. Energy from soy products has been reported to be inversely associated with prostate cancer mortality (Hebert et al., 1998). The increase in the incidence of prostate cancer in the Asia Pacific region has also been attributed to the influence of Western lifestyle habits and strong economic growth that has led to higher average family incomes. The diet shifted from a traditional high fiber and carbohydrate diet based on vegetable foods to a diet rich in processed or red meat and total fat content. This change was accompanied by adoption of a sedentary lifestyle and lack of physical activity. Together, these factors can contribute to increased risk of developing cancer (Baade et al., 2013).

Smoking has been negatively correlated to risk and prognosis of prostate cancer. It has a strong association with prostate cancer–associated mortality. Reasons hypothesized for this include suppression of immune cells (T cells) by cigarette smoking that may lead to poor elimination of cancer cells by the immune system, enhanced progression of prostate cancer by carcinogens from tobacco, angiogenesis induced by nicotine, and complications in chemotherapy due to smoking (Polesel et al., 2015).

2.4 DIAGNOSIS AND TREATMENT

2.4.1 Staging and Grading of Prostate Cancer

Prostate cancer is graded by the Gleason grading system (Falconer, 2013). In this system, the tissue from biopsy samples are stained with hematoxylin and eosin (H&E) and then viewed at low magnification (10´–40´) in an optical microscope. Then, based on the growth pattern and extent of differentiation, the nine observed growth patterns are divided into five grades (Humphrey, 2004). For staging of prostate cancer, the data obtained from digital rectal examination (DRE) or transrectal ultrasound (TRUS) is used. The most widely used method for staging of prostate cancer is the tumor, node, and metastasis (TNM) staging system by the American Joint Committee on Cancer/ Union Internationale Contre le Cancer (Cheng et al., 2011).

2.4.2 Diagnosis

Benign and malignant tumors in the prostate can be diagnosed by various invasive and noninvasive techniques. Noninvasive diagnostic methods include PSA testing, MRI, CT scan, and TRUS. Invasive techniques for prostate cancer diagnosis include DRE and needle biopsy.

In PSA testing, the patient's blood is tested for PSA levels. PSA is produced by the prostate glands. The cut-off value for abnormal PSA levels has not been determined but it is generally considered that higher levels of circulating PSA correlate with a greater chance of prostate cancer. However, high levels of PSA do not necessarily indicate the presence of prostate cancer (Bastian et al. 2014). In fact, PSA testing is leading to overdiagnosis of prostate cancer, and therefore use of alternate methods of diagnosis for prostate cancer has become necessary. MRI is one such alternative. MRI scans of the prostate are becoming increasingly accurate in identifying the prostatic tumors, mostly because of the advent of diffusion-weighted imaging (DWI) (Rosenkrantz and Taneja, 2015).

DRE involves insertion of a gloved and lubricated finger into the rectum followed by feeling the gland to examine for a palpable tumor. Tumors detected by DRE are usually advanced (Hoffman, 2015). Biopsy is performed currently by ultrasound-guided transrectal or transperineal lateral-directed 18G core biopsy. However, biopsy should not be performed if only the PSA levels are high, unless the DRE, patient's age, and potential comorbidities also indicate its requirement (Bastian et al., 2014).

2.4.3 Treatment

Treatment options for prostate cancer include radical prostatectomy, radiation therapy with low-dose rate brachytherapy, hormonal therapy, and chemotherapy. The treatment chosen by the physician depends on the stage of the disease. Surveillance, prostatectomy, and radiation therapy are suitable for stage I to stage III cancers, while for stage IV disease and high-risk stage III cancers, androgen ablation is the preferred treatment. Androgen ablation is carried out by surgical or chemical castration. If castration resistance develops in stage IV cancer patients due to certain genetic mutations in the androgen receptor (AR), the prognosis is poor. In such cases, further treatment necessitates the administration of docetaxel (Trewartha and Carter, 2013).

Radiation or external beam radiation therapy (EBRT) is the standard treatment implemented for localized cancers, carried out by irradiation of the prostate tissue with a conventional radiation of 64-72 Gy, so as to kill the cancer cells. EBRT may also be given postoperatively and as palliative treatment. If the prostate cancer has metastasized to the bone, the sharp pain is completely eliminated in 20–50% of patients by single-fraction radiotherapy with a dose of 8 Gy. Fifty to eighty percent of patients who receive the same therapy experience partial pain relief (Lumen et al., 2013). Radiation therapy can cause significant toxicity to the tissues surrounding the prostate, such as the rectum and bladder, and this problem can be overcome by administering brachytherapy rather than EBRT. Prostate brachytherapy involves implantation of a radioactive source such as I^{125}, Pd^{103}, Au^{198}, or Yb^{169} (permanent implantation) or Ir^{192} (temporary implantation) into the malignant prostate tissue. This implant gives extreme radiation at a low dose with high precision to the prostate such that the cytotoxic effect to nearby normal organs including bladder, urethra, and rectum is negligible (Porter et al., 1995; Chang et al., 2014). Brachytherapy has become possible with the development of TRUS, which is used to guide the transperineal placement of the implant (Morton and Hoskin, 2013).

Apart from this, androgen deprivation therapy (ADT) has become the linchpin for treatment of prostate cancer since Huggins and Hodges showed in the 1950s that metastatic prostate cancer responds to testosterone deprivation (Kirby, 2015). The size of the tumor is shrunk by giving agonists and antagonists of gonadotropin-releasing hormone (GnRH) which severely reduce the levels of circulating testosterone (referred to as "castrate levels of testosterone"). While this approach may seem innocuous, it is associated with a range of toxic symptoms including reduced bone density, metabolic changes leading to weight gain, decreased muscle mass with increased insulin resistance, anemia, fatigue, hot flashes, loss of libido, sexual dysfunction, and reduced testicle size (Iacovelli et al., 2015). Hormonal therapy for prostate cancer, known as combined androgen blockade (CAB) therapy, involves a combination of chemical or surgical castration with anti-androgen molecules (Matsumoto et al., 2013). After a few months to years of ADT or CAB, tumors become resistant to ADT and yield what is called castration-resistant prostate cancer (CRPC) or hormone-refractory prostate cancer. Metastatic CRPC (mCRPC) is difficult to control, and recent studies on treatment of prostate cancer have focused on this particular type of cancer as a target for therapy. The novel molecules developed against this type of cancer include chemotherapeutic agents and hormonal agents such as docetaxel, cabazitaxel, enzalutamide, and abiraterone (Afshar et al., 2015; Iacovelli et al., 2015),

Docetaxel chemotherapy along with ADT has been shown to increase recurrence-free survival in patients with high-risk prostate cancer compared to ADT alone (Fizazi et al., 2015). Abiraterone acetate is often given in combination with prednisone before or after docetaxel treatment (Attard et al., 2015; Brasso et al., 2015). Enzalutamide, like abiraterone, is also usually given in combination with prednisone. It may be given as pre- or post-docetaxel–based therapy.

Although the above agents have been approved by the FDA as the primary treatment for patients with CRPC, they are associated with toxicities such as edema, neutropenia, sensory neuropathy, hyperkalemia, transaminase increases, hot flashes, and cardiovascular toxicity including hypertension, atrial fibrillation, and cardiac events. The toxic effects of these agents necessitate development of less toxic treatment methods and contribute to a reduced quality of life for patients (Iacovelli et al., 2015; Shigeta et al., 2015).

2.5 CONCLUSION

Prostate cancer contributes to 6.6% of deaths due to cancer in the world. It affects primarily the elderly and is predominant in the black population. Its incidence is increasing, and recent studies have shown that lifestyle factors may contribute greatly to this increase. In addition, the increasing trend of employing PSA testing for prostate cancer diagnosis is leading to a rise in incidence rates due to overdiagnosis. There is an urgent need for more accurate diagnostic tests to precisely calculate the burden of prostate cancer in the world. The available treatment options, though effective, do not improve the quality of life of the patient. They cause toxicity in one form or another, and thus there is an urgent need for newer and less toxic therapy options, such as alternative medicine– and personalized medicine–based therapies. Research is being conducted across the world to understand the true potential of these modalities of therapy for prostate cancer. The personalized medicine approach requires identification of novel prostatic biomarkers to provide highly individualized treatment, tailored to the patient's physiology. Research is also under way for finding these biomarkers. Alternative medicine involves prevention and treatment of prostate cancer using nutraceuticals, special diets, yoga, Ayurvedic medicines, and so forth, and these are being extensively explored. They show great promise in providing safe treatment but need to be publicized more zealously so that more people can benefit from them.

REFERENCES

Afshar, M. Evison, F. James, N.D. et al. 2015. Shifting paradigms in the estimation of survival for castration-resistant prostate cancer: a tertiary academic center experience. *Urol Oncol* 33(8): 338.

Attard, G. de Bono, J.S. Logothetis, C.J. et al. 2015. Improvements in radiographic progression-free survival stratified by ERG gene status in metastatic castration-resistant prostate cancer patients treated with abiraterone acetate. *Clin Cancer Res* 21(7): 1621–1627.

Baade, P.D. Youlden, D.R. Cramb, S.M. et al. 2013. Epidemiology of prostate cancer in the Asia-Pacific Region. *Prostate Int* 1(2): 47–58.

Bastian, P.J. Bellmunt, J. Bolla, M. et al. 2014. EAU guidelines on prostate cancer. Part 1: screening, diagnosis, and local treatment with curative intent – update 2013. *Eur Urol* 65(1): 124–137.

Brasso, K. Thomsen, F.B. Schrader, A.J. et al. 2015. Enzalutamide antitumour activity against metastatic castration-resistant prostate cancer previously treated with docetaxel and abiraterone: A multicentre analysis. *Eur Urol* 68(2): 317–324.

Bray, F. Ren, J.S. Masuyer, E. et al. 2012. Global estimates of cancer prevalence for 27 sites in the adult population in 2008. *Int J Cancer* 132(5): 1133–1145.

Center, M.M. Jemal, A. Lortet-Tieulent, J. et al. 2012. International variation in prostate cancer incidence and mortality rates. *Eur Urol* 61(6): 1079–1092.

Chang, A.J. Autio, K.A. Roach, M. et al. 2014. High-risk prostate cancer – classification and therapy. *Nat Rev Clin Oncol* 11(6): 308–323.

Cheng, L. Montironi, R. Bostwick, D.G. et al. 2011. Staging of prostate cancer. *Histopathology* 60(1): 87–117.

Cuzick, J. Thorat, M.A. Andriole, G. et al. 2014. Review prevention and early detection of prostate cancer. *Lancet Oncol* 15(11): 484–492.

Falconer, N. 2013. *Dealing with Prostate Cancer: The Complete Guide to Prevention, Symptoms, Diagnosis, Treatment and Care*. Raleigh: Lulu Press.

Ferlay J. Soerjomataram, I. Ervik, M. et al. GLOBOCAN 2012 v1.0, Cancer incidence and mortality worldwide: IARC cancer base no. 11 [Internet]. Lyon, France. Available from: http://globocan.iarc.fr (accessed 26 August, 2015). International Agency for Research on Cancer; 2013.

Fizazi, K. Faivre, L. Lesaunier, F. et al. 2015. Androgen deprivation therapy plus docetaxel and estramustine versus androgen deprivation therapy alone for high-risk localised prostate cancer (GETUG 12): a phase 3 randomised controlled trial. *Lancet Oncol* 16: 787–794.

Hebert, J.R. Hurley, T.G. Olendzki, B.C. et al. 1998. Nutritional and socioeconomic factors in relation to prostate cancer mortality: a cross-national study. *J Natl Cancer Inst* 90(21): 1637–1647.

Hoffman, R.M. Screening for Prostate Cancer. Last updated on 24 July 2015. http://www.uptodate.com/contents/screening-for-prostate-cancer (accessed 25 November, 2015).

Humphrey, P.A. 2004. Gleason grading and prognostic factors in carcinoma of the prostate. *Mod Pathol* 17 (3): 292–306.

Hussein, S. Satturwar, S. der-Kwast, T.V. 2015. Young-age prostate cancer. *J Clin Pathol* 68 (7): 511–515.

Iacovelli, R. Verri, E. Rocca, M.C. et al. 2015. The incidence and relative risk of cardiovascular toxicity in patients treated with new hormonal agents for castration-resistant prostate cancer. *Eur J Cancer* 51 (14): 1970–1977.

Jain, S. Saxena, S. Anup, K. 2010. Epidemiology of prostate cancer in India. *Mgene* 2: 596–605.

Kirby, R. 2015. Revolution in prostate cancer treatment. *Trends in Urology Men's Health* 6(4): 5, July–August 2015.

Lumen, N. Ost, P. Praet, C.V. et al. 2013. Developments in external beam radiotherapy for prostate cancer. *Urology* 82(1): 5–10.

Matsumoto, K. Tanaka, N. Hayakawa, N. et al. 2013. Efficacy of estramustine phosphate sodium hydrate (EMP) monotherapy in castration-resistant prostate cancer patients: report of 102 cases and review of literature. *Med Oncol* 30(4): 717–724.

Morton, G.C. Hoskin, P.J. 2013. Brachytherapy: current status and future strategies – can high dose rate replace low dose rate and external beam radiotherapy? *Clin Oncol* 25(8): 474–482.

Polesel, J. Andrea, G. Maso, L.D. et al. 2015. The negative impact of tobacco smoking on survival after prostate cancer diagnosis. *Cancer Cause Control* 26(9): 1299–1305.

Porter, A.T. Blasko, J.C. Grimm, P.D. et al. 1995. Brachytherapy for prostate cancer. *CA Cancer J Clin* 45(3): 165–178.

Powell, I.J. Vigneau, F.D. Bock, C.H. et al. 2014. Reducing prostate cancer racial disparity: evidence for aggressive early prostate cancer PSA testing of African American men. *Cancer Epidemiol Biomarkers Prev* 23(8): 1505–1511.

Rosenkrantz, A.B. Taneja, S.S. 2015. Prostate MRI can reduce overdiagnosis and overtreatment of prostate cancer. *Academic Radiol* 22(8): 1000–1006.

Schaid, D.J. 2004. The complex genetic epidemiology of prostate cancer. *Hum Mol Gen* 13: R103–R121.

SEER Cancer Statistics Factsheets: Prostate Cancer. National Cancer Institute. Bethesda, MD. http://seer.cancer.gov/statfacts/html/prost.html (accessed 25 November, 2015).

Sharma, G. Sharma, S. Sehgal, P. 2014. Emerging trends in epidemiology of breast, prostate and gall-bladder cancer. *IJPSR* 5(7): 329–337.

Shigeta, K. Kosaka, T. Yazawa, S. et al. 2015. Predictive factors for severe and febrile neutropenia during docetaxel chemotherapy for castration-resistant prostate cancer. *Int J Clin Oncol* 20: 605–612.

Siegel, R. Ma, J. Zou, Z. et al. 2014. Cancer statistics, 2014. *CA Cancer J Clin* 64(1): 1–21.

Smith, C.V. Bauer, J.J. Connelly, R.R. et al. 2000. Prostate cancer in men age 50 years or younger: a review of the Department of Defense Center for Prostate Disease Research multicenter prostate cancer database. *J Urol* 164(6): 1964–1967.

Torre, L.A. Bray, F. Siegel, R.L. et al. 2015. Global cancer statistics, 2012. *CA Cancer J Clin* 65(2): 87–108.

Trewartha, D. Carter, K. 2013. Advances in prostate cancer treatment. *Nat Rev Drug Discov* 12: 823–824.

CHAPTER 3

Medicinal Plants with Anticancer Activity against Prostate Cancer: Compilation of Data Published 2010–2015

Roland Hardman

Prostate cancer is emerging as one of the leading causes of death worldwide for men. There is increasing evidence to support the notion that dietary habits and lifestyle play a crucial role in prostate cancer pathogenesis. Studies conducted in the past few decades have successfully identified several medicinal plants and have isolated various compounds with their respective molecular mechanisms of action against prostate cancer both *in vitro* and *in vivo*. The molecular mechanism action varies among different plant extracts or isolated compounds. Among other things, it can be cell growth inhibition, cell cycle arrest, suppression of angiogenesis and metastasis, inhibition of survival signaling cascade, inducing apoptosis or autophagy or both. In this chapter we have compiled the studies of anticancer activity of various medicinal plants reported against prostate cancer (both *in vitro* and *in vivo*) during 2010–2015.

Abstract No.	Species	Prostate Cancer Cells	Title of Research	First Named Author	Journal Reference
		2015 (Year published in Cabi Citations)			
3026255	*Solanum glabratum* Dunal var. *sepicula* (2 new saponin glycosides: 23-β-D glucopyranosyl (23S, 25R)-spirost-5-en-3, 23 diol 3-O-α-L-rhamnopyranosyl-(1→2)-O-[α-L-rhamnopyranosyl-(1→4)]-β-D-glucopyranoside (2) and (25R)-spirost-5-en-3-ol 3-O-α-L-rhamnopyranosyl-(1→2)-O-[β-D-galactopyranoside (3), plus 2 known)	PC-3	Chemical constituents from *Solanum glabratum* Dunal var. *sepicula*.	Abdel-Sattar, E. et al.	*Records of Natural Products*, 2015, 9, 1, 94–104.
3026441	*Dendrobium nobile* Denbinobin, a phenanthrene	CXCL-12-induced PC-3	Denbinobin, a phenanthrene from *Dendrobium nobile*, impairs prostate cancer migration by inhibiting Rac1 activity.	TeLing, L. et al.	*Journal of Chinese Medicine*, 2014, 42, 6, 1539–1554.
3026683	Conjugated linoleic acid, oleic acid, safflower oil and taxol, synergistic effects	PC-3	*In vitro* synergistic efficacy of conjugated linoleic acid, oleic acid, safflower oil and taxol cytotoxicity on PC3 cells.	Kizılşahin, S. et al.	*Natural Product Research*, 2015, 29, 4, 378–382.
3028965	*Zingiber zerumbet* Zerumbone	DU-145 PC-3	Zerumbone inhibits growth of hormone refractory prostate cancer cells by inhibiting JAK2/STAT3 pathway and increases paclitaxel sensitivity.	Jorvig, J.E.	*Anti-Cancer Drugs*, 2015, 26, 2, 160–166.
3029761	Botanical compound LCS101	PC-3, DU-145	Selective anticancer effects and protection from chemotherapy by the botanical compound LCS101: implications for cancer treatment.	Cohen, Z. et al.	*International Journal of Oncology*, 2015, 46, 1, 308–316.
3035096	*Pleurotus cystidiosus* O. K. Mill. (Chinese edible fungus) (2 new bisabolane-type sesquiterpenoids, pleuroton A and pleuroton B (apoptosis), and clitocybulol derivatives: D, E & F)	DU-145, C42B	New apoptosis-inducing sesquiterpenoids from the mycelial culture of Chinese edible fungus *Pleurotus cystidiosus*.	Zheng YongBiao et al.	*Journal of Agricultural and Food Chemistry*, 2015, 63, 2, 545–551.

Abstract No.	Species	Prostate Cancer Cells	Title of Research	First Named Author	Journal Reference
3035903	*Hygrophorus penarius* (Hygrophoraceae) (Basidiomycetes) (fruiting bodies) Penarines A-F, (nor-) sesquiterpene carboxylic acids	PC-3	Penarines A-F, (nor-)sesquiterpene carboxylic acids from *Hygrophorus penarius* (Basidiomycetes).	Otto, A. et al.	*Phytochemistry*, 2014, 108, 229–233.
3137497	*Melampodium leucanthum* (Texas) (leaves and branches) meleucanthin New tricyclic sesquiterpene, and 4 known germacranolide sesquiterpene lactones	PC-3 DU-145	*Melampodium leucanthum*, a source of cytotoxic sesquiterpenes with antimitotic activities.	Robles, A.J. et al.	*Journal of Natural Products*, 2015, 78, 3, 388–395.
3141049	Solanaceous plants, eggplants, potatoes, and tomatoes (glycoalkaloids)		Chemistry and anticarcinogenic mechanisms of glycoalkaloids produced by eggplants, potatoes, and tomatoes.	Friedman, M.	*Journal of Agricultural and Food Chemistry*, 2015, 63, 13, 3323–3337.
3129311	*Annona muricata* L. (soursop: seed and pulp)	PC-3	An analysis *in-vitro* of the cytotoxic, antioxidant and antimicrobial activity of aqueous and alcoholic extracts of *Annona muricata* L. seed and pulp.	Raybaudi-Massilia, R. et al.	*Journal of Applied Science & Technology*, 2015, 5, 4, 333N341.
3130076	*Hymenodictyon excelsum*, anthraquinones and coumarins		Evaluation of *Hymenodictyon excelsum* phytochemical's therapeutic value against prostate cancer by molecular docking study.	Rahman, M.M. et al.	*Jundishapur Journal of Natural Pharmaceutical Products*, 2015, 10, 1, e18216.
3121989	Ojeok-san – oriental herbal formula		Cytotoxicity and subacute toxicity in Crl:CD (SD) rats of traditional herbal formula Ojeok-san.	Jeong SooJin et al.	*BMC Complementary and Alternative Medicine*, 2015, 15, 38.
3114309	*Dionysia aucheri*	PC-3	Preliminary study for the effect of *Dionysia aucheri* methanolic extract on the viability of some cell lines.	Alsamarrae, K.W. et al.	*World Journal of Pharmaceutical Research*, 2015, 4, 2, 35–42.
3102444	*Jatropha ribifolia* (Pohl) Baill (Euphorbiaceae) (root essential oil)	PC-3	Chemical composition and cytotoxic activity of the root essential oil from *Jatropha ribifolia* (Pohl) Baill (Euphorbiaceae).	Silva, C.E.L. da. et al.	*Journal of the Brazilian Chemical Society*, 2015, 26, 2, 233–238.
3089036	Coumarin derivative complexes with Cu(II) and Ni(II) (apoptosis)	PC-3	Anticancer activity and DNA-binding investigations of the Cu(II) and Ni(II) complexes with coumarin derivative.	Zhu TaoFeng et al.	*Chemical Biology and Drug Design*, 2015, 85, 3, 385–393.

Abstract No.	Species	Prostate Cancer Cells	Title of Research	First Named Author	Journal Reference
3089694	Pleurotus djamor var. roseus, silver nanoparticles (apoptosis)	PC-3	Mycosynthesis and characterization of silver nanoparticles from Pleurotus djamor var. roseus and their in vitro cytotoxicity effect on PC3 cells.	Jegadeesh Raman et al.	Process Biochemistry, 2015, 50, 1, 140–147.
3091342	Tinospora cordifolia (Menispermaceae) (stem)		Ferric reducing, anti-radical and cytotoxic activities of Tinospora cordifolia stem extracts.	Sharma, A.K. et al.	Biochemistry and Analytical Biochemistry, 2014, 3, 2, 153.
3091453	Nymphoides peltata (wetland)	PC-3	Antitumor constituents of the wetland plant Nymphoides peltata: a case study for the potential utilization of constructed wetland plant resources.	Du YuanDa et al.	Natural Product Communications, 2015, 10, 2, 233–236.
3091479	Solanum macaonense Macaocerebroside A (new cerebroside and 15 known compounds)	DU-145	Anti-inflammatory and cytotoxic compounds from Solanum macaonense	Lee ChiaLin et al.	Natural Product Communications, 2015, 10, 2, 345–348.
3092924	Schisandra grandiflora (fruits) (sesquiterpenes: 3 new & 3 known)	DU-145	Novel sesquiterpenes from Schisandra grandiflora: isolation, cytotoxic activity and synthesis of their triazole derivatives using "click" reaction.	Poornima, B. et al.	European Journal of Medicinal Chemistry, 2015, 92, 449–458.
3084881	Citrus (Rutaceae) Obacunone and obacunone glucoside	LNCaP	Cytotoxicity of obacunone and obacunone glucoside in human prostate cancer cells involves Akt-mediated programmed cell death.	Murthy, K.N.C. et al.	Toxicology, 2015, 329, 88–97.
3081621	Orthosiphon stamineus (cat's whiskers tea, leaves) aromatic sesquiterpenes etc.	PC-3	Optimization of cat's whiskers tea (Orthosiphon stamineus) using supercritical carbon dioxide and selective chemotherapeutic potential against prostate cancer cells.	Al-Suede, F.S.R. et al.	Evidence-based Complementary and Alternative Medicine, 2014, Article ID 396016, 2014.
3066210	Solanum nigrum (leaves and stems; Sudan)	PC-3	In vitro anticancer activity and cytotoxicity of Solanum nigrum on cancers and normal cell lines.	Moglad, E.H.O. et al.	International Journal of Cancer Research (USA), 2014, 10, 2, 74–80.

Abstract No.	Species	Prostate Cancer Cells	Title of Research	First Named Author	Journal Reference
3071743	*Valeriana jatamansi* (10 new valepotriates, jatamanvaltrates P–Y and a known one, nardostachin, from whole plants)	PC-3 M	Minor valepotriates from *Valeriana jatamansi* and their cytotoxicity against metastatic prostate cancer cells.	Lin Sheng et al.	*Planta Medica*, 2015, 81, 1, 56–61.
3064507	*Denhamia celastroides* (8 new dihydro-β-agarofurans, denhaminols A–H from leaves) (Australian rainforest)	LNCaP	Denhaminols A–H, dihydro-β-agarofurans from the endemic Australian rainforest plant *Denhamia celastroides*.	Levrier, C. et al.	*Journal of Natural Products*, 2015, 78, 1, 111–119.
3064682	*Euodia rutaecarpa* (fruits) (4 quinolone alkaloids and 3 indole alkaloids, 30 known alkaloids)	PC-3	Quinolone and indole alkaloids from the fruits of *Euodia rutaecarpa* and their cytotoxicity against two human cancer cell lines.	Zhao Nan et al.	*Phytochemistry*, 2015, 109, 133–139.
3175610	*Silybum marianum* (L) Gaertn. (milk thistle, using fungal endophytes from plant)	PC-3	Phylogenetic and chemical diversity of fungal endophytes isolated from *Silybum marianum* (L) Gaertn. (milk thistle).	Raja, H.A. et al.	*Mycology – An International Journal on Fungal Biology*, 2015, 6, 1, 8–27.
3164346	*Croton membranaceus* (aqueous root extract)	Benign prostatic hyperplasia (BPH-1) and prostate cancer	Mitochondria-dependent apoptogenic activity of the aqueous root extract of *Croton membranaceus* against human BPH-1 cells.	Afriyie, D.K. et al.	*FUNPEC, Brazil, Genetics and Molecular Research*, 2015, 14, 1, 149–162.
3164805	Aloe emodin derivatives (synthesized)	PC-3	Synthesis and antitumor activity of natural compound aloe emodin derivatives.	Thimmegowda, N.R. et al.	*Chemical Biology and Drug Design*, 2015, 85, 5, 638–644.
3167393	Egyptian: juniper, thyme, and clove oils (α-pinene, thymol, and eugenol) reference drug, doxorubicin	PC-3	Essential oils from Egyptian aromatic plants as antioxidant and novel anticancer agents in human cancer cell lines.	Ramadan, M.M. et al.	*Grasas y Aceites (Sevilla)*, 2015, 66, 2, e080.
3158646	Curcumin, asymmetric analogues, synthesized	PC-3	Synthesis and assessment of the antioxidant and antitumor properties of asymmetric curcumin analogues.	Li QingYong et al.	*European Journal of Medicinal Chemistry*, 2015, 93, 461–469.
3235077	*Hibiscus sabdariffa* leaves	PC-3	In vitro antioxidant, anti-inflammatory, cytotoxic activities against prostate cancer of extracts from *Hibiscus sabdariffa* leaves.	Worawattananutai, P. et al.	*Journal of the Medical Association of Thailand*, 2014, 97, 8 Supplement 8, 81–87.

Abstract No.	Species	Prostate Cancer Cells	Title of Research	First Named Author	Journal Reference
3235080	Sung Yod rice bran oil	PC-3	Biological activities and chemical content of Sung Yod rice bran oil extracted by expression and soxhlet extraction methods.	Uttama, S. et al.	*Journal of the Medical Association of Thailand*, 2014, 97, 8 Supplement 8, 125–132.
3236712	Taxol from *Taxus* spp. Trees Endophytic fungi		Use of endophytic fungi in the taxol anticancer drug production.	Barrales-Cureño, H.J. et al.	*Biotecnología Vegetal*, 2014, 14, 1, 3–13.
3220263	Lupiwighteone (Isoflavone) e.g. from *Glycyrrhiza glabra, Lupinus, and Lotus pedunculatus*	DU-145	Isoflavone lupiwighteone induces cytotoxic, apoptotic, and antiangiogenic activities in DU-145 prostate cancer cells.	Ren Jie et al.	*Anti-Cancer Drugs*, 2015, 26, 6, 599–611.
3226135	*Madhuca pasquieri* (Dubard) (leaves)		Anti-inflammatory activity of pyrrolizidine alkaloids from the leaves of *Madhuca pasquieri* (Dubard).	Le Son Hoang et al.	*Chemical & Pharmaceutical Bulletin*, 2015, 63, 6, 481–484.
3214657	*Ferula assafoetida* Galbanic acid	PC-9	Apoptotic effect of galbanic acid via activation of caspases and inhibition of Mcl-1 in H460 non-small lung carcinoma cells.	Oh BumSeok et al.	*Phytotherapy Research*, 2015, 29, 6, 844–849.
3218760	*Calliandra portoricensis* (root)	LNCaP PC-3	Antioxidant, antiangiogenic and antiproliferative activities of root methanol extract of *Calliandra portoricensis* in human prostate cancer cells.	Adaramoye, O. et al.	*Journal of Integrative Medicine*, 2015, 13, 3, 185–193.
3219349	*Stillingia lineata* (endemic Mascarene species) (flexibilane and tigliane)	PC-3	Antiviral activity of flexibilane and tigliane diterpenoids from *Stillingia lineata*.	Olivon, F. et al.	*Journal of Natural Products*, 2015, 78, 5, 1119–1128.
3219359	*Bursera microphylla* (diterpenoids and triterpenoids from resin) (15 compounds isolated, of which 3 new: malabaricatrienone, malabaricatrienol, and microphyllanin)	PC-3	Diterpenoids and triterpenoids from the resin of *Bursera microphylla* and their cytotoxic activity.	Messina, F. et al.	*Journal of Natural Products*, 2015, 78, 5, 1184–1188.
3219405	Bamboo species leaf	PC-3	Phytofabrication of biomolecule-coated metallic silver nanoparticles using leaf extracts of *in vitro* – raised bamboo species and its anticancer activity against human PC3 cell lines.	Kalamegam Kalaiarasi et al.	*Turkish Journal of Biology*, 2015, 39, 2, 223–232.

Abstract No.	Species	Prostate Cancer Cells	Title of Research	First Named Author	Journal Reference
3211043	Bursera species (Mexico) *B. ariensis* (Kunth) McVaugh and Rzed. Kew Bull (two populations) *B. bicolor* Engl., *B. lancifolia* Engl., *B. glabrifolia* Engl. (2 populations) *B. fagaroides* (La Llave) Rez., Calderón and Medina, *B. linanoe* (La Llave) Rez., Calderón and Medina, *B. galeottiana* Engl., *B. kerberi* Engl., and *B. excelsa* Engl.	PC-3	Cytotoxic and anti-inflammatory activities of Bursera species from Mexico.	Acevedo, M. et al.	*Journal of Clinical Toxicology*, 2015, 5, 1, 232.
3197545	Guttiferone F (sensitizes prostate cancer to starvation-induced apoptosis)	LNCaP PC-3 (xenografts in mice)	The natural compound Guttiferone F sensitizes prostate cancer to starvation-induced apoptosis via calcium and JNK elevation.	Li Xin et al.	*BMC Cancer*, 2015, 15, 254.
3203768	Baliospermum montanum		Effect of *Baliospermum montanum* nanomedicine apoptosis induction and anti-migration of prostate cancer cells.	Cherian, A.M. et al.	*Biomedicine & Pharmacotherapy*, 2015, 71, 201–209.
3189801	Ageratum conyzoides (leaf)	LNCap PNT2	*In vitro* antioxidant and anticancer properties of hydroethanolic extracts and fractions of *Ageratum conzoides*.	Acheampong, F. et al.	*European Journal of Medicinal Plants*, 2015, 7, 4, 205–214.
3190089	(Gürarslan) of *Trigonella foenum graecum* L. (seeds)	Mat-LyLu rat prostate carcinoma	*In vitro* antitumor effects of a new cultivar (Gürarslan) of *Trigonella foenum graecum* L.	Aktas, H.G. et al.	*African Journal of Traditional, Complementary and Alternative Medicines*, 2015, 12, 3, 113–119.
3196765	Garcinia oligantha (3-methoxy-5-methoxycarbonyl-4-hydroxy-biphenyl)	PC-3	A new biphenyl from *Garcinia oligantha* and its cytotoxicity.	Liu GuiYou et al.	*Asian Journal of Chemistry*, 2015, 27, 7, 2731–2732.
3196766	Desmodium renifolium (2',5-dihydroxy-4,4'-dimethoxy-3-prenyl-chalcone)	PC-3	A new cytotoxic prenylated chalcone from *Desmodium renifolium*.	Yang JuanXia et al.	*Asian Journal of Chemistry*, 2015, 27, 7, 2733–2734.
3187440	Acanthopanax trifoliatus (L.) Merr. (apoptosis)	PC-3	Potent inhibitory effect of terpenoids from *Acanthopanax trifoliatus* on growth of PC-3 prostate cancer cells *in vitro* and *in vivo* is associated with suppression of NF-κB and STAT3 signalling.	Li DongLi et al.	*Journal of Functional Foods*, 2015, 15, 274–283.

Abstract No.	Species	Prostate Cancer Cells	Title of Research	First Named Author	Journal Reference
3188322	Saw palmetto (seeds) (new: chalcanonol glycoside-bis-O-[(I-4') -> (II-6')]-α-hydroxyphloretin-2'-O-β-glucoside plus 6 known compounds)	PC-3	New chalcanonol glycoside from the seeds of saw palmetto: antiproliferative and antioxidant effects.	Abdel Bar, F.M.	Natural Product Research, 2015, 29, 10, 926–932.
3241697	Saponaria officinalis L. (Caryophyllaceae) roots		Antiproliferative quillaic acid and gypsogenin saponins from Saponaria officinalis L. roots.	Lu YuPing et al.	Phytochemistry, 2015, 113, 108–120.
3240053	Phyllanthus spp. (P. amarus, P. niruri, P. urinaria and P. watsonii)	PC-3	Phyllanthus spp. exerts anti-angiogenic and antimetastatic effects through inhibition on matrix metalloproteinase enzymes.	Tang YinQuan et al.	Nutrition and Cancer, 2015, 67, 5, 783–795.
3255767	Pittosporum venulosum (new monoterpene glycosides – venulosides C and D)	LNCaP	LAT transport inhibitors from Pittosporum venulosum identified by NMR fingerprint analysis.	Grkovic, T. et al.	Journal of Natural Products, 2015, 78, 6, 1215–1220.
3264552	Croton membranaceus (aqueous root extract)	BPH-1	Genotoxic and cytotoxic activity of aqueous extracts of Croton membranaceus in rodent bone marrow and human benign prostate hyperplasic cells.	Asare, G.A. et al.	European Journal of Medicinal Plants, 2015, 9, 2.
3263288	Ocimum sanctum Linn. Tulsi. (holy basil)	LNCaP	Apoptosis induction by Ocimum sanctum extract in LNCaP prostate cancer cells.	Dhandayuthapa-ni, S. et al.	Journal of Medicinal Food, 2015, 18, 7, 776–785.
3258506	Curcumin-loaded pH-sensitive redox nanoparticles		Redox nanoparticles inhibit curcumin oxidative degradation and enhance its therapeutic effect on prostate cancer.	Thangavel, S. et al.	Journal of Controlled Release, 2015, 209, 110–119.
3277901	Valeriana jatamansi	PC-3 M	Three decomposition products of valepotriates from Valeriana jatamansi and their cytotoxic activity.	Lin Sheng et al.	Journal of Asian Natural Products Research, 2015, 17, 5, 455–461.
3277858	Rosa rugosa (flowers) rugosaquinone A (a new dihydronaphthoquinone)	PC-3	A new dihydronaphthoquinone from the flowers of Rosa rugosa and its cytotoxicities.	Dong Wei et al.	Asian Journal of Chemistry, 2015, 27, 10, 3917–3918.
3277857	Aspergillus versicolor (endophytic fungus) versicoumarin D (a new isocoumarin)	PC-3	A new isocoumarin from fermentation products of endophytic fungus of Aspergillus versicolor.	Ji Bing Kun et al.	Asian Journal of Chemistry, 2015, 27, 10, 3915–3916.

Abstract No.	Species	Prostate Cancer Cells	Title of Research	First Named Author	Journal Reference
3277680	*Eucalyptus camaldulensis* (essential oil) Egypt	Oil showed cytotoxicity against prostate, colon, and breast cancer	Antioxidant, antiproliferated activities and GC/MS analysis of *Eucalyptus camaldulensis* essential oil.	El-Baz, F.K. et al.	*International Journal of Pharma and Bio Sciences*, 2015, 6, 2, B-883–B-892.
3298506	*Withania somnifera*	DU-145	Hedgehog inhibitors from *Withania somnifera*.	Yoneyama, T. et al.	*Bioorganic & Medicinal Chemistry Letters*, 2015, 25, 17, 3541–3544.
3289777	Gallotannin	DU-145, PC-3, M-2182	Inhibition of myeloid cell leukemia 1 and activation of caspases are critically involved in gallotannin-induced apoptosis in prostate cancer cells.	Park EunKyung et al.	*Phytotherapy Research*, 2015, 29, 8, 1225–1236.
3303253	*Foeniculum vulgare*	DU-145	Cytotoxicity of syringin and 4-methoxycinnamyl alcohol isolated from *Foeniculum vulgare* on selected human cell lines.	Lall, N. et al.	*Natural Product Research*, 2015, 29, 18, 1752–1756.
3302987	*Arum palaestinum* Boiss (roots)	Verified prostate cancer cells were plated as 3D spheroids	*Arum palaestinum* with isovanillin, linolenic acid and β-sitosterol inhibits prostate cancer spheroids and reduces the growth rate of prostate tumors in mice.	Cole, C. et al.	*BMC Complementary and Alternative Medicine*, 2015, 15, 264.
3300923	*Solanum seaforthianum* Andr. and *S. macrocarpon* L (Egypt)	PC-3	Impact of certain *Solanum* species' natural products as potent cytotoxic and anti-inflammatory agents.	Alsherbiny, M.A. et al.	*Journal of Medicinal Plants Research*, 2015, 9, 29, 779–786.
3341940	Qianlie Xiaozheng Tang (a Chinese herbal decoction)	Castration-resistant prostate cancer	Effect of Qianlie Xiaozheng Tang, a Chinese herbal decoction, on castration-resistant prostate cancer: a pilot study.	Pang Ran et al.	*African Journal of Traditional, Complementary and Alternative Medicines*, 2015, 12, 6, 21–26.
3342272	*Chresta sphaerocephala*	Ten human cancer cells, VERO (no cancer cell)	Antiproliferative activity, antioxidant capacity and chemical composition of extracts from the leaves and stem of *Chresta sphaerocephala*.	Da Costa, L.S. et al.	*Revista Brasileira de Farmacognosia*, 2015, 25, 4, 369–374.

Abstract No.	Species	Prostate Cancer Cells	Title of Research	First Named Author	Journal Reference
3343986	No plant material mentioned	PC-3 DU-145	Synthesis and biological evaluation of 6H-1-benzopyrano[4,3-b]quinolin-6-one derivatives as inhibitors of colon cancer cell growth.	Li TieLing et al.	*Bangladesh Journal of Pharmacology*, 2015, 10, 3, 660–671.
3345796	No plant material mentioned	No prostate cancer cell types mentioned	VEGFA SNPs (rs34357231 & rs35569394), transcriptional factor binding sites and human disease.	Buroker, N.E.	*British Journal of Medicine and Medical Research*, 2015, 10, 12.
3345829	No plant material mentioned	No prostate cancer cell types mentioned	Mortality through tumors in Bihor/ Hajdu-Bihar counties.	Daina, L. et al.	*Analele Universităţii din Oradea, Fascicula: Ecotoxicologie, Zootehnie şi Tehnologii de Industrie Alimentară*, 2013, 12, A, 108–113.
3337638	*Angelica gigas* Nakai root	Mouse model	Chemopreventive effects of Korean Angelica versus its major pyranocoumarins on two lineages of transgenic adenocarcinoma of mouse prostate carcinogenesis.	Tang, S.N. et al.	*Cancer Prevention Research*, 2015, 8, 9, 835–844.
3338370	*Crinum asiaticum*	DU-145	Hedgehog/GLI-mediated transcriptional activity inhibitors from *Crinum asiaticum*.	Arai, M.A. et al.	*Journal of Natural Medicines*, 2015, 69, 4, 538–542.
3326278	Tetrandrine, a traditional Chinese medicine	DU-145 PC-3	Tetrandrine suppresses proliferation, induces apoptosis, and inhibits migration and invasion in human prostate cancer cells.	Liu Wei et al.	*Asian Journal of Andrology*, 2015, 17, 5, 850–853.
3327304	*Agaricus bisporus*	PSA levels, myeloid-derived suppressor cells	A phase I trial of mushroom powder in patients with biochemically recurrent prostate cancer: roles of cytokines and myeloid-derived suppressor cells for *Agaricus bisporus*-induced prostate-specific antigen responses.	Twardowski, P. et al.	*Cancer*, 2015, 121, 17, 2942–2950.

Abstract No.	Species	Prostate Cancer Cells	Title of Research	First Named Author	Journal Reference
3327583			Resveratrol 2014 – The 3rd International Conference on Resveratrol and Health, Hawaii, USA, 30 November-3 December 2014. (contains 18 papers)	Vang, O. et al.	Annals of the New York Academy of Sciences, 2015, 1348, 1–179.
3329100	Abelia triflora R. Br. (Caprifoliaceae) leaves (new phenolic glucoside, abeliaside)	PC-3	Abeliaside, a new phenolic glucoside from Abelia triflora.	Al-Taweel, A.M. et al.	Natural Product Research, 2015, 29, 21, 1978–1984.
3315639	Sugiol (a naturally occurring diterpene)	DU-145 Signal transducer and activator of transcription 3 (STAT3)	Sugiol inhibits STAT3 activity via regulation of transketolase and ROS-mediated ERK activation in DU145 prostate carcinoma cells.	Jung SeungNam et al.	Biochemical Pharmacology, 2015, 97, 1, 38–50.
3312563	Dietary flavonoid fisetin	PCa	Dietary flavonoid fisetin binds to β-tubulin and disrupts microtubule dynamics in prostate cancer cells.	Mukhtar, E. et al.	Cancer Letters, 2015, 367, 2, 173–183.
3312726	Silibinin	PrSCs-prostate stromal cells PCA PC-3	Silibinin prevents prostate cancer cell-mediated differentiation of naïve fibroblasts into cancer-associated fibroblast phenotype by targeting TGF β2.	Ting, H.J. et al.	Molecular Carcinogenesis, 2015, 54, 9, 730–741.
3312927	Genistein	LNCaP, LAPC-4 PC-3	Genistein increases estrogen receptor beta expression in prostate cancer via reducing its promoter methylation.	Mahmoud, A.M. et al.	Journal of Steroid Biochemistry and Molecular Biology, 2015, 152, 62–75.
3313506		Benign prostatic hyperplasia	Relationship between benign prostatic hyperplasia and International Prostatic Symptom Score.	Iffat Raza et al.	British Journal of Medicine and Medical Research, 2015, 10, 5.
3314212	Brusatol from the Chinese traditional medicine, Fructus bruceae	DU-145 PC-3	Inhibitory effects of brusatol on human prostate cancer cells DU145 and its molecular mechanism.	Tan YaFang et al.	Science Press, Beijing, China, Guangxi Zhiwu / Guihaia, 2015, 35, 3, 431–436.
3353153	A mixture of polyherbal extracts	CWR22Rv1 PC-3	Zyflamend, a polyherbal mixture, inhibits lipogenesis and mTORC1 signalling via activation of AMPK.	Zhao, Y. et al.	Journal of Functional Foods, 2015, 18, Part A, 147–158.

Abstract No.	Species	Prostate Cancer Cells	Title of Research	First Named Author	Journal Reference
3354442	Palmatine and Nexrutine; are protoberberine alkaloids found in several plants including *Phellodendron amurense* (bark extract)		Palmatine inhibits growth and invasion in prostate cancer cell: potential role for rpS6/NFκB/FLIP.	Hambright, H.G. et al.	*Molecular Carcinogenesis*, 2015, 54, 10, 1227–1234.
3267258	*Asclepias subulata Decne* a shrub occurring in Sonora, Arizona desert (Mexico–USA)	PC-3	Antiproliferative activity of cardenolide glycosides from *Asclepias subulata*.	Rascón-Valenzuela, L. et al.	*Journal of Ethnopharmacology*, 2015, 171, 280–286.
3389672	*Coelastrella oocystiformis* (microalgae) from Mumbai, India	DU-145	Characterization of high carotenoid producing *Coelastrella oocystiformis* and its anticancer potential.	Ganesh Iyer. et al.	*International Journal of Current Microbiology and Applied Sciences*, 2015, 4, 10, 527–536.
3390044	*Achillea teretifolia* Wiild (Turkish name: Beyaz civanperÇemi)	DU-145 PC-3	*In vitro* antioxidant, cytotoxic and pro-apoptotic effects of *Achillea teretifolia* Wiild extracts on human prostate cancer cell lines.	Bali, E.B. et al.	*Pharmacognosy Magazine*, 2015, 11, 44 (Suppl.), 308–315.
3377162	Resveratrol tetramer r-viniferin	LNCaP	The resveratrol tetramer r-viniferin induces a cell cycle arrest followed by apoptosis in the prostate cancer cell line LNCaP.	Empl, M.T. et al.	*Phytotherapy Research*, 2015, 29, 10, 1640–1645.
3382816	*Garcinia indica* (Garcinol, isolated from fruit rinds, a polyisoprenylated benzophenone)	PC-3	Antitumor activity of garcinol in human prostate cancer cells and xenograft mice.	Wang, Y. et al.	*Journal of Agricultural and Food Chemistry*, 2015, 63, 41, 9047–9052.
3383072	*Dioclea reflexa* (Hook F)	None specified	Flavonoids from the roots of *Dioclea reflexa* (Hook F).	Oladimeji, A.O. et al.	*Bulletin of the Chemical Society of Ethiopia*, 2015, 29, 3, 441–448.
3373389	*Manilkara zapota* (Sapotaceae) A Cameroonian medicinal plant (Taraxastane and lupane triterpenoids from the bark)	PC-3	Taraxastane and lupane triterpenoids from the bark of *Manilkara zapota*.	Toze, F.A.A. et al.	*International Research Journal of Pure and Applied Chemistry*, 2015, 7, 4, 157–164.
3421467			Plant-derived SAC domain of PAR-4 (prostate apoptosis response 4) exhibits growth inhibitory effects in prostate cancer cells.	Shayan Sarkar et al.	*Frontiers in Plant Science*, 2015, 6, October, 822.

Abstract No.	Species	Prostate Cancer Cells	Title of Research	First Named Author	Journal Reference
3414460	Cantinoa stricta (Benth.) Harley & J.F.B. Pastore (Lamiaceae) essential oils from flowers and leaves	PC-3	Chemical composition and cytotoxic activity of the essential oils of Cantinoa stricta (Benth.) Harley & J.F.B. Pastore (Lamiaceae).	Scharf, D.R. et al.	Records of Natural Products, 2016, 10, 2, 257–261.
3414731	Juglans regia (root)	PC-3 DU-145	Activity guided isolation and modification of juglone from Juglans regia as potent cytotoxic agent against lung cancer cell lines.	Zhang XueBang et al.	BMC Complementary and Alternative Medicine, 2015, 15, 396.
3402102	Zingiber zerumbet Smith (Zerumbone, a natural monocyclic sesquiterpene)	PC-3 DU-145	Zerumbone, a ginger sesquiterpene, induces apoptosis and autophagy in human hormone-refractory prostate cancers through tubulin binding and crosstalk between endoplasmic reticulum stress and mitochondrial insult.	Chan MeiLing et al.	Naunyn-Schmiedeburgs Archives of Pharmacology, 2015, 388, 11, 1223–1236.
3403386	Cruciferous vegetables Brassinin, a type of indole compound Chili pepper: Capsaicin, an alkaloid	PC-3	Brassinin combined with capsaicin enhances apoptotic and antimetastatic effects in PC-3 human prostate cancer cells.	Kim Sung Moo et al.	Phytotherapy Research, 2015, 29, 11, 1828–1836.
3403916			Tapping botanicals for essential oils: progress and hurdles in cancer mitigation.	Seema Patel	Industrial Crops and Products, 2015, 76, 1148–1163.
3441429	Radix Stephaniae tetrandrae S. Moore (Fangchinoline, a bisbenzylisoquinoline alkaloid)	PC-3	Inhibition on proteasome β1 subunit might contribute to the anticancer effects of fangchinoline in human prostate cancer cells.	Li Dong et al.	PLoS ONE, 2015, 10, 10, e0141681.
3444431	Ganoderma lucidum (A new gymnomitrane-type sesquiterpenoid, gymnomitrane-3α,5α,9β,15-tetrol, was isolated from the fruiting body)	PC-3	A new cytotoxic gymnomitrane sesquiterpene from Ganoderma lucidum fruiting bodies.	Pham Thanh Binh et al.	Natural Product Communications, 2015, 10, 11, 1911–1912.
3434180	Celastrol	PC-3	Inhibiting inducible miR-223 further reduces viable cells in human cancer cell lines MCF-7 and PC3 treated by celastrol.	Cao Lu et al.	BMC Cancer, 2015, 15, 873.

Abstract No.	Species	Prostate Cancer Cells	Title of Research	First Named Author	Journal Reference
3435383	*Gynostemma pentaphyllum* (Gypensapogenin H is a novel dammarane-type triterpene)	DU145 22RV-1	Gypensapogenin H, a novel dammarane-type triterpene, induces cell cycle arrest and apoptosis on prostate cancer cells.	Zhang XiaoShu et al.	*Steroids*, 2015, 104, 276–283.
			2014 (Year published in Cabi Citations)		
3003460	*Castilleja tenuiflora* Benth. (Orobanchaceae)	PC-3	*In vivo* anti-inflammatory and anti-ulcerogenic activities of extracts from wild growing and *in vitro* plants of *Castilleja tenuiflora* Benth. (Orobanchaceae).	Sanchez, P.M. et al.	*Journal of Ethnopharmacology*, 2013, 150, 3, 1032–1037.
3011753	*Garcina epunctata*	PC-3	Ethyl acetate fraction of *Garcina epunctata* induces apoptosis in human promyelocytic cells (HL-60) through the ROS generation and G0/G1 cell cycle arrest: a bioassay-guided approach.	Anatole, P.C. et al.	*Environmental Toxicology and Pharmacology*, 2013, 36, 3, 865–874
3031992	*Piper sarmentosum*	DU-145	Dichamanetin inhibits cancer cell growth by affecting ROS-related signaling components through mitochondrial-mediated apoptosis.	Yong, Y.J. et al.	*Anticancer Research*, 2013, 33, 12, 5349–5356.
3028759	*Holoptelea integrifolia* (Roxb.) Planch (Ulmaceae)	DU-145	Antineoplastic activity of *Holoptelea integrifolia* (Roxb.) Planch bark extracts (*in vitro*).	Guo HuiQin	*Journal of Pharmaceutical Sciences*, 2013, 26, 6, 1151–1156.
3043772	*Alpania galangal*	DU-145	Design, synthesis and cytotoxic evaluation of o-carboxamido stilbene analogues.	Mohamad Nurul Azmi et al.	*International Journal of Molecular Sciences*, 2013, 14, 12, 23369–23389.
3043236	*Alpania galangal*	PC-3	Isolation, synthesis and biological evaluation of phenylpropanoids from the rhizomes of *Alpania galangal*.	Chourasiya, S. et al.	*Natural Product Communications*, 2013, 8, 12, 1741–1746.

Abstract No.	Species	Prostate Cancer Cells	Title of Research	First Named Author	Journal Reference
3043225	*Lysimachia thyrsiflora* L.	PC-3	Minor triterpene saponins from underground parts of *Lysimachia thyrsiflora*: structure elucidation, LC-ESI-MS/MS quantification, and biological activity.	Podolak, I. et al.	*Natural Product Communications*, 2013, 8, 12, 1691–1696.
3051945	*Viscum album*	DU-145	Interaction of standardized mistletoe (*Viscum album*) extracts with chemotherapeutic drugs regarding cytostatic and cytotoxic effects *in vitro*.	Weissenstein, U. et al.	*BMC Complementary and Alternative Medicine*, 2014, 14, 6.
3060247	Lycopene-containing fruits and vegetables		Multiple molecular and cellular mechanisms of action of lycopene in cancer inhibition.	Trejo-Solís, C. et al.	*Evidence-based Complementary and Alternative Medicine*, 2013, 2013.
3060160	*Phyllanthus* (*P. amarus, P. niruri, P. urinaria,* and *P. watsonii*)	PC-3	*Phyllanthus* suppresses prostate cancer cell, PC-3, proliferation and induces apoptosis through multiple signaling pathways (MAPKs, PI3K/Akt, NFκB, and hypoxia).	Tang YinQuan et al.	*Evidence-Based Complementary and Alternative Medicine*, 2013, 2013.
3059871	Pomegranate juice	DU-145 and PC-3 androgen-independent PCa cells	Pomegranate juice metabolites, ellagic acid and urolithin A, synergistically inhibit androgen-independent prostate cancer cell growth via distinct effects on cell cycle control and apoptosis.	Vicinanza, R. et al.	*Evidence-Based Complementary and Alternative Medicine*, 2013.
3054720	*Aegle marmelos* (L.) Correa leaves	PC-3	Pharmacognostic standardization and antiproliferative activity of *Aegle marmelos* (L.) Correa leaves in various human cancer cell lines.	Rajbir Bhatti et al.	*Indian Journal of Pharmaceutical Sciences*, 2013, 75, 6, 628–634.
3054433	*Psoralea corylifolia* (Leguminosae)		Neobavaisoflavone sensitizes apoptosis via the inhibition of metastasis in TRAIL-resistant human glioma U373MG cells.	Kim YoungJoo et al.	*Life Sciences*, 2014, 95, 2, 101–107.
3062091	Piper longum plant		Piperlongumine inhibits NF-κB activity and attenuates aggressive growth characteristics of prostate cancer cells.	Ginzburg, S. et al.	*Prostate*, 2014, 74, 2, 177–186.

Abstract No.	Species	Prostate Cancer Cells	Title of Research	First Named Author	Journal Reference
3077018	*Tillandsia recurvata* (Jamaican ball moss)		Cycloartanes with anticancer activity demonstrate promising inhibition of the Mrckα and Mrckβ kinases.	Lowe, H.I.C. et al.	*British Journal of Medicine and Medical Research*, 2014, 4, 9, 1802–1811.
3090846	*Magnolia officinalis*	LNCaP	Honokiol inhibits androgen receptor activity in prostate cancer cells.	Hahm, E.R. et al.	*Prostate*, 2014, 74, 4, 408–420.
3086617	*Ficus pseudopalma*	PRST2 cancer cell line	Cytotoxicity and apoptotic activity of *Ficus pseudopalma* Blanco leaf extracts against human prostate cancer cell lines.	Llagas, M.C. de las et al.	*Tropical Journal of Pharmaceutical Research*, 2014, 13, 1, 93–100.
3108243	Zyflamend, a mixture containing extracts of 10 herbs	CWR22Rv1 cells, a castrate-resistant prostate cancer cell line	Zyflamend, a polyherbal mixture, down regulates class I and class II histone deacetylases and increases p21 levels in castrate-resistant prostate cancer cells.	Huang, E.C. et al.	*BMC Complementary and Alternative Medicine*, 2014, 14, 68.
3114047	*Garcinia bracteata*	PC3	Antiproliferative activities of *Garcinia bracteata* extract and its active ingredient, isobractatin, against human tumor cell lines.	Shen Tao et al.	*Archives of Pharmacal Research*, 2014, 37, 3, 412–420.
3113603	*Campomanesia adamantium* (Myrtaceae)	PC-3	Antiproliferative activity and induction of apoptosis in PC-3 cells by the Chalcone cardamonin from *Campomanesia adamantium* (Myrtaceae) in a bioactivity-guided study.	Pascoal, A.C.R.F. et al.	*Molecules*, 2014, 19, 2, 1843–1855.
3127019	*Neofusicoccum australe* endophytic in (*Myrtus communis*)	DU-145, PC-3	Myrtucommulone production by a strain of *Neofusicoccum australe* endophytic in myrtle (*Myrtus communis*).	Nicoletti, R. et al.	*World Journal of Microbiology & Biotechnology*, 2014, 30, 3, 1047–1052.
3119759	Pomegranate extract	PCa	Pomegranate extract inhibits the bone metastatic growth of human prostate cancer cells and enhances the *in vivo* efficacy of docetaxel chemotherapy.	Wang, Y.R. et al.	*Prostate*, 2014, 74, 5, 497–508.

Abstract No.	Species	Prostate Cancer Cells	Title of Research	First Named Author	Journal Reference
3115734	*Salviae miltiorrhizae*	PC-3	Tanshinone IIA induces autophagic cell death via activation of AMPK and ERK and inhibition of mTOR and p70 S6K in KBM-5 leukemia cells.	Yun SunMi et al.	*Phytotherapy Research*, 2014, 28, 3, 458–464.
3115729	Brassinin (cabbage)	PC-3	Brassinin induces apoptosis in PC-3 human prostate cancer cells through the suppression of PI3K/Akt/mTOR/S6K1 signaling cascades.	Kim SungMoo et al.	*Phytotherapy Research*, 2014, 28, 3, 423–431.
3135760	Silibinin	PCA PC3MM2, PC-3, and C4-2 B)	Silibinin inhibits prostate cancer cells- and RANKL-induced osteoclastogenesis by targeting NFATc1, NF-κB, and AP-1 activation in RAW264.7 cells.	Kavitha, C.V. et al.	*Molecular Carcinogenesis*, 2014, 53, 3, 169–180.
3135510	Root of *Reevesia formosana*	Human hormone-refractory prostate cancers	Reevesioside A, a cardenolide glycoside, induces anticancer activity against human hormone-refractory prostate cancers through suppression of c-myc expression and induction of G1 arrest of the cell cycle.	Leu WohnJenn et al.	*PLoS ONE*, 2014, 9, 1, e87323.
3133152	*Withania somnifera* L. Dunal leaves	PC-3	5,6-De-epoxy-5-en-7-one-17-hydroxy withaferin A, a new cytotoxic steroid from *Withania somnifera* L. Dunal leaves.	Siddique, A.A. et al.	*Natural Product Research*, 2014, 28, 6, 392–398.
3141220	*Bauhinia kockiana* Korth.	DU-145 PC-3	Bioactivity-guided isolation of anticancer agents from *Bauhinia kockiana* Korth.	Chew YikLing et al.	*African Journal of Traditional, Complementary and Alternative Medicines*, 2014, 11, 3, 291–299.
3149236	*Incarvillea emodi*	PC-3	Comparative studies for screening of bioactive constituents from various parts of *Incarvillea emodi*.	Ajay Rana et al.	*Natural Product Research*, 2014, 28, 8, 593–596.
3168473	Silibinin (milk thistle)	PC-3	Silibinin down-regulates expression of secreted phospholipase A_2 enzymes in cancer cells.	Hagelgans, A. et al.	*Anticancer Research*, 2014, 34, 4, 1723–1729.

Abstract No.	Species	Prostate Cancer Cells	Title of Research	First Named Author	Journal Reference
3168052	Beta vulgaris L. extract (B)	PC-3 PaCa	Synergistic cytotoxicity of red beetroot (Beta vulgaris L.) extract with doxorubicin in human pancreatic, breast, and prostate cancer cell lines.	Kapadia, G.J. et al.	Journal of Complementary & Integrative Medicine, 2013, 10, 1, 113–122.
3165307	Panax ginseng		Recent progress in research on anticancer activities of ginsenoside-Rg3.	Nam KiYeul et al.	Korean Journal of Pharmacognosy, 2014, 45, 1, 1–10.
3162215	Nimbolide constituent of neem	PC-3	Antiproliferative and apoptosis inducing effect of nimbolide by altering molecules involved in apoptosis and IGF signaling via PI3K/Akt in prostate cancer (PC-3) cell line.	Singh, P.R. et al.	Cell Biochemistry and Function, 2014, 32, 3, 217–228.
3181279	Curcumin and genistein combination	PC-3	Antiangiogenic effect of combined treatment with curcumin and genistein on human prostate cancer cell line.	Aditya, N.P. et al.	Journal of Functional Foods, 2014, 8, 204–213.
3180679	Zanthoxylum simullans Hance	PC-3M LNCaP	Acridone alkaloids with cytotoxic and antimalarial activities from Zanthoxylum simullans Hance.	Wang Chao et al.	Pharmacognosy Magazine, 2014, 10, 37, 73–76.
3193942	Tripterygium wilfordii Hook F.	PC-3	Celastrol blocks interleukin-6 gene expression via downregulation of NF-κB in prostate carcinoma cells.	Chiang KunChun et al.	PLoS ONE, 2014, 9, 3, e93151.
3193694	Essential oils from leaves Ocimum basilicum, O. americanum, Hyptis spicigera, Lippia multiflora, Ageratum conyzoides, Eucalyptus camaldulensis and Zingiber officinale	LNCaP PC-3	Chemical composition, antioxidant, anti-inflammatory, and antiproliferative activities of essential oils of plants from Burkina Faso.	Bayala, B. et al.	PLoS ONE, 2014, 9, 3, e92122.
3193532	Apigenin	LNCaP, PC-3 DU-145	Plant flavone apigenin binds to nucleic acid bases and reduces oxidative DNA damage in prostate epithelial cells.	Sharma, H. et al.	PLoS ONE, 2014, 9, 3, e91588.

Abstract No.	Species	Prostate Cancer Cells	Title of Research	First Named Author	Journal Reference
3193317	*Tephrosia apollinea*		Crystal structure elucidation and anticancer studies of (−)-Pseudosemiglabrin: a flavanone isolated from the aerial parts of *Tephrosia apollinea*.	Loiy Elsir, A.H. et al.	*PLoS ONE*, 2014, 9, 3, e90806.
3193106	*Rosmarinus officinalis*	22Rv1, LNCaP, prostate epithelial cells	Rosemary (*Rosmarinus officinalis*) extract modulates CHOP/GADD153 to promote androgen receptor degradation and decreases xenograft tumor growth.	Petiwala, S.M. et al.	*PLoS ONE*, 2014, 9, 3, e89772.
3193032	*Tribulus terrestris* L.		Terrestrosin D, a steroidal saponin from *Tribulus terrestris* L., inhibits growth and angiogenesis of human prostate cancer *in vitro* and *in vivo*.	Wei, S. et al.	*Pathobiology*, 2014, 81, 3, 123–132.
3191014	*Ochrophyta*	LNCaP	Bioprospecting of brown seaweed (Ochrophyta) from the Yucatan Peninsula: cytotoxic, antiproliferative, and antiprotozoal activities.	Caamal-Fuentes, E. et al.	*Journal of Applied Phycology*, 2014, 26, 2, 1009–1017.
3190873	*Ligularia fischeri*	Prostate carcinoma (Bc3)	Petasins from the rhizomes of *Ligularia fischeri* and its derivatives.	Wang CaiFang et al.	*Records of Natural Products*, 2014, 8, 2, 156–164.
3188674	Anethole	DU-145	CXCR4 and PTEN are involved in the antimetastatic regulation of anethole in DU145 prostate cancer cells.	Rhee YunHee et al.	*Biochemical and Biophysical Research Communications*, 2014, 447, 4, 557–562.
3201605	*Helleborus thibetanus*		Two new bufadienolides from the rhizomes of *Helleborus thibetanus* with inhibitory activities against prostate cancer cells.	Cheng Wei et al.	*Natural Product Research*, 2014, 28, 12, 901–908.
3199491	*Piper aduncum* L. (matico)	DU-145	*Piper aduncum* L. (matico) essential oil *in vitro* antitumoral effect and oral toxicity in mice.	Arroyo, J. et al.	*Anales de la Facultad de Medicina*, 2014, 75, 1, 13–18.
3223055	Pao Pereira	CRPC PC-3	Pao Pereira extract suppresses castration-resistant prostate cancer cell growth, survival, and invasion through inhibition of NFκB signaling.	Chang CunJie et al.	*Integrative Cancer Therapies*, 2014, 13, 3, 249–258.

Abstract No.	Species	Prostate Cancer Cells	Title of Research	First Named Author	Journal Reference
3221743	*Annona muricata*	PC-3	Three new anti-antiproliferative *Annonaceous acetogenins* with mono-tetrahydrofuran ring from graviola fruit (*Annona muricata*).	Sun, S. Liu et al.	*Bioorganic & Medicinal Chemistry Letters*, 2014, 24, 12, 2773–2776.
3219202	*Campomanesia pubescens*	PC-3	Evaluation of antioxidant and antiproliferative activities in fruits of *Campomanesia pubescens*.	Cardoso, C.A.L. et al.	*Revista do Instituto Adolfo Lutz*, 2013, 72, 4, 324–330.
3216709	Pumpkin 2S albumin	PC-3 and DU-145	Characterization of anticancer, DNase and antifungal activity of pumpkin 2S albumin.	Tomar, P.P.S. et al.	*Biochemical and Biophysical Research Communications*, 2014, 448, 4, 349–354.
3214244	*Pancratium maritimum* L.	PC-3 M	Non-alkaloidal compounds from the bulbs of the Egyptian plant *Pancratium maritimum*.	Ibrahim, S.R. M. et al.	*Zeitschrift für Naturforschung. Section C, Biosciences*, 2014, 69, 3/4, 92–98.
3213945	*Cyamopsis tetragonoloba*	PC-3	Evaluation of anticancer, antimycoplasmal activities and chemical composition of guar (*Cyamopsis tetragonoloba*) seeds extract.	Badr, S.E.A. et al.	*Research Journal of Pharmaceutical, Biological and Chemical Sciences*, 2014, 5, 3, 413–423.
3212365	*Urtica dioica*	LNCaP	*Urtica dioica* induces cytotoxicity in human prostate carcinoma LNCaP cells: involvement of oxidative stress, mitochondrial depolarization and apoptosis.	Levy, A. et al.	*Tropical Journal of Pharmaceutical Research*, 2014, 13, 5, 711–717.
3229589	Cucumbers and other vegetables	PC-3 LNCaP PrEC	Inactivation of ATP citrate lyase by cucurbitacin B: a bioactive compound from cucumber, inhibits prostate cancer growth.	Gao, Y.J. et al.	*Cancer Letters*, 2014, 349, 1, 15–25.
3227418		PC-3	Oleanolic acid induces metabolic adaptation in cancer cells by activating the AMP-activated protein kinase pathway.	Liu Jia et al.	*Journal of Agricultural and Food Chemistry*, 2014, 62, 24, 5528–5537.
3226857	*Tillandsia recurvata* (ball moss)	PC-3 DU-145	Unearthing the medicinal properties of *Tillandsia recurvata* (ball moss): a mini review.	Lowe, H.I.C. et al.	*European Journal of Medicinal Plants*, 2014, 4, 9, 1138–1149.

Abstract No.	Species	Prostate Cancer Cells	Title of Research	First Named Author	Journal Reference
3225671	Matrine	PC-3M	Effect of matrine on cell cycle and apoptosis of human prostate cancer PC-3M.	Wang GuiQiu	Practical Pharmacy and Clinical Remedies, 2014, 17, 5, 528–531.
3237097	Tillandsia recurvata (ball moss)	PC-3	In vitro and in vivo anticancer effects of Tillandsia recurvata (ball moss) from Jamaica.	Lowe, H.I.C. et al.	West Indian Medical Journal, 2013, 62, 3, 177–180.
3236485	Zingiber officinale Roscoe	LNCaP, DU-145, and PC-3 HMVP2 (mouse)	6-Shogaol from dried ginger inhibits growth of prostate cancer cells both in vitro and in vivo through inhibition of STAT3 and NF-κB signaling.	Saha, A. et al.	Cancer Prevention Research, 2014, 7, 6, 627–638.
3244451	Cichorium intybus	LNCaP	Anticancer activity of n-hexane extract of Cichorium intybus on lymphoblastic leukemia cells (Jurkat cells).	Mohammad Saleem et al.	African Journal of Plant Science, 2014, 8, 6, 315–319.
3244236	Commiphora opobalsamum	DU-145 and PC-3	Myrrhanolide D and myrrhasin A, new germacrane-type sesquiterpenoids from the resin of Commiphora opobalsamum.	Shen Tao et al.	Helvetica Chimica Acta, 2014, 97, 6, 881–886.
3261942	Curcurbita pepo	LNCaP	Cytotoxic effect of pumpkin (Curcurbita pepo) seed extracts in LNCaP prostate cancer cells is mediated through apoptosis.	Rathinavelu, A. et al.	Current Topics in Nutraceutical Research, 2013, 11, 4, 137–144.
3256566	Heteroscyphus tener	PCa	Diterpenoids from the Chinese liverwort Heteroscyphus tener and their antiproliferative effects.	Lin ZhaoMin et al.	Journal of Natural Products, 2014, 77, 6, 1336–1344.
3273348	Salvia officinalis	PC-3	Evaluation of antioxidative and cytotoxic properties of ethanolic extract of Salvia officinalis on PC3 human prostate cancer and Hela cervical cancer cell lines.	Sarmast, P. et al.	Journal of Advanced Biological and Biomedical Research, 2014, 2, 4, 956–965.
3272572.	Scutellaria baicalensis	DU-145	Oroxylin A inhibits hypoxia-induced invasion and migration of MCF-7 cells by suppressing the Notch pathway.	Cheng Yao et al.	Anti-Cancer Drugs, 2014, 25, 7, 778–789.
3265836	Sapindus mukorossi Gaertn	PC-3	A new triterpenoid saponin and an oligosaccharide isolated from the fruits of Sapindus mukorossi.	Zhang XuanMing et al.	Natural Product Research, 2014, 28, 14, 1058–1064.

Abstract No.	Species	Prostate Cancer Cells	Title of Research	First Named Author	Journal Reference
3264897	Ginger extract	Human prostate tumor xenografts	Enterohepatic recirculation of bioactive ginger phytochemicals is associated with enhanced tumor growth-inhibitory activity of ginger extract.	Gundala, S.R. et al.	Carcinogenesis, 2014, 35, 6, 1320–1329.
3276319	Tripterygium wilfordii		Evaluation of anticancer activity of celastrol liposomes in prostate cancer cells.	Wolfram, J. et al.	Journal of Microencapsulation, 2014, 31, 5, 501–507.
3276084	Silibinin	DU-145	Fabrication, characterization, and bioevaluation of silibinin-loaded chitosan nanoparticles.	Deep Pooja et al.	International Journal of Biological Macromolecules, 2014, 69, 267–273.
3275006	Cibotium barometz, Heteropterys chrysophylla, and Sideroxylon obtusifolium (=Bumelia sartorum)	LNCaP and PC-3	Multiple readout assay for hormonal (androgenic and antiandrogenic) and cytotoxic activity of plant and fungal extracts based on differential prostate cancer cell line behavior.	Bobach, C. et al.	Journal of Ethnopharmacology, 2014, 155, 1, 721–730.
3286876	Ledebouria hyderabadensis	DU-145	Anticancer active homoisoflavone from the underground bulbs of Ledebouria hyderabadensis.	Yakaiah Chinthala et al.	Pharmacognosy Research, 2014, 6, 4, 303–305.
3298975	Taverniera spartea	PC-3 and Du-145	Cytotoxicity evaluation of Taverniera spartea on human cancer cell lines.	Khalighi-Sigaroodi, F. et al.	Journal of Medicinal Plants, 2014, 13, 50, Pe114–Pe128.
3297614	Cannabis sativa L.	LNCaP, DU-145, PC-3	In vitro anticancer activity of plant-derived cannabidiol on prostate cancer cell lines.	Sharma, M. et al.	Pharmacology and Pharmacy, 2014, 5, 8, 806–820.
3297460	Calotropis procera	PC-3	Proceraside A, a new cardiac glycoside from the root barks of Calotropis procera with in vitro anticancer effects.	Ibrahim, S.R.M. et al.	Natural Product Research, 2014, 28, 17, 1322–1327.
3296776	Magnolia officinalis	PC-3 LNCaP Myc-CaP PC-3 tumor xenografts	Honokiol activates reactive oxygen species-mediated cytoprotective autophagy in human prostate cancer cells.	Hahm, E.R. et al.	Prostate. 2014, 74, 12, 1209–1221.

Abstract No.	Species	Prostate Cancer Cells	Title of Research	First Named Author	Journal Reference
3316322	*Eurycoma longifolia*	PCa PCas	Phytoandrogenic properties of *Eurycoma longifolia* as natural alternative to testosterone replacement therapy.	George, A. et al.	*Andrologia*, 2014, 46, 7, 708–721.
3419341	*Pterodon pubescens*	PC-3	Antitumor screening of *Pterodon pubescens* terpenic fraction indicates high sensitivity for lymphocytic leukemia cells.	Martino, T. et al.	*Natural Product Communications*, 2014, 9, 11, 1547–1551.
3419343	*Syzygium kusukusense*	PC-3	Anti-tumor activities of triterpenes from *Syzygium kusukusense*.	Bai LiYuan et al.	*Natural Product Communications*, 2014, 9, 11, 1557–1558.
3423307	Corn silk, *Zea mays* L.	PC-3	Corn silk maysin induces apoptotic cell death in PC-3 prostate cancer cells via mitochondria-dependent pathway.	Lee JiSun et al.	*Life Sciences*, 2014, 119, 1/2, 47–55.
3411712	*Allium* species		Compounds from *Allium* species with cytotoxic and antimicrobial activity.	Lanzotti, V. et al.	*Phytochemistry Reviews*, 2014, 13, 4, 769–791.
3411713			Oleanane triterpenoids in the prevention and therapy of breast cancer: current evidence and future perspectives.	Parikh, N.R. et al.	*Phytochemistry Reviews*, 2014, 13, 4, 793–810.
3399207	*Dioscorea membranacea*	PC-3	Isolation and characterization of a new cytotoxic dihydrophenanthrene from *Dioscorea membranacea* rhizomes and its activity against five human cancer cell lines.	Itharat, A. et al.	*Journal of Ethnopharmacology*, 2014, 156, 130–134.
3403584	*Echinophora platyloba* DC (Apiaceae)	PC-3	*Echinophora platyloba* DC (Apiaceae) crude extract induces apoptosis in human prostate adenocarcinoma cells (PC 3).	Shahneh, F.Z. et al.	*Biomedical Journal*, 2014, 37, 5, 298–304.
3405177	*Rubus coreanus* Miquel	PC-3 DU-145	Unripe *Rubus coreanus* Miquel suppresses migration and invasion of human prostate cancer cells by reducing matrix metalloproteinase expression.	Kim Yesl et al.	*Biotechnology and Biochemistry*, 2014, 78, 8, 1402–1411.

Abstract No.	Species	Prostate Cancer Cells	Title of Research	First Named Author	Journal Reference
3387843	Artocarpus incisa (breadfruit) seeds		Recombinant production of plant lectins in microbial systems for biomedical application – the frutalin case study.	Oliveira, C. et al.	Frontiers in Plant Science, 2014, 5, August, 390.
3389581	Erythrophleum fordii	PC-3	In vitro apoptotic effect of cassaine-type diterpene amides from Erythrophleum fordii on PC-3 prostate cancer cells.	Hung TranManh et al.	Bioorganic & Medicinal Chemistry Letters, 2014, 24, 21, 4989–4994.
3389732	Potentilla fulgens L.	PC-3	In vitro cytotoxicity of the polar extracts of Potentilla fulgens L. against human cancer cell lines: detection and isolation of bioactive phenolics.	Anal, J.M.H. et al.	Journal of Chemical and Pharmaceutical Research, 2014, 6, 9, 89–95.
3390454	Laurencia pacifica	Du-145	Cytotoxic compounds from Laurencia pacifica.	Zaleta-Pinet, D.A. et al.	Organic and Medicinal Chemistry Letters, 2014, 4, 8.
3390600	Rhodosorus marinus	22Rv-1	Antiproliferative and antibacterial activity evaluation of red microalgae Rhodosorus marinus.	Garcia-Galaz, A. et al.	African Journal of Biotechnology, 2014, 13, 43, 4169–4175.
3390616	Asclepias curassavica	DU-145	Structures, chemotaxonomic significance, cytotoxic and Na$^+$, K$^+$-ATPase inhibitory activities of new cardenolides from Asclepias curassavica.	Zhang RongRong et al.	Organic & Biomolecular Chemistry, 2014, 12, 44, 8919–8929.
3376038	Escin	PC-3 DU-145	Cytotoxic effects of escin on human castration-resistant prostate cancer cells through the induction of apoptosis and G2/M cell cycle arrest.	Piao SongZhe et al.	Urology, 2014, 84, 4, 982.e1–982.e7.
3376183	Betel leaf Hydroxychavicol	PC-3	Hydroxychavicol, a betel leaf component, inhibits prostate cancer through ROS-driven DNA damage and apoptosis.	Gundala, S.R. et al.	Toxicology and Applied Pharmacology, 2014, 280, 1, 86–96.

Abstract No.	Species	Prostate Cancer Cells	Title of Research	First Named Author	Journal Reference
3379670	*Magnolia officinalis* (roots and bark)	DU-145 PC-3	Magnolol causes alterations in the cell cycle in androgen insensitive human prostate cancer cells *in vitro* by affecting expression of key cell cycle regulatory proteins.	McKeown, B.T. et al.	*Nutrition and Cancer*, 2014, 66, 7, 1154–1164.
3371187	*Phyllostachys bambusoides and P. pubescens*	PC-3	Evaluation of antioxidant and anticancer activity of steam extract from the bamboo species.	Kim JiSu et al.	*Journal of the Korean Wood Science and Technology*, 2014, 42, 5, 543–554.
3374182	*Ganoderma lucidum* (Curt. Fr.) P. Karst.		Collection, identification, phytochemical analysis and phyto toxicity test of wood inhabiting fungi *Ganoderma lucidum* (Curt. Fr.) P. Karst.	Nithya, M. et al.	*Hygeia – Journal for Drugs and Medicine*, 2014, 6, 1, 31–39.
3360847	Pristimerin	LNCaP PC-3	Ubiquitin-proteasomal degradation of antiapoptotic surviving facilitates induction of apoptosis in prostate cancer cells by pristimerin.	Liu, Y.B. et al.	*International Journal of Oncology*, 2014, 45, 4, 1735–1741.
3366756	Phytol (diterpene alcohol)	PC-3	An insight into the cytotoxic activity of phytol at *in vitro* conditions.	Pejin, B. et al.	*Natural Product Research*, 2014, 28, 22, 2053–2056.
3366951	*Annona squamosa* Linn	DU-145	*Annona squamosa* Linn: cytotoxic activity found in leaf extract against human tumor cell lines.	Wang DeShen et al.	*Pakistan Journal of Pharmaceutical Sciences*, 2014, 27, 5, 1559–1563.
3351983	β-caryophyllene oxide from e.g. *Psidium guajava* (guava) and *Origanum vulgare* L. (oregano) essential oils		β-Caryophyllene oxide inhibits constitutive and inducible STAT3 signaling pathway through induction of the SHP-1 protein tyrosine phosphatase.	Kim ChulWon et al.	*Molecular Carcinogenesis*, 2014, 53, 10, 793–806.
3336280	*Hypericum riparium* A. Chev. Biscoumarin derivatives (rare) and flavonoids	PC-3	Rare biscoumarin derivatives and flavonoids from *Hypericum riparium*.	Tanemossu, S.A. et al.	*Phytochemistry*, 2014, 105, 171–177.
3338005	*Phyllanthus niruri* (Nanoparticules)		Enhanced delivery of *Phyllanthus niruri* nanoparticles for prostate cancer therapy.	Unni, R.T. et al.	*Journal of Bionanoscience*, 2014, 8, 2, 101–107.

Abstract No.	Species	Prostate Cancer Cells	Title of Research	First Named Author	Journal Reference
3324446	*Thermopsis turcica*		Antimicrobial activity against periodontopathogenic bacteria, antioxidant, and cytotoxic effects of various extracts from endemic *Thermopsis turcica*.	Bali, E.B. et al.	*Asian Pacific Journal of Tropical Biomedicine*, 2014, 4, 7, 505–514.
		2013 (Year published in Cabi Citations)			
3413499	Tomato	PC-3	Alpha-tomatine synergises with paclitaxel to enhance apoptosis of androgen-independent human prostate cancer PC-3 cells *in vitro* and *in vivo*.	Lee SuiTing et al.	*Phytomedicine*, 2013, 20, 14, 1297–1305.
3413500	*Cimicifuga racemosa*		Attenuation of nucleoside and anticancer nucleoside analog drug uptake in prostate cancer cells by *Cimicifuga racemosa* extract BNO-1055.	Dueregger, A. et al.	*Phytomedicine*, 2013, 20, 14, 1306–1314.
3414787	Corn silk varieties: (Denghai6702, Delinong988, Tunyu808, Zhongdan909, Liangyu208, Jingke968)	PC-3	Comparative studies on the constituents, antioxidant and anticancer activities of extracts from different varieties of corn silk.	Tian JingGe et al.	*Food and Function*, 2013, 4, 10, 1526–1534.
3415868	Emodin	LNCaP (androgen-sensitive) and PC-3 (androgen-refractory), as well as the pro-metastatic low-density lipoprotein receptor-related protein 1 (LRP1)	Exploration of effects of emodin in selected cancer cell lines: enhanced growth inhibition by ascorbic acid and regulation of LRP1 and AR under hypoxia-like conditions.	Shashank Masaldan et al.	*Journal of Applied Toxicology*, 2014, 34, 1, 95–104.
3410746	2'-Hydroxyflavanone	LNCaP PC-3 and DU-145	Repression of cell proliferation and androgen receptor activity in prostate cancer cells by 2'-Hydroxyflavanone.	Ofude, M. et al.	*Anticancer Research*, 2013, 33, 10, 4453–4462.

Abstract No.	Species	Prostate Cancer Cells	Title of Research	First Named Author	Journal Reference
3401115	Vernonia guineensis Benth. (Asteraceae) tuber extract (VGDE)	PC-3	In vivo antiprostate tumor potential of Vernonia guineensis Benth. (Asteraceae) tuber extract (VGDE) and the cytotoxicity of its major compound pentaisovaleryl sucrose.	Toyang, N.J. et al.	Journal of Ethnopharmacology, 2013, 150, 2, 724–728.
3401870	Jacaranda puberula Cham. (Bignoniacea)	PC-3	Anti-tumor potential and acute toxicity of Jacaranda puberula Cham. (Bignoniacea).	De Almeida, M.R.A. et al.	Pakistan Journal of Pharmaceutical Sciences, 2013, 26, 5, 881–892.
3403225	Zanthoxylum schinifolium	PC-3	Coumarins and lignans from Zanthoxylum schinifolium and their anticancer activities.	Li Wei et al.	Journal of Agricultural and Food Chemistry, 2013, 61, 45, 10730–10740.
3390748	Artemisia amygdalina Decne	PC-3	Isolation, cytotoxicity evaluation and HPLC-quantification of the chemical constituents from Artemisia amygdalina Decne.	Lone, S.H. et al.	Journal of Chromatography, B, 2013, 940, 135–141.
3392086	Withania somnifera	PC-3 DU-145	Withaferin A, a steroidal lactone from Withania somnifera, induces mitotic catastrophe and growth arrest in prostate cancer cells.	Roy, R.V. et al.	Journal of Natural Products, 2013, 76, 10, 1909–1915.
3397063	Lupeol and casearin G	PC-3	In vitro effect of lupeol and casearin G on peripheral blood mononuclear and tumor cells.	Dupuy L.O.A. et al.	Revista Médica de Chile, 2013, 141, 9.
3381895	Taxoid SBT-1214 and a novel polyenolic zinc-binding curcuminoid, CMC2.24	PPT2 cells and highly metastatic PC3MM2	Prostate cancer stem cell-targeted efficacy of a new-generation taxoid, SBT-1214 and novel polyenolic zinc-binding curcuminoid, CMC2.24.	Botchkina, G.I. et al.	PLoS ONE, 2013, 8, 9, e69884.
3382832	Lysimachia ciliata	DU-145 PC-3	Triterpene saponosides from Lysimachia ciliata differentially attenuate invasive potential of prostate cancer cells.	Koczurkiewicz, P. et al.	Chemico-Biological Interactions, 2013, 206, 1, 6–17.
3382894	Sweet potato greens		Polar biophenolics in sweet potato greens extract synergize to inhibit prostate cancer cell proliferation and in vivo tumor growth.	Gundala, S.R. et al.	Carcinogenesis, 2013, 34, 9, 2039–2049.

Abstract No.	Species	Prostate Cancer Cells	Title of Research	First Named Author	Journal Reference
3372092	*Pancratium maritimum*	PC-3	New alkaloids from *Pancratium maritimum*.	Ibrahim, S.R. M. et al.	*Planta Medica*, 2013, 79, 15, 1480–1484.
3372259	*Cedrus deodara* (Roxb.) ex Lamb. *Berberis aristata* (Roxb.) ex DC *Withania somnifera* Dunal. *Picrorhiza kurroa* Royle ex Benth. and *Piper longum L.*		Evaluation of some plant extracts for standardization and anticancer activity.	Gaidhani, S.N. et al.	*Indian Journal of Traditional Knowledge*, 2013, 12, 4, 682–687.
3360325	*Brucea mollis* Wall. ex Kurz.	LNCaP	Cytotoxic compounds from *Brucea mollis*.	Mai Hung Thanh Tung et al.	*Scientia Pharmaceutica*, 2013, 81, 3, 819–831.
3360755	*Laminaria japonica*	PC-3M LNCaP	Cytotoxic compounds from *Laminaria japonica*.	Wang Chao et al.	*Chemistry of Natural Compounds*, 2013, 49, 4, 699–701.
3361563	*Schisandra chinensis*	PC-3	Antioxidant and antiproliferative activities of five compounds from *Schisandra chinensis* fruit.	Zhang LiKang et al.	*Industrial Crops and Products*, 2013, 50, 690–693.
3366352	*Crocus sativus* (Saffron)	PC-3	DNA fragmentation and apoptosis induced by safranal in human prostate cancer cell line.	Samarghandian, S. et al.	*Indian Journal of Urology*, 2013, 29, 3, 177–183.
3354659	*Guettarda pohliana* Müll. Arg. (Rubiaceae)	PCO-3	Cytotoxic activity of *Guettarda pohliana* Müll. Arg. (Rubiaceae).	de Oliveira, P.R.N. et al.	*Natural Product Research*, 2013, 27, 18, 1677–1681.
3357261	Licorice extract	PTEN-deleted human prostate cancer cells	CDK2 and mTOR are direct molecular targets of isoangustone A in the suppression of human prostate cancer cell growth.	Lee EunJung et al.	*Toxicology and Applied Pharmacology*, 2013, 272, 1, 12–20.
3345219	*Croton dichrous* Müll. Arg., *C. erythroxyloides* Baill., *C. myrianthus* Müll. Arg. and *C. splendidus* Mart. ex Colla	PC-3	Antiproliferative activity of methanol extracts of four species of *Croton* on different human cell lines.	Savietto, J.P. et al.	*Revista Brasileira de Farmacognosia*, 2013, 23, 4, 662–667.
3348131	*Dorstenia psilurus*	PC-3	Induction of mitochondrial dependent apoptosis and cell cycle arrest in human promyelocytic leukemia HL-60 cells by an extract from *Dorstenia psilurus*, a spice from Cameroon.	Pieme, C.A. et al.	*BMC Complementary and Alternative Medicine*, 2013, 13, 223.
3318853	Blackberry	LNCaP	The protective effect of blackberry anthocyanins against free radical-induced oxidative stress and cytotoxicity.	Elisia, I. et al.	*Current Topics in Phytochemistry*, Volume 11, 2012, 35–45.

Abstract No.	Species	Prostate Cancer Cells	Title of Research	First Named Author	Journal Reference
3333850	*Veratrum sp.*	PC-3	The *Veratrum* alkaloids jervine, veratramine, and their analogues as prostate cancer migration and proliferation inhibitors: biological evaluation and pharmacophore modeling.	Khanfar, M.A. et al.	*Medicinal Chemistry Research*, 2013, 22, 10, 4775–4786.
3323247	Grape seed extracts	PC-3	Modulation of the antioxidant/ pro-oxidant balance, cytotoxicity and antiviral actions of grape seed extracts.	Ignea, C. et al.	*Food Chemistry*, 2013, 141, 4, 3967–3976.
3326224	Bearberry leaf extract	DU-145 (androgen receptor-negative prostate carcinoma)	Inhibition of proliferation of human carcinoma cell lines by phenolic compounds from a bearberry-leaf crude extract and its fractions.	Amarowicz, R. et al.	*Journal of Functional Foods*, 2013, 5, 2, 660–667.
3312139	Licorice (*Glycyrrhiza glabra* L.)	PC-3	Licorice (*Glycyrrhiza glabra* L.): chemical composition and biological impacts.	Badr, S.E.A. et al.	*Research Journal of Pharmaceutical, Biological and Chemical Sciences*, 2013, 4, 3, 606–621.
3317127	Satsuma-mandarin and Changshan-huyou	PC-3	Preparation of low-molecular-weight citrus pectin from citrus pomace and evaluation of their anticancer activities.	Yin Ying et al.	*Acta Agriculturae Zhejiangensis*, 2013, 25, 3, 614–618.
3310095	Lignan polyphenols		The antitumor lignan nortrachelogenin sensitizes prostate cancer cells to TRAIL-induced cell death by inhibition of the Akt pathway and growth factor signaling.	Peuhu, E. et al.	*Biochemical Pharmacology*, 2013, 86, 5, 571–583.
3300306	Caffeic acid phenethyl ester	PC-3, DU-145 and LNCaP	Caffeic acid phenethyl ester synergistically enhances docetaxel and paclitaxel cytotoxicity in prostate cancer cells.	Tolba, M.F. et al.	*IUBMB Life*, 2013, 65, 8, 716–727.

Abstract No.	Species	Prostate Cancer Cells	Title of Research	First Named Author	Journal Reference
301986	*Eurya emarginata* (stems), *Gleditsia japonica* var. *koraiensis* (leaves), *Photinia glabra* (leaves) and *Elaeagnus macrophylla* (leaves) *Styrax japonica* (fruits), *Aralia continentalis* (leaves), *Fagus crenata* var. *multinervis* (stems), *Thuja orientalis* (stems) and *Poncirus trifoliate* (branches) (leaves)	LNCaP, DU145	Antiproliferative effects of native plants on prostate cancer cells.	Kim HanHyuk et al.	*Natural Product Sciences*, 2013, 19, 2, 192–200.
3304997	*Crinum latifolium*		Extracts of *Crinum latifolium* inhibit the cell viability of mouse lymphoma cell line EL4 and induce activation of antitumor activity of macrophages *in vitro*.	Nguyen, H.Y.T. et al.	*Journal of Ethnopharmacology*, 2013, 149, 1, 75–83.
3306867	*Pteridium aquilinum*	PC-3	A novel bihomoflavanonol with an unprecedented skeleton from *Pteridium aquilinum*.	Chen NaiDong et al.	*Chinese Herbal Medicines*, 2013, 5, 2, 96–100.
3309265	*Pimenta dioica* (allspice) berries	CWR22RV1, PC-3 or DU145	Ericifolin: a novel antitumor compound from allspice that silences androgen receptor in prostate cancer.	Shamaladevi, N. et al.	*Carcinogenesis*, 2013, 34, 8, 1822–1832.
3289594	*Ocimum sanctum* Linn. (holy basil)		*Ocimum sanctum* Linn. (holy basil): pharmacology behind its anticancerous effect.	Baby Joseph et al.	*International Journal of Pharma and Bio Sciences*, 2013, 4, 2, P-556-P-575.
3281098	Pomegranate peel	PC-3	The proliferation and apoptosis effects of polyphenols of pomegranate peel on human prostate cancer PC-3 cells.	Wang ChunMei et al.	*Northwest Pharmaceutical Journal*, 2013, 28, 3, 271–274.
3281178	*Salvia miltiorrhiza* bunge	PC-3 LNCaP	Synergistic antitumor effects of tanshinone IIA in combination with cisplatin via apoptosis in the prostate cancer cells.	Hou LiLi et al.	*Acta Pharmaceutica Sinica*, 2013, 48, 5, 675–679.

Abstract No.	Species	Prostate Cancer Cells	Title of Research	First Named Author	Journal Reference
3268234	Garlic	PC-3 and noncancerous human prostate epithelial cells PNT1A PC-3 prostate cancer and noncancerous human prostate epithelial cells PNT1A	Diallyl trisulfide is more cytotoxic to prostate cancer cells PC-3 than to noncancerous epithelial cell line PNT1A: a possible role of p66Shc signaling axis.	Borkowska, A. et al.	*Nutrition and Cancer*, 2013, 65, 5, 711–717.
3272452	*Clematis mandshurica*	PC-3	Triterpene saponins from *Clematis mandshurica* and their antiproliferative activity	Gong YiXi et al.	*Planta Medica*, 2013, 79, 11, 987–994.
3259232	Ellagic acid	LnCap	Effects of ellagic acid on angiogenic factors in prostate cancer cells.	Vanella, L. et al.	*Cancers*, 2013, 5, 2, 726–738.
3251357	*Camellia sinensis* (seeds)	PC-3	*In vitro* cytotoxicity, antimicrobial, and metal-chelating activity of triterpene saponins from tea seed grown in the Kangra Valley, India.	Robin Joshi et al.	*Medicinal Chemistry Research*, 2013, 22, 8, 4030–4038.
3257454	*Annona pickelii* and *A. salzmannii* (Annonaceae)		Chemical composition of the essential oils of *Annona pickelii* and *Annona salzmannii* (Annonaceae), and their antitumor and trypanocidal activities.	Costa, E.V. et al.	*Natural Product Research*, 2013, 27, 11, 997–1001.
3257476	*Hedyotis chrysotricha*	PC-3	24S)-Ergostane-3β,5α,6β-triol from *Hedyotis chrysotricha* with inhibitory activity on migration of SK-HEP-1 human hepatocarcinoma cells.	Ye Miao et al.	*Natural Product Research*, 2013, 27, 12, 1136–1140.
3256944	Curcumin	LNCaP PC-3	Curcumin induces cell cycle arrest and apoptosis of prostate cancer cells by regulating the expression of IκBα, c-Jun and androgen receptor.	Guo Hui et al.	*Pharmazie*, 2013, 68, 6, 431–434.

Abstract No.	Species	Prostate Cancer Cells	Title of Research	First Named Author	Journal Reference
3244455	Jacaric acid and its octadecatrienoic acid geoisomers	Hormone-dependent (LNCaP) and -independent (PC-3) human prostate cancer cells, and normal human prostate epithelial cells (RWPE-1)	Jacaric acid and its octadecatrienoic acid geoisomers induce apoptosis selectively in cancerous human prostate cells: a mechanistic and 3D structure-activity study.	Gasmi, J. et al.	*Phytomedicine*, 2013, 20, 8/9, 734–742.
3240623	*Anthocephalus cadamba* Miq. (Rubiaceae)	PC-3, CNS (SF-295)	Cytotoxic effect of *Anthocephalus cadamba* Miq. leaves on human cancer cell lines.	Satyajit Singh et al.	*Pharmacognosy Journal*, 2013, 5, 3, 127–129.
3233568	*Lysimachia nummularia* L.	DU-145 PC-3	A new cytotoxic triterpene saponin from *Lysimachia nummularia* L.	Podolak, I. et al.	*Carbohydrate Research*, 2013, 375, 16–20.
3236350	*Hypericum hircinum* L. subsp. *majus* (Aiton)	PC-3	Antioxidant and antiproliferative activity of *Hypericum hircinum* L. subsp. *majus* (Aiton) N. Robson essential oil.	Quassinti, L. et al.	*Natural Product Research*, 2013, 27, 10, 862–868.
3236369	*Epilobium angustifolium* L., *E. parviflorum* Schreb., and *E. hirsutum* L.	LNCaP	Extracts from *Epilobium* sp. herbs induce apoptosis in human hormone–dependent prostate cancer cells by activating the mitochondrial pathway.	Stolarczyk, M. et al.	*Journal of Pharmacy and Pharmacology*, 2013, 65, 7, 1044–1054.
3236481	Camalexin (phytoalexin)	LNCaP and ARCaP-Neo cells, respectively, (PrEC) normal prostate epithelial cells	The phytoalexin camalexin mediates cytotoxicity towards aggressive prostate cancer cells via reactive oxygen species.	Smith, B.A. et al.	*Journal of Natural Medicines*, 2013, 67, 3, 607–618.
3228604	Pseudolaric acid B (terpenoid)	LNCaP androgen-dependent PC-3 and DU-145 androgen-independent prostate cancer cells	Pseudolaric acid B induces caspase-dependent apoptosis and autophagic cell death in prostate cancer cells.	Tong Jing et al.	*Phytotherapy Research*, 2013, 27, 6, 885–891.

Abstract No.	Species	Prostate Cancer Cells	Title of Research	First Named Author	Journal Reference
3230498	*Curcuma longa*	PC-3	Biological studies of turmeric oil: selective *in vitro* anticancer activity of turmeric oil (TO) and TO-paclitaxel combination.	Jacob, J.N. et al.	*Natural Product Communications*, 2013, 8, 6, 807–810.
3220658	*Corylopsis coreana* Uyeki (phenolic compounds)	DU-145 LNCaP	Anti-oxidative and antiproliferative activity on human prostate cancer cells lines of the phenolic compounds from *Corylopsis coreana* Uyeki.	Kim ManhHeun et al.	*Molecules*, 2013, 18, 5, 4876–4886.
3221223	*Jatropha ribifolia* (roots) (hexanic extract, cyperenoic acid, and jatrophone terpenes)	PC-3	Isolation, structural identification and cytotoxic activity of hexanic extract, cyperenoic acid, and jatrophone terpenes from *Jatropha ribifolia* roots.	Fernandes, E. de S. et al.	*Revista Brasileira de Farmacognosia*, 2013, 23, 3, 441–446.
3207802			Nanoformulation of natural products for prevention and therapy of prostate cancer.	Sanna, V. et al.	*Cancer Letters*, 2013, 334, 1, 142–151.
3207992	*Juglans mandshurica* Maxim (Juglone)	LNCaP	Juglone, isolated from *Juglans mandshurica* Maxim., induces apoptosis via downregulation of AR expression in human prostate cancer LNCaP cells.	Xu HuaLi et al.	*Bioorganic & Medicinal Chemistry Letters*, 2013, 23, 12, 3631–3634.
3202123	Curcumin	DU-145	Crosstalk from survival to necrotic death coexists in DU-145 cells by curcumin treatment.	Kang DongXu et al.	*Cellular Signalling*, 2013, 25, 5, 1288–1300.
3206232	*Aerva lanata* L. (flowering aerial part)		*In vitro* anticancer activity of ethanol extract fractions of *Aerva lanata* L.	Abhishek Bhanot et al.	*Pakistan Journal of Biological Sciences*, 2013, 16, 22, 1612–1617.
3206769	*Punica granatum*		Usefulness of pomegranate in prostate cancer.	Chéchile Toniolo, G.E. et al.	*Options Méditerranéennes. Série A, Séminaires Méditerranéens*, 2012, 103, 311–320.

Abstract No.	Species	Prostate Cancer Cells	Title of Research	First Named Author	Journal Reference
3191584	*Maytenus royleanus* (Wall. ex M. A. Lawson)	PC-3	Ficusonic acid: a new cytotoxic triterpene isolated from *Maytenus royleanus* (Wall. ex M. A. Lawson) Cufodontis.	Ala-ud-din et al.	*Journal of the Brazilian Chemical Society*, 2013, 24, 4, 663–668.
3180497	*Eugenia jambolana*		Anticancer activity of the extracts of *Eugenia jambolana*.	Satyanarayana Rentala et al.	*International Journal of Pharma and Bio Sciences*, 2013, 4, 1, B-601–B-608.
3182949	*Artocarpus camans*	PC-3	Chemical constituents of *Artocarpus camansi*.	Tsai PoWei et al.	*Pharmacognosy Journal*, 2013, 5, 2, 80–82.
3172471	*Polygonum perfoliatum* L.	PC-3	A new lignan with antitumor activity from *Polygonum perfoliatum* L.	Wang KuiWu et al.	*Natural Product Research*, 2013, 27, 6, 568–573.
3167323	Flaxseed-derived enterolignans		Flaxseed-derived enterolactone is inversely associated with tumor cell proliferation in men with localized prostate cancer.	Azrad, M. et al.	*Journal of Medicinal Food*, 2013, 16, 4, 357–360.
3163050	*Horsfieldia superba*	PC-3	New flavan and alkyl α,β-lactones from the stem bark of *Horsfieldia superba*.	Al-Mekhlafi, N.A. et al.	*Natural Product Communications*, 2013, 8, 4, 447–451.
3163230	*Garcina lucida, Fagara heitzii* and *Hymenocardia lyrata* (barks, seeds, leaves and roots)	PC-3	Cytotoxic and antimicrobial activity of selected Cameroonian edible plants.	Dzoyem, J.P. et al.	*BMC Complementary and Alternative Medicine*, 2013, 13, 78.
3150274	Sulforaphane (SFN) in cruciferous vegetable		Sulforaphane enhances Nrf2 expression in prostate cancer TRAMP C1 cells through epigenetic regulation.	Zhang ChengYue et al.	*Biochemical Pharmacology*, 2013, 85, 9, 1398–1404.
3139795	Z-Ligustilide and radix *Angelica sinensis*	TRAMP C1	Epigenetic reactivation of Nrf2 in Murine prostate cancer TRAMP C1 cells by natural phytochemicals Z-Ligustilide and radix *Angelica sinensis* via promoter CpG demethylation.	Su, Z.Y.et al.	*Chemical Research in Toxicology*, 2013, 26, 3, 477–485.

Abstract No.	Species	Prostate Cancer Cells	Title of Research	First Named Author	Journal Reference
3140203	Apigenin		Apigenin sensitizes prostate cancer cells to Apo2L/TRAIL by targeting adenine nucleotide translocase-2.	Oishi, M. et al.	*PLoS ONE*, 2013, 8, 2, e55922.
3140284	Betulinic acid	TRAMP	Betulinic acid selectively increases protein degradation and enhances prostate cancer-specific apoptosis: possible role for inhibition of deubiquitinase activity.	Reiner, T. et al.	*PLoS ONE*, 2013, 8, 2, e56234.
3144692	*Oenothera paradoxa*	DU-145 immortalized prostate epithelial cells (PNT1A)	Flavanols from evening primrose (*Oenothera paradoxa*) defatted seeds inhibit prostate cells invasiveness and cause changes in *Bcl-2/Bax* mRNA ratio.	Lewandowska, U. et al.	*Journal of Agricultural and Food Chemistry*, 2013, 61, 12, 2987–2998.
3146382	*Myricaria germanica* (Tamaricaceae)	PC-3	Cytotoxic isoferulic acidamide from *Myricaria germanica* (Tamaricaceae).	Nawwar, M.A. et al.	*Plant Signaling and Behavior*, 2013, 8, 1, e22642.
3146506	*Cucumis sativus* (cucumber), *Benincasa hispida* (ash gourd), *Coccinia indica*, *Cucurbita maxima* (pumpkin), and *Luffa acutangula* (ridge gourd) of Cucurbitaceae family	HeLa cell line (human cervix carcinoma)	Comparative cytotoxic efficacies of five *Cucurbitaceous* plant extracts on HeLa cell line.	Varalakshmi, K.N. et al.	*Journal of Pharmacy Research*, 2012, 5, 12, 5310–5313.
3147638	Cisplatin and Anvirzel™		Anvirzel™ in combination with cisplatin in breast, colon, lung, prostate, melanoma, and pancreatic cancer cell lines.	Apostolou, P. et al.	*BMC Pharmacology and Toxicology*, 2013, 14, 18.
3143253	*Inonotus obliquus*	PC-3	Anti-inflammatory and anticancer activities of extracts and compounds from the mushroom *Inonotus obliquus*.	Ma LiShuai et al.	*Food Chemistry*, 2013, 139, 1/4, 503–508.
3138118	*Trichilia hirta* extracts (Jubabán)		Ethnopharmacological evaluation of *Trichilia hirta* L. as anticancer source in traditional medicine of Santiago de Cuba.	Hernández, E. et al.	*Boletín Latinoamericano y del Caribe de Plantas Medicinales y Aromáticas*, 2013, 12, 2, 176–185.

Abstract No.	Species	Prostate Cancer Cells	Title of Research	First Named Author	Journal Reference
3126459	*Absidia corymbifera.* AS 3.3387	DU-145 PC-3	Microbial transformation of 20(S)-protopanaxadiol by *Absidia corymbifera*. Cytotoxic activity of the metabolites against human prostate cancer cells.	Chen GuangTong et al.	*Fitoterapia*, 2013, 84, 6–10.
3126917	*Vernonia guineensis* Benth. (Asteraceae) (leaves)	PC-3 DU-145	Cytotoxic sesquiterpene lactones from the leaves of *Vernonia guineensis* Benth. (Asteraceae).	Toyang, N.J. et al.	*Journal of Ethnopharmacology*, 2013, 146, 2, 552–556.
3112413	*Magnolia officinalis*	PC-3 LNCap cells.	4-O-methylhonokiol, a PPARγ agonist, inhibits prostate tumor growth: p21-mediated suppression of NF-κB activity.	Lee, N.J. et al.	*Journal of Pharmacology*, 2013, 168, 5, 1133–1145.
3113565	*Achillea millefolium* (flowers)	PC-3	Cytotoxic flavonoids from the flowers of *Achillea millefolium*.	Huo ChangHong et al.	*Chemistry of Natural Compounds*, 2013, 48, 6, 958–962.
3113772	*Nardostachys jatamansi* (rhizomes)	DU-145	Two new sesquiterpenoids from the rhizomes of *Nardostachys jatamansi*.	Rekha, K. et al.	*Journal of Asian Natural Products Research*, 2013, 15, 2, 111–116.
3115324	*Apios americana* Medik	LNCaP	Novel isoflavone glucosides in groundnut (*Apios americana* Medik) and their antiandrogenic activities.	Ichige, M. et al.	*Journal of Agricultural and Food Chemistry*, 2013, 61, 9, 2183–2187.
3116065	*Puerariae thomsonii* Flos.		Application of an efficient strategy for discovery and purification of bioactive compounds from Chinese herbal medicines, a case study on the *Puerariae thomsonii* Flos.	Wang Qi et al.	*Journal of Pharmaceutical and Biomedical Analysis*, 2013, 75, 25–32.
3103833	*Lasienthera africanum*	PC-3	Antiproliferative effects of *Lasienthera africanum* on prostate epithelial cancer cells.	Matheen, A. et al.	*Journal of Bio Innovation*, 2012, 1, 6, 186–196.
3089205	*Valeriana jatamansi* (syn. *Valeriana wallichii* DC.)	PC-3M (metastatic prostate cancer)	Characterization of chlorinated valepotriates from *Valeriana jatamansi*.	Lin Sheng et al.	*Phytochemistry*, 2013, 85, 185–193.
3082018	Caribbean propolis Caribbean propolis [3] (natural source)		Flavonoids isolated from Caribbean propolis show cytotoxic activity in human cancer cell lines.	Acikelli, A.H. et al.	*International Journal of Clinical Pharmacology and Therapeutics*, 2013, 51, 1, 51–53.

Abstract No.	Species	Prostate Cancer Cells	Title of Research	First Named Author	Journal Reference
3082019	*Clusia* sp. Cuban propolis [1] [2,3]		Multi-targeted polycyclic polyprenylated acylphloroglucinols are major constituents of Cuban propolis and contributors to its anticancer activity.	Díaz-Carballo, D. et al.	*International Journal of Clinical Pharmacology and Therapeutics*, 2013, 51, 1, 54–55.
3079609	*Physalis angulata*	DU-145	Physangulidine A, a withanolide from *Physalis angulata*, perturbs the cell cycle and induces cell death by apoptosis in prostate cancer cells.	Reyes-Reyes, E.M. et al.	*Journal of Natural Products*, 2013, 76, 1, 2–7.
3079617	*Hyptis brevipes*		Absolute configuration and conformational analysis of brevipolides, bioactive 5,6-dihydro-α-pyrones from *Hyptis brevipes*.	Suárez-Ortiz, G.A. et al.	*Journal of Natural Products*, 2013, 76, 1, 72–78.
3069309	*Juglans regia* L (green husk)	PC-3	Validation of the antiproliferative effects of organic extracts from the green husk of *Juglans regia* L. on PC-3 human prostate cancer cells by assessment of apoptosis-related genes.	Alshatwi, A.A. et al.	*Evidence-based Complementary and Alternative Medicine*, 2012, 2012.
3069667	*Clausena excavata* Burm. F	PC-3 LNCaP	Dentatin induces apoptosis in prostate cancer cells via Bcl-2, Bcl-xL, survivin downregulation, caspase-9, -3/7 activation, and NF-κB inhibition.	Ismail Adam Arbab et al.	*Evidence-based Complementary and Alternative Medicine*, 2012, 2012.
3050872	*Ilex hainanensis* Merr.	induce apoptosis of human prostatic carcinoma	Inhibiting effects of ilexgenin A from *Ilex hainanensis* Merr. on tumor cell HepG2.	Ding YeChun et al.	*Medicinal Plant*, 2012, 3, 11, 91–94.
3055769	*Piper longum* Linn.	PC-3	Pipernonaline from *Piper longum* Linn. induces ROS-mediated apoptosis in human prostate cancer PC-3 cells.	Lee Wan et al.	*Biochemical and Biophysical Research Communications*, 2013, 430, 1, 406–412.
3058084	*Euglena viridis*	PC-3, DU-145	*In vitro* cytotoxic and antibacterial activity of ethanolic extract of *Euglena viridis*.	Das, B.K. et al.	*International Journal of Pharma and Bio Sciences*, 2012, 3, 4, B-321–B-331.

Abstract No.	Species	Prostate Cancer Cells	Title of Research	First Named Author	Journal Reference
3043138	*Lycopodium clavatum* spores	LnCaP PC-3	Lycopodine triggers apoptosis by modulating 5-lipoxygenase, and depolarizing mitochondrial membrane potential in androgen sensitive and refractory prostate cancer cells without modulating p53 activity: signaling cascade and drug-DNA interaction.	Kausik Bishayee et al.	*European Journal of Pharmacology*, 2013, 698, 1/3, 110–121.
3047693	Cucurbitacin II b	PC-3	Inhibitory effect of Cucurbitacin II b on proliferation of human prostate cancer PC-3 cells through disruption of microfilaments and upregulation of p21^{Cip1} expression.	Ren Shuai et al.	*Chinese Journal of Pharmacology and Toxicology*, 2012, 26, 6, 835–841.
3036399	*Clusia rosea*	LNCaP	7-epi-nemorosone from *Clusia rosea* induces apoptosis, androgen receptor down-regulation and dysregulation of PSA levels in LNCaP prostate carcinoma cells.	Diaz-Carballo, D. et al.	*Phytomedicine*, 2012, 19, 14, 1298–1306.
3036583	*Aglaia exima* (Meliaceae)	DU-145	Triterpenes and steroids from the leaves of *Aglaia exima* (Meliaceae).	Khalijah Awang et al.	*Fitoterapia*, 2012, 83, 8, 1391–1395.
3037574	*Chrysanthemum indicum* L.	DU-145	*Chrysanthemum indicum* L. extract induces apoptosis through suppression of constitutive STAT3 activation in human prostate cancer DU145 cells.	Kim ChulWon et al.	*Phytotherapy Research*, 2013, 27, 1, 30–38.
3028376	*Cannabis sativa* (marijuana)		Towards the use of non-psychoactive cannabinoids for prostate cancer.	Pacher, P.	*British Journal of Pharmacology*, 2013, 168, 1, 76–78.
3032611	*Centipeda minima* (Asteraceae)	PC-3	Phytochemical screening, antimicrobial and antiproliferative properties of *Centipeda minima* (Asteraceae) on prostate epithelial cancer cells.	Pradeep, B.V. et al.	*Journal of Pharmacy Research*, 2012, 5, 9, 4804–4807.
3018378	*Piper longum*		Piperlongumine induces rapid depletion of the androgen receptor in human prostate cancer cells.	Golovine, K.V. et al.	*Prostate*, 2013, 73, 1, 23–30.

Abstract No.	Species	Prostate Cancer Cells	Title of Research	First Named Author	Journal Reference
3018461	*Plumbago zeylanica* L.		Plumbagin inhibits prostate cancer development in TRAMP mice via targeting PKCε, Stat3, and neuroendocrine markers.	Hafeez, B. et al.	*Carcinogenesis*, 2012, 33, 12, 2586–2592.
3022003	*Menispermum dauricum*	PC-3M	Dauricine can inhibit the activity of proliferation of urinary tract tumor cells.	Wang Jun et al.	*Asian Pacific Journal of Tropical Medicine*, 2012, 5, 12, 973–976.
3012482	Emodin	DU-145	Emodin inhibits invasion and migration of prostate and lung cancer cells by downregulating the expression of chemokine receptor CXCR4.	Ok SooHo et al.	*Immunopharmacology and Immunotoxicology*, 2012, 34, 5/6, 768–778.
3015132	*Odyendyea gabonensis*	PC-3	Oxidative burst inhibitory and cytotoxic activity of constituents of the fruits of *Odyendyea gabonensis*.	Donkwe, S.M.M. et al.	*Planta Medica*, 2012, 78, 18, 1949–1956.
3015449	*Annona muricata*	PC-3	Acetogenins from *Annona muricata*.	Ragasa, C.Y. et al.	*Pharmacognosy Journal*, 2012, 4, 32, 32–37.
3001240	*Ganoderma lucidum* and other related fungi, such as *Poria cocos, Laetiporus sulphureus, Inonotus obliquus, Antrodia camphorata, Daedalea dickinsii,* and *Elfvingia applanata*		Lanostanoids from fungi: a group of potential anticancer compounds.	Ríos, J.L. et al.	*Journal of Natural Products*, 2012, 75, 11, 2016–2044.
3006680	Triptolide, a Chinese medicine		Triptolide sensitizes TRAIL-induced apoptosis in prostate cancer cells via p53-mediated DR5 upregulation.	Hu XiaoWen et al.	*Molecular Biology Reports*, 2012, 39, 9, 8763–8770.
2012 (Year published in Cabi Citations)					
3406280	*Scutellaria* flavones (wogonin, wogonoside, baicalein, and baicalin)		Current state-of-the-art research on pharmacological activity of *Scutellaria* flavones.	Wilczańska-Barska, A. et al.	*Postepy Fitoterapii*, 2012, 1, 28–34.
3394787	*Scoparia dulcis* (sweet broomweed)	DU-145	Benzoxazinoids from *Scoparia dulcis* (sweet broomweed) with antiproliferative activity against the DU-145 human prostate cancer cell line.	Wu WanHsun et al.	*Phytochemistry*, 2012, 83, 110–115.

Abstract No.	Species	Prostate Cancer Cells	Title of Research	First Named Author	Journal Reference
3395809	Qianliening capsule	Human prostate stromal cell line WPMY-1 (benign prostatic hyperplasia)	Qianliening capsule inhibits human prostate cell growth via induction of mitochondrion-dependent cell apoptosis.	Hong ZhenFeng et al.	Chinese Journal of Integrative Medicine, 2012, 18, 11, 824–830.
3398207	Brassinosteroids (a group of polyhydroxylated sterol derivatives)	LNCaP DU-145	Mechanisms of natural brassinosteroid-induced apoptosis of prostate cancer cells.	Steigerová, J. et al.	Food and Chemical Toxicology, 2012, 50, 11, 4068–4076.
3391503	Tillandsia recurvata L. (Jamaican ball moss)	PC-3	Kinase inhibition by the Jamaican ball moss, Tillandsia recurvata L.	Lowe, H.I.C. et al.	Anticancer Research, 2012, 32, 10, 4419–4422.
3379834			Traditional West African pharmacopeia, plants, and derived compounds for cancer therapy.	Sawadogo, W.R. et al.	Biochemical Pharmacology, 2012, 84, 10, 1225–1240.
3383150	Mahkota Dewa (Phaleria macrocarpa [Scheff.] Boerl) (benzophenone glucopyranosides)		Isolation, characterization, and cytotoxic activity of benzophenone glucopyranosides from Mahkota Dewa (Phaleria macrocarpa [Scheff.] Boerl).	Zhang SaiYang et al.	Bioorganic & Medicinal Chemistry Letters, 2012, 22, 22, 6862–6866.
3383332	Saccharina japonica (brown macro-alga)	267B1/K-ras (human prostate cancer cells)	The anticancer effects of Saccharina japonica on 267B1/K-ras human prostate cancer cells.	Jo MiJeong et al.	International Journal of Oncology, 2012, 41, 5, 1789–1797.
3364781	Quercetin		A review of quercetin: antioxidant and anticancer properties.	Baghel, S.S. et al.	Journal of Pharmacy and Pharmaceutical Sciences (WJPPS), 2012, 1, 1, 146–160.
3344216	Reaumuria vermiculata L.	PC-3	Cytotoxic ellagitannins from Reaumuria vermiculata.	Nawwar, M.A. et al.	Fitoterapia, 2012, 83, 7, 1256–1266.
3299310	Capparis deciduas (stachydrine)	PC-3 LNcaP	In vitro anticancer activity of stachydrine isolated from Capparis decidua on prostate cancer cell lines.	Permender Rathee et al.	Natural Product Research, 2012, 26, 18, 1737–1740.
3300554	Curcumin (Demethoxycurcumin bisdemethoxycurcumin)	PC-3	Demethoxycurcumin modulates prostate cancer cell proliferation via AMPK-induced downregulation of HSP70 and EGFR.	Hung ChaoMing et al.	Journal of Agricultural and Food Chemistry, 2012, 60, 34, 8427–8434.

Abstract No.	Species	Prostate Cancer Cells	Title of Research	First Named Author	Journal Reference
3287741	*Boesenbergia rotunda* L. (fingerroot) (boesenbergin A, a chalcone)	PC-3	*In vitro* anti-inflammatory, cytotoxic, and antioxidant activities of boesenbergin A, a chalcone isolated from *Boesenbergia rotunda* (L.) (fingerroot).	Isa, N.M. et al.	*Brazilian Journal of Medical and Biological Research*, 2012, 45, 6, 524–530.
3288288	Aloe-emodin (phosphatidylinositol 3-kinase, phosphatase and tensin homolog).	PC-3	Aloe-emodin suppresses prostate cancer by targeting the mTOR complex 2.	Liu KangDong et al.	*Carcinogenesis*, 2012, 33, 7, 1406–1411.
3288989	*Lagenaria siceraria* (Cucurbitaceae)	DU-145	Evaluation of *in vitro* anticancer activity of fruit *Lagenaria siceraria* against MCF7, HOP62, and DU145 cell lines.	Kishor Kothawade et al.	*International Journal of Pharmacy and Technology*, 2012, 4, 1, 3909–3924.
3281935	*Tagetes erecta* (roots)	PC-3	Antioxidant and cytotoxic potential of a new thienyl derivative from *Tagetes erecta* roots.	Pankaj Gupta et al.	*Pharmaceutical Biology*, 2012, 50, 8, 1013–1018.
3284658	*Leonotis nepetifolia* (L.) R. Br. (aerial parts)	DU-145	Preliminary phytochemical and biological screening of methanolic and acetone extracts from *Leonotis nepetifolia* (L.) R. Br.	Sobolewska, D. et al.	*Journal of Medicinal Plants Research*, 2012, 6, 30, 4582–4585.
3285030	*Acronychia pedunculata* (prenylated acetophenone dimers)	DU-145	Cytotoxic prenylated acetophenone dimers from *Acronychia pedunculata*.	Kouloura, E. et al.	*Journal of Natural Products*, 2012, 75, 7, 1270–1276.
3267056	*Sinningia allagophylla* (Mart.) (benzochromene 8-methoxylapachenol)	PC-3	Chemical study of *Sinningia allagophylla* guided by antiproliferative activity assays.	Riva, D. et al.	*Química Nova*, 2012, 35, 5, 974–977.
3271275	*Cuphea aequipetala* Cav. (Lythraceae)	DU-145	Ethnobotany, analytical micrograph of leaves and stems and phytochemistry of *Cuphea aequipetala* Cav. (Lythraceae): a contribution to the Herbal Pharmacopoeia of the United Mexican States (FHEUM).	Aguilar-Rodríguez, S. et al.	*Plantas Medicinales y Aromáticas*, 2012, 11, 4, 316–330.
3272255	*Yangzheng Xiaoji*		Impact of *Yangzheng Xiaoji* on the adhesion and migration of human cancer cells: the role of the AKT signaling pathway.	Ye Lin et al.	*Anticancer Research*, 2012, 32, 7, 2537–2543.

Abstract No.	Species	Prostate Cancer Cells	Title of Research	First Named Author	Journal Reference
3272262	*Antrodia camphorate* (triterpenoids)	PC-3	Anticancer effects of eleven triterpenoids derived from *Antrodia camphorata*.	Lee YiPang et al.	*Anticancer Research*, 2012, 32, 7, 2727–2734.
3265425	Apigenin (plant flavone)	Mouse (prostate cancer model)	Apigenin attenuates insulin-like growth factor-I signaling in an autochthonous mouse prostate cancer model.	Shukla, S. et al.	*Pharmaceutical Research*, 2012, 29, 6, 1506–1517.
3265426	*Salvia miltiorrhiza* Bunge (Chinese herb – Danshen) (Tanshinones)	LNCaP, PCa androgen-independent	Tanshinones from Chinese medicinal herb Danshen (*Salvia miltiorrhiza* Bunge) suppress prostate cancer growth and androgen receptor signaling.	Zhang, Y. et al.	*Pharmaceutical Research*, 2012, 29, 6, 1595–1608.
3265755	Berberine (genotoxic alkaloid)	RM-1 (murine prostate cancer cell line)	Berberine, a genotoxic alkaloid, induces ATM-Chk1 mediated G2 arrest in prostate cancer cells.	Wang Yu et al.	*Mutation Research, Fundamental and Molecular Mechanisms of Mutagenesis*, 2012, 734, 1/2, 20–29.
3263005	*Laurencia microcladia* (red algae) (Elatol) – marine derivative compound	Mouse model (C57Bl6 mice bearing B16F10 cells)	Antitumor effects of elatol, a marine derivative compound obtained from red algae *Laurencia microcladia*.	Campos, A. et al.	*Journal of Pharmacy and Pharmacology*, 2012, 64, 8, 1146–1154.
3251997	*Gochnatia polymorpha* (Less) Cabr. ssp. *floccosa* Cabr. (trunk bark) (sesquiterpene lactones)	PC-3	Bioactivity-guided isolation of cytotoxic sesquiterpene lactones of *Gochnatia polymorpha* ssp. *floccosa*.	Strapasson, R.L.B. et al.	*Phytotherapy Research*, 2012, 26, 7, 1053–1056.
3257241	*Commiphora mukul* (steroids)	PC-3 DU-145	Steroids from *Commiphora mukul* display antiproliferative effect against human prostate cancer PC3 cells via induction of apoptosis.	Shen Tao et al.	*Bioorganic & Medicinal Chemistry Letters*, 2012, 22, 14, 4801–4806.
3257381	Flavonoid ampelopsin	LNCaP (androgen-sensitive) PC-3 (androgen-independent)	Flavonoid ampelopsin inhibits the growth and metastasis of prostate cancer *in vitro* and in mice.	Ni Feng et al.	*PLoS ONE*, 2012, 7, 6, e38802.
3257914	*Gnaphalium elegans, Achyrocline bogotensis* (flavone isomers)	PC-3, LNCaP	Anti-neoplastic activity of two flavone isomers derived from *Gnaphalium elegans* and *Achyrocline bogotensis*.	Thomas, C.M. et al.	*PLoS ONE*, 2012, 7, 6, e39806.

Abstract No.	Species	Prostate Cancer Cells	Title of Research	First Named Author	Journal Reference
3242676	*Tydemania expeditionis* (marine alga) (diketosteroid)	DU-145, PC-3, LNCaP	Steroids with inhibitory activity against the prostate cancer cells and chemical diversity of marine alga *Tydemania expeditionis*.	Zhang JianLong et al.	*Fitoterapia*, 2012, 83, 5, 973–978.
3247598	*Tripterygium wilfordii* Hook.F (Chinese herb)	DU-145	Triptolide-induced apoptosis of androgen-independent prostatic cancer (AIPC) via modulation of histone methylation.	Zhao KaiLiang et al.	*Drug Development Research*, 2012, 73, 4, 222–228.
3240113	*Fortunella margarita* (Nagami kumquats)	LNCaP	Inhibition of prostate cancer (LNCaP) cell proliferation by volatile components from Nagami kumquats.	Jayaprakasha, G.K. et al.	*Planta Medica*, 2012, 78, 10, 974–980.
3230701	*Arisaema utile*	PC-3	Antimicrobial, cytotoxic and antioxidant activites of *Arisaema utile*.	Sofi Mubashir et al.	*Journal of Pharmacy Research*, 2012, 5, 3, 1368–1370.
3216552	*Casearia capitellata, Baccaurea motleyana, Phyllanthus pulcher and Strobilanthus crispus*	DU-145	Anticancer properties and phenolic contents of sequentially prepared extracts from different parts of selected medicinal plants indigenous to Malaysia.	Maznah Ismail et al.	*Molecules*, 2012, 17, 5, 5745–5756.
3203470	*Cirsium oleraceum* (L.) Scop (flavonoids, phenolic acids, sterols, triterpenes, lignans, isoflavones)		*Cirsium oleraceum* (L.) Scop.-active substances and possible usage.	Parus, A.	*Postepy Fitoterapii*, 2011, 2, 100–105.
3189361	*Polygonum limbatum*	PC-3	Cytotoxicity and antimicrobial activity of the methanol extract and compounds from *Polygonum limbatum*.	Dzoyem, J.P. et al.	*Planta Medica*, 2012, 78, 8, 787–792.
3190087	Ginsenoside Rg3 (ginseng root)	PC-3M	Ginsenoside Rg3 attenuates cell migration via inhibition of aquaporin 1 expression in PC-3M prostate cancer cells.	Pan XueYang et al.	*European Journal of Pharmacology*, 2012, 683, 1/3, 27–34.
3181781	*Erythrina vespertilio* Benth (alkaloids and isoflavonoids) glucoalkaloid-vespertilioside	PC-3	Cytotoxic evaluation of alkaloids and isoflavonoids from the Australian tree *Erythrina vespertilio*.	Iranshahi, M. et al.	*Planta Medica*, 2012, 78, 7, 730–736.

Abstract No.	Species	Prostate Cancer Cells	Title of Research	First Named Author	Journal Reference
3183006	*Paepalanthus geniculatus* Kunth (phenolics) (flowers)	PC-3	HPLC-ESIMS^n profiling, isolation, structural elucidation, and evaluation of the antioxidant potential of phenolics from *Paepalanthus geniculatus*.	do Amaral, F.P. et al.	*Journal of Natural Products*, 2012, 75, 4, 547–556.
3183021	*Callicarpa longissima*	PC-3	Bioactive diterpenes from *Callicarpa longissima*.	Liu YuanWei et al.	*Journal of Natural Products*, 2012, 75, 4, 689–693.
3174364	β-carotene	PC-3 (mouse model)	Diverse effects of β-carotene on secretion and expression of VEGF in human hepatocarcinoma and prostate tumor cells.	Chen HueiYan et al.	*Molecules*, 2012, 17, 4, 3981–3988.
3162161	Gambogic acid	PC-3	Gambogic acid inhibits TNF-α–induced invasion of human prostate cancer PC3 cells *in vitro* through PI3K/Akt and NF-κB signaling pathways.	LüLei Tang Dong et al.	*Acta Pharmacologica Sinica*, 2012, 33, 4, 531–541.
3163001	Phenoxodiol (isoflavone)	LNCaP, DU-145 PC-3	Cytotoxic effects of the novel isoflavone, phenoxodiol, on prostate cancer cell lines.	Mahoney, S. et al.	*Journal of Biosciences*, 2012, 37, 1, 73–84.
3167561	Pseudolaric acid B (diterpene acid from Chinese herb Tu-Jin-Pi)	DU-145	Pseudolaric acid B induces apoptosis via proteasome-mediated Bcl-2 degradation in hormone-refractory prostate cancer DU145 cells.	Zhao DanDan et al.	*Toxicology in Vitro*, 2012, 26, 4, 595–602.
3168238	Luteolin (a polyphenolic flavone)	LNCaP	Upregulation of prostate-derived Ets factor by luteolin causes inhibition of cell proliferation and cell invasion in prostate carcinoma cells.	Tsui KeHung et al.	*International Journal of Cancer*, 2012, 130, 12, 2812–2823.
3158236	Anti-androgens (for example, spearmint tea, red reishi, licorice, Chinese peony, green tea, black cohosh, chaste tree, and saw palmetto extract)		An update on plant derived anti-androgens.	Grant, P.	*International Journal of Endocrinology and Metabolism*, 2012, 10, 2, 497–502.
3145658	*Digitalis ciliata* (seeds) (steroidal glycosides) (A new furostanol glycoside, and a new pregnane glycoside, with 8 known spirostanes, pregnanes, and cardenolide glycosides)	PC-3	Antiproliferative steroidal glycosides from *Digitalis ciliata*.	Perrone, A. et al.	*Fitoterapia*, 2012, 83, 3, 554–562.

Abstract No.	Species	Prostate Cancer Cells	Title of Research	First Named Author	Journal Reference
3149563	Tomato δ-Tomatine and Tomatidine (glycoalkaloids)	PC-3	Structure-activity relationships of α-, β₁-, γ-, and δ-Tomatine and Tomatidine against human breast (MDA-MB-231), gastric (KATO-III), and prostate (PC3) cancer cells.	Choi SukHyun et al.	*Journal of Agricultural and Food Chemistry*, 2012, 60, 15, 3891–3899.
3149811	*Momordica charantia* leaf extract (bitter melon) Kuguacin J, (triterpeniod)	PC-3	Kuguacin J, a triterpeniod from *Momordica charantia* leaf, modulates the progression of androgen-independent human prostate cancer cell line, PC3.	Pitchakarn, P. et al.	*Food and Chemical Toxicology*, 2012, 50, 3/4, 840–847.
3140323	*Gleditsia caspia* (flavanone glycosides, 2 new)	DU-145	Flavanone glycosides from *Gleditsia caspia*.	Ragab, E.A. et al.	*Journal of Natural Products (India)*, 2010, 3, 35–46.
3140532	*Amyris madrensis* (Amyrisins A-C, O-prenylated flavonoids)	PC-3 DU-145	Amyrisins A-C, O-prenylated flavonoids from *Amyris madrensis*.	Peng, J.N. et al.	*Journal of Natural Products*, 2012, 75, 3, 494–496.
3135875	*Ficus glumosa* Del. (Moraceae) (fig, stem bark) Ceramides (2 new)	PC-3	Ceramides and cytotoxic constituents from *Ficus glumosa* Del. (Moraceae).	Nana, F. et al.	*Journal of the Brazilian Chemical Society*, 2012, 23, 3, 482–487.
3081295	*Inula viscosa*, (wild watermelon) *Citrullus colocynthis*, figs, spinach (natural antioxidants)		Natural antioxidants: just free radical scavengers or much more?	Grossman, S. et al.	*Research Trends, Trivandrum, India, Trends in Cancer Research*, Volume 7, 2011, 57–73.
3111044	*Psidium guajava* L. (guava leaves) (60 compounds)	PC-3	A hexane fraction of guava leaves (*Psidium guajava* L.) induces anticancer activity by suppressing AKT/mammalian target of rapamycin/ribosomal p70 S6 kinase in human prostate cancer cells.	Ryu NaeHyung et al.	*Journal of Medicinal Food*, 2012, 15, 3, 231–241.
3098080	*Prangos uloptera* roots (aviprin and aviprin-3''-O-D-glucopyranoside)	LNCaP	Antioxidant activity and cytotoxic effect of aviprin and aviprin-3''-O-D-glucopyranoside on LNCaP and HeLa cell lines.	Zahri, S. et al.	*Natural Product Research*, 2012, 26, 6, 540–547.
3090590	*Adenema hyssopifolium* G. Don. (flavones and iridoids)	PC-3	Pharmacognostic profile and *in vitro* cytotoxic activity of *Adenema hyssopifolium* G. Don.	Rajasekaran, A. et al.	*Journal of Pharmacy and Bioresources*, 2009, 6, 1.

Abstract No.	Species	Prostate Cancer Cells	Title of Research	First Named Author	Journal Reference
3094430	*Salvia leriaefolia* (diterpenoids including Salvialeriafone, a novel diterpene-norditerpene conjugate, 2 new abietane-type diterpenoids, salvialerial and salvialerione, as well as 4 known compounds, sugiol, salvicanaric acid, dehydroroyleanone, and cariocal)	PC-3	Diterpenoids including a novel dimeric conjugate from *Salvia leriaefolia*.	Choudhary, M.I. et al.	*Planta Medica*, 2012, 78, 3, 269–275.
3081762	*Luehea candicans* Mart. et Zucc. (Tiliaceae) ("açoita-cavalo") (branches & leaves) Lupeol, betulin, epicatechin, vitexin, and liriodendrin (steroids)	PC-3	Antiproliferative activity of *Luehea candicans* Mart. et Zucc. (Tiliaceae).	da Silva, D.A. et al.	*Natural Product Research*, 2012, 26, 4, 364-369.
3073045	Celastrol	PC-3	Paraptosis accompanied by autophagy and apoptosis was induced by celastrol, a natural compound with influence on proteasome, ER stress, and Hsp90.	Wang WenBo et al.	*Journal of Cellular Physiology*, 2012, 227, 5, 2196–2206.
3074535	*Lantana Camara* (leaf and flower)	PC-3	Anti proliferative effects of *Lantana Camara* on prostate epithelial cancer cells.	Devi, K.R. et al.	*Agricultural & Biological Research*, 2012, 28, 1, 1–11.
3077771	*Citrus grandis* Osbeck "*Dangyuja*" Nobiletin (leaves)	DU-145	Antiproliferative effects of *Dangyuja* (*Citrus grandis* Osbeck) leaves through suppression of constitutive signal transducer and activator of transcription 3 activation in human prostate carcinoma DU145 cells.	Chiang ShuYuan et al.	*Journal of Medicinal Food*, 2012, 15, 2, 152–160.
3067941	*Salvia miltiorrhiza* Bunge (tanshen root) (15,16-dihydrotanshinone)	DU-145	15,16-dihydrotanshinone I, a compound of *Salvia miltiorrhiza* Bunge, induces apoptosis through inducing endoplasmic reticular stress in human prostate carcinoma cells.	Chuang MaoTe et al.	*Evidence-based Complementary and Alternative Medicine*, 2011, 2011.
3068105	*Garcinia xanthochymus* (stem bark) Xanthones (2 new compounds, garcinenones X and Y, along with 5 known xathones)	PC-3	Xanthones with antiproliferative effects on prostate cancer cells from the stem bark of *Garcinia xanthochymus*.	Ji Feng et al.	*Natural Product Communications*, 2012, 7, 1, 53–56.

Abstract No.	Species	Prostate Cancer Cells	Title of Research	First Named Author	Journal Reference
3068649	*Morinda lucida* Benth. (Rubiaceae) (leaves) (β-Sitosterol)	PNT2A (normal prostate cells) DU-145, PC-3 LNCAP AS	*In vitro* anti-trypanosomal activity of *Morinda lucida* leaves.	Nweze, N.E.	*African Journal of Biotechnology*, 2012, 11, 7, 1812–1817.
3055840	*Nigella sativa* Thymoquinone (murine model)		Thymoquinone: potential cure for inflammatory disorders and cancer.	Woo ChernChiuh et al.	*Biochemical Pharmacology*, 2012, 83, 4, 443–451.
3052872	Cryptotanshinone	AR-positive PCa cells, AR-negative PC-3 cells, non-malignant prostate epithelial cells Androgen-responsive PCa LNCaP cells and castration-resistant CWR22rv1 cells	Cryptotanshinone suppresses androgen receptor-mediated growth in androgen-dependent and castration-resistant prostate cancer cells.	Xu DeFeng et al.	*Cancer Letters*, 2012, 316, 1, 11–22.
3035836	Mexican species from Lamiales order: *Limosella aquatica* L. (Scrophulariaceae), *Mimulus glabratus* Kunth. (Phrymaceae), *Pedicularis mexicana* Zucc. ex Benth. (Orobanchaceae), *Penstemon campanulatus* (Cav.), Willd. (Plantaginaceae), *Veronica americana* (Raf.), Schwein (Plantaginaceae)	PC-3	Cytotoxic and antioxidant activities of selected Lamiales species from Mexico.	Moreno-Escobar, J.A. et al.	*Pharmaceutical Biology*, 2011, 49, 12, 1243–1248.
3043479	*Oricia renieri* (3 new β-indoloquinazoline alkaloids, orirenierine A, B, and C [stems])	PC-3	Bioactive β-indoloquinazoline alkaloids from *Oricia renieri*.	Wansi, J.D. et al.	*Planta Medica*, 2012, 78, 1, 71–75.
3044015	*Colocasia esculenta* (taro) (edible root)		Antimetastatic activity isolated from *Colocasia esculenta* (taro).	Kundu, N. et al.	*Anti-Cancer Drugs*, 2012, 23, 2, 200–211.
3044454	Alternol-compound purified from the fermentation products of *Alternaria alternata* var. *monosporus*, a microorganism from the bark of the yew tree	C4-2 RWPE-1 (prostate epithelial)	Alternol exerts prostate-selective antitumor effects through modulations of the AMPK signaling pathway.	Yeung, E.D. et al.	*Prostate*, 2012, 72, 2, 165–172.

Abstract No.	Species	Prostate Cancer Cells	Title of Research	First Named Author	Journal Reference
3026112	Apogossypolone gossypol derivative, ApoG$_2$	PC-3	Apogossypolone induces autophagy of PC-3 prostate cancer cells *in vitro*.	Yuan Qing et al.	*Cancer Research on Prevention and Treatment*, 2011, 38, 9, 1006–1011.
3016234	Triphala (polyherbal Ayurvedic formulation) Gallic acid	LNCaP	Differential cytotoxicity of triphala and its phenolic constituent gallic acid on human prostate cancer LNCaP and normal cells.	Russell, L.H., Jr. et al.	*Anticancer Research*, 2011, 31, 11, 3739–3746.
3010006	Sanguinarine (benzophenanthridine alkaloid) (bloodroot)	DU145, C4-2 B, LNCaP	Inhibition of Stat3 activation by sanguinarine suppresses prostate cancer cell growth and invasion.	Sun, M. et al.	*Prostate*, 2012, 72, 1, 82–89.
3003308	*Thamnolia vermicularis* (Sw.) Ach. ex Schaerer (lichen) (3 new phenolic compounds: thamnoliadepsides A, B, and thamnolic acid A, and 7 known compounds: everninic acid, baeomycesic acid, β-orcinol, β-resorcylic acid, ethylorsellinate, squamatic acid, and vermicularin)		Three new phenolic compounds from the lichen *Thamnolia vermicularis* and their antiproliferative effects in prostate cancer cells.	Guo Jia et al.	*Planta Medica*, 2011, 77, 18, 2042–2046.
			2011 (Year published in Cabi Citations)		
3403676	*Vitex negundo* (chrysoplenetin and chrysosplenol D)	PC-3	Identification of chrysoplenetin from *Vitex negundo* as a potential cytotoxic agent against PANC-1 and a panel of 39 human cancer cell lines (JFCR-39).	Awale, S. et al.	*Phytotherapy Research*, 2011, 25, 12, 1770–1775.
3390786	Silibinin (E-cadherin)	PCAPC-3, PC3MM2, C4-2B	Role of E-cadherin in antimigratory and antiinvasive efficacy of silibinin in prostate cancer cells.	Deep, G. et al.	*Cancer Prevention Research*, 2011, 4, 8, 1222–1232.
3386325	*Ferula assafoetida* (resin) Galbanic acid	LNCaP and LNCaP C4-2 vs. DU145 PC-3 PCa	Galbanic acid decreases androgen receptor abundance and signaling and induces G$_1$ arrest in prostate cancer cells.	Zhang, Y. et al.	*Journal of Cancer*, 2012, 130, 1, 200–212.

Abstract No.	Species	Prostate Cancer Cells	Title of Research	First Named Author	Journal Reference
3355109	Zeyheria montana Mart. (Bignoniaceae) (leaves) (3 methoxylated flavonoids: 4',5,7-trimethoxy-luteolin and 6-hydroxy-5,7-dimethoxyflavone and the flavanone 5-hydroxy-6,7-dimethoxyflavanone)	PC-3	Antiproliferative activity of three methoxylated flavonoids isolated from Zeyheria montana Mart. (Bignoniaceae) leaves.	Seito, L.N. et al.	Phytotherapy Research, 2011, 25, 10, 1447–1450.
3354557	Myrcia laruotteana Camb. (Myrtaceae) (unripe fruits) α-bisabolol and α-bisabolol oxide B	PC-3	Chemical composition and cytotoxic activity of essential oil from Myrcia laruotteana fruits.	Stefanello, M.É.A. et al.	Journal of Essential Oil Research, 2011, 23, 5, 7–10.
3355841	Ocimum sanctum Linn or Tulsi flavonoid vicenin (2 alone & with docetaxel)	PC-3, DU-145 LNCaP	Anti-cancer effects of novel flavonoid vicenin-2 as a single agent and in synergistic combination with docetaxel in prostate cancer.	Nagaprashantha L.D. et al.	Biochemical Pharmacology, 2011, 82, 9, 1100–1109.
3359451	Celastrol (triterpene)		Celastrol inhibits tumor cell proliferation and promotes apoptosis through the activation of c-Jun N-terminal kinase and suppression of PI3 K/Akt signaling pathways.	Radhamani Kannaiyan et al.	Apoptosis, 2011, 16, 10, 1028–1041.
3347617	Physalisalkekengi var. franchetii, Physalins A and B (secosteriods)	AI-PCa (androgen-independent prostate cancer) C42B	Physalins A and B inhibit androgen-independent prostate cancer cell growth through activation of cell apoptosis and downregulation of androgen receptor expression.	Han HuiYing et al.	Biological & Pharmaceutical Bulletin, 2011, 34, 10, 1584–1588.
3335508	Casearia lasiophylla Eichler, Salicaceae (leaves, essential oil), germacrene D, and β-caryophyllene	PC-03	Chemical composition and cytotoxic activity of the essential oil from the leaves of Casearia lasiophylla.	Salvador, M.J. et al.	Revista Brasileira de Farmacognosia, 2011, 21, 5, 864–868.
3315600	Lycopene and apo-10'-lycopenal	LNCaP	Lycopene and apo-10'-lycopenal do not alter DNA methylation of GSTP1 in LNCaP cells.	Liu, A.G. et al.	Biochemical and Biophysical Research Communications, 2011, 412, 3, 479–482.
3319184	Angelica gigas Nakai (Decursin)	RC-58T/h/SA#4	Decursin from Angelica gigas Nakai induces apoptosis in RC-58T/h/SA#4 primary human prostate cancer cells via a mitochondria-related caspase pathway.	Choi SaRa et al.	Food and Chemical Toxicology, 2011, 49, 10, 2517–2523.

Abstract No.	Species	Prostate Cancer Cells	Title of Research	First Named Author	Journal Reference
3320338	Gambogic acid	PC-3	Gambogic acid inhibits cell proliferation and induces apoptosis of human prostate cancer PC-3 cells in vitro.	Tang Dong et al.	Tumor, 2011, 31, 8, 688–692.
3302190	Piper regnellii (Miq.) C. DC. var. regnellii leaves (eupomatenoid-5, neolignan)	PC-3	In vitro and in vivo anticancer activity of extracts, fractions, and eupomatenoid-5 obtained from Piper regnellii leaves.	Longato, G.B. et al.	Planta Medica, 2011, 77, 13, 1482–1488.
3302591	Ardisia brevicaulis, roots (resorcinol derivatives 2 new: 2-methoxy-4-hydroxy-6-(8Z-pentadecenyl)-benzene-1-O-acetate and 2-methoxy-4-hydroxy-6-pentadecyl-benzene-1-O-acetate and 4 known)	PC-3	Antitumor effect of resorcinol derivatives from the roots of Ardisia brevicaulis by inducing apoptosis.	Chen LiPing. et al.	Journal of Asian Natural Products Research, 2011, 13, 7/8, 734–743.
3303031	Gossypol, in synergistic action with valproic acid	DU-145	Valproic acid synergistically enhances the cytotoxicity of gossypol in DU145 prostate cancer cells: an iTRTAQ-based quantitative proteomic analysis.	Ouyang DongYun et al.	Journal of Proteomics, 2011, 74, 10, 2180–2193.
3291282	(+)-Spongistatin 1 (marine)	DU-145	In vitro and in vivo anticancer activity of (+)-spongistatin 1.	Xu, Q.L. et al.	Anticancer Research, 2011, 31, 9, 2773–2780.
3274991	18α-glycyrrhetinic acid (triterpenoid metabolite of glycyrrhizin in licorice roots)	DU-145	18α-glycyrrhetinic acid targets prostate cancer cells by down-regulating inflammation-related genes.	Shetty, A.V. et al.	International Journal of Oncology, 2011, 39, 3, 635–640.
3264410	Sulforaphane (a isothiocyanate derived from cruciferous vegetables e.g. broccoli)	LnCap PC-3	Differential effects of sulforaphane on histone deacetylases, cell cycle arrest and apoptosis in normal prostate cells versus hyperplastic and cancerous prostate cells.	Clarke, J.D. et al.	Molecular Nutrition & Food Research, 2011, 55, 7, 999–1009.
3234337	Resveratrol (3,5,4'-trans-trihydroxystilbene, RV) (a phytoalexin) and its analogue 3,5,4'-trans-trimethoxystilbene (a natural stilbene)	DU-145	Chemotherapeutic effects of resveratrol and its analogue 3,5,4'-trans-trimethoxystilbene on DU145 cells.	Malfa, G. et al.	Trends in Cancer Research, Volume 6, 2010, 45–54.

Abstract No.	Species	Prostate Cancer Cells	Title of Research	First Named Author	Journal Reference
3246592	Salvia miltiorrhiza (cryptotanshinone tanshinone IIA and tanshinone I)	DU-145	Bioactive tanshinones in Salvia miltiorrhiza inhibit the growth of prostate cancer cells in vitro and in mice.	Gong, Y. et al.	International Journal of Cancer, 2011, 129, 5, 1042–1052.
3248570	Patrinia heterophylla Bunge, (Caprifoliaceae)	PC-3	Preliminary evaluation of antitumor effect and induction apoptosis in PC-3 cells of extract from Patrinia heterophylla.	Yang Bo et al.	Revista Brasileira de Farmacognosia, 2011, 21, 3, 471–476.
3240664	Extra-virgin olive oil yielding (-)-Oleocanthal (secoiridoid)	PC-3	(-)-Oleocanthal as a c-met inhibitor for the control of metastatic breast and prostate cancers.	Elnagar, A.Y. et al.	Planta Medica, 2011, 77, 10, 1013–1019.
3228596	Vallaris glabra Acoschimperoside P, 2'-acetate (leaves)	DU-145	Acoschimperoside P, 2'-acetate: a Hedgehog signaling inhibitory constituent from Vallaris glabra.	Rifai, Y. et al.	Journal of Natural Medicines, 2011, 65, 3/4, 629–632.
3231731	Ceratonia siliqua L. (carob tree, leaves) (gallic acid, (+)-catechin and quercetin)	DU-145	In vitro cytotoxic effects and apoptosis induction by a methanol leaf extract of carob tree (Ceratonia siliqua L.).	Custódio, L. et al.	Journal of Medicinal Plants Research, 2011, 5, 10, 1987–1996.
3225793	Ursolic acid	Mice, nude DU-145 LNCaP	Ursolic acid inhibits multiple cell survival pathways leading to suppression of growth of prostate cancer xenograft in nude mice.	Shanmugam, M.K. et al.	Journal of Molecular Medicine, 2011, 89, 7, 713–727.
3219494	Saururus chinensis (aerial parts)	LNCaP	A methylene chloride fraction of Saururus chinensis induces apoptosis through the activation of caspase-3 in prostate and breast cancer cells.	Kim HanYoung et al.	Phytomedicine, 2011, 18, 7, 567–574.
3222029	Glechoma hederacea L. (whole plant) (3 new sesquiterpene lactones: 1α,10β-epoxy-4-hydroxy-glechoma-5-en-olide (1), 1β,10α-epoxy-4,8-dihydroxy-glechoma-5-en-olide (2), and 1β,10α;4α,5β-diepoxy-8-methoxy-glechoman-8α,12-olide (3), and 4 known sesquiterpene lactones)	DU-145	New sesquiterpene lactones from Glechoma hederacea L. and their cytotoxic effects on human cancer cell lines.	Kim JinPyo et al.	Planta Medica, 2011, 77, 9, 955–957.

Abstract No.	Species	Prostate Cancer Cells	Title of Research	First Named Author	Journal Reference
3222387	*Funalia trogii* (mycelial extract)	LNCaP, PC3	A study of anticancer effects of *Funalia trogii in vitro* and *in vivo*.	Rashid, S. et al.	*Food and Chemical Toxicology*, 2011, 49, 7, 1477–1483.
3216713	*Languas galangal* (Siamese ginger) 1'-Acetoxychavicol acetate	PC-3 Also ACA-treated mice	1'-Acetoxychavicol acetate suppresses angiogenesis-mediated human prostate tumor growth by targeting VEGF-mediated Src-FAK-Rho GTPase-signaling pathway.	Pang XiuFeng et al.	*Carcinogenesis*, 2011, 32, 6, 904–912.
3202578	*Vitis coignetiae* Rhapontigenin	Hypoxic PC-3 LNCaP	Rhapontigenin inhibited hypoxia inducible factor 1 alpha accumulation and angiogenesis in hypoxic PC-3 prostate cancer cells.	Jung DeokBeom et al.	*Biological & Pharmaceutical Bulletin*, 2011, 34, 6, 850–855.
3203611	*Phyllanthus pulcher* Wall. ex Müll. Arg. (Euphorbiaceae) (dried powdered roots) (5 pentacyclic triterpenes)	DU-145	Isolation and cytotoxicity of triterpenes from the roots of *Phyllanthus pulcher* Wall. ex Müll. Arg. (Euphorbiaceae).	Gururaj Bagalkotkar et al.	*Journal of Pharmacy and Pharmacology*, 2011, 5, 2, 183–188.
3203618	*Andrographis paniculata* (Andrographolide, a major constituent)	PC-3 DU-145	Andrographolide induces cell cycle arrest and apoptosis in PC-3 prostate cancer cells.	Wong HuiChyn et al.	*African Journal of Pharmacy and Pharmacology*, 2011, 5, 2, 225–233.
3208901	Silybin (nanosuspension)	PC-3	*In vitro* antitumor activity of silybin nanosuspension in PC-3 cells.	Zheng DanDan et al.	*Cancer Letters*, 2011, 307, 2, 158–164.
3194222	21 plants used in Mayan traditional medicine including: *Aeschynomene fascicularis* (root bark extract), *Bonellia macrocarpa* (stem and root bark extracts)	PC-3	Screening of plants used in Mayan traditional medicine to treat cancer-like symptoms.	Caamal-Fuentes, E. et al.	*Journal of Ethnopharmacology*, 2011, 135, 3, 719–724.
3170402	*Typhonium blumei* Nicolson & Sivadasan – Chinese traditional medicine, herb	LNCaP	*Typhonium blumei* extract inhibits proliferation of human lung adenocarcinoma A549 cells via induction of cell cycle arrest and apoptosis.	Hsu HsiaFen et al.	*Journal of Ethnopharmacology*, 2011, 135, 2, 492–500.
3174189	*Momordica charantia* (leaf) Kuguacin J, a triterpenoid	LNCaP	Induction of G1 arrest and apoptosis in androgen-dependent human prostate cancer by Kuguacin J, a triterpenoid from *Momordica charantia* leaf.	Pitchakarn, P. et al.	*Cancer Letters*, 2011, 306, 2, 142–150.

Abstract No.	Species	Prostate Cancer Cells	Title of Research	First Named Author	Journal Reference
3144842	Soyabean (SE Asia) (phytoestrogens)		Phytoestrogens and tumorigenesis.	Briese, V.	*Zeitschrift für Phytotherapie*, 2010, 31, 6, 285–287.
3155546	*Valeriana jatamansi* and *V. officinalis* (2 new chlorinated iridoids: 1,5-dihydroxy-3,8-epoxyvalechlorine, volvaltrate B, and valeriotetrate C)	PC-3M (metastatic)	Revision of the structures of 1,5-dihydroxy-3,8-epoxyvalechlorine, volvaltrate B, and valeriotetrate C from *Valeriana jatamansi* and *V. officinalis*.	Lin Sheng et al.	*Journal of Natural Products*, 2010, 73, 10, 1723–1726.
3155605	*Poria cocos* (6 lanostane-type triterpene acids, methyl ester [1b–6b], and hydroxy derivatives [1c–6c])	DU-145	Cytotoxic and apoptosis-inducing activities of triterpene acids from *Poria cocos*.	Kikuchi, T. et al.	*Journal of Natural Products*, 2011, 74, 2, 137–144.
3155615	*Mammea americana* (tropical/subtropical plant) (14 mammea-type coumarins including 3 new compounds: mammea F/ BB [1], mammea F/BA [2], and mammea C/AA [3])	PC-3	Natural and semisynthetic mammea-type isoprenylated dihydroxycoumarins uncouple cellular respiration.	Du, L. et al.	*Journal of Natural Products*, 2011, 74, 2, 240–248.
3158188	*Punica granatum* (Pomegranate) extracts (13 pure compounds found) (4 active compounds: epigallocatechin gallate, delphinidin chloride, kaempferol, and punicic acid)	LNCaP	Growth inhibitory, antiandrogenic, and pro-apoptotic effects of punicic acid in LNCaP human prostate cancer cells.	Gasmi, J.	*Journal of Agricultural and Food Chemistry*, 2010, 58, 23, 12149–12156.
3137365	Geraniol (monoterpene) and Docetaxel	PC-3 (tumor grafted mice)	Geraniol inhibits prostate cancer growth by targeting cell cycle and apoptosis pathways.	Kim SuHwa et al.	*Biochemical and Biophysical Research Communications*, 2011, 407, 1, 129–134.
3124659	*Bergenia ciliata* (Haw.) Sternb. (rhizome)	PC-3	Anti-neoplastic activities of *Bergenia ciliata* rhizome.	Venkatadri Rajkumar et al.	*Journal of Pharmacy Research*, 2011, 4, 2, 443–445.
3117226	*Kadsura oblongifolia* (roots and stems) Lignans (4 new dibenzocyclooctane-type: Kadsufolin A (1), kadsufolin D (4), angeloylbinankadsurin A, and heteroclitin B, and 11 known)	DU-145	Kadsufolins A–D and related cytotoxic lignans from *Kadsura oblongifolia*.	Huang ZeHao et al.	*Helvetica Chimica Acta*, 2011, 94, 3, 519–527.

Abstract No.	Species	Prostate Cancer Cells	Title of Research	First Named Author	Journal Reference
3121523	*Nicotiana tabacum* (tobacco cembranoids, (1*S*,2*E*,4*R*,6*R*,7*E*,11*E*)-2,7,11-cembratriene-4,6-diol (1) and its C-4 epimer)	PC-3M-CT+ (spheroid disaggregation assay) and PC-3 (wound-healing assay)	Bioactive natural, biocatalytic, and semisynthetic tobacco cembranoids.	Baraka, H.N. et al.	*Planta Medica*, 2011, 77, 5, 467–476.
3113422	Diallyl disulfide on Ca^{2+}	PC-3	Effect of diallyl disulfide on Ca^{2+} movement and viability in PC3 human prostate cancer cells.	Chen WeiChuan et al.	*Toxicology in Vitro*, 2011, 25, 3, 636–643.
3100033	*Artemisia vulgaris, Cichorium intybus, Smilax glabra, Solanum nigrum* and *Swertia chirayta*		Evaluation of anticancer properties of medicinal plants from the Indian subcontinent.	Nawab, A. et al.	*Molecular and Cellular Pharmacology*, 2011, 3, 1, 21–29.
3097319	*Commiphora mukul* (Ayurvedic plant) (Gugulipid extract)	LNCaP	Reactive oxygen species-dependent apoptosis by gugulipid extract of ayurvedic medicine plant *Commiphora mukul* in human prostate cancer cells is regulated by c-Jun N-terminal kinase.	Xiao, D. et al.	*Molecular Pharmacology*, 2011, 79, 3, 499–507.
3083610	"Thunder god vine" (Chinese) (triptolide)		Inhibition of tumor cellular proteasome activity by triptolide extracted from the Chinese medicinal plant "Thunder god vine."	Lu L. et al.	*Anticancer Research*, 2011, 31, 1, 1–10.
3083835	*Ruta graveolens*		*Ruta graveolens* extract induces DNA damage pathways and blocks Akt activation to inhibit cancer cell proliferation and survival.	Fadlalla, K. et al.	*Anticancer Research*, 2011, 31, 1, 233–241.
3068904	*Pygeum africanum*		The natural compounds atraric acid and N-butylbenzene-sulfonamide as antagonists of the human androgen receptor and inhibitors of prostate cancer cell growth.	Roell, D. et al.	*Molecular and Cellular Endocrinology*, 2011, 332, 1/2, 1–8.
3071026	Used over 50 different Chinese medicinal herbs and plants (extracted β-Elemene)	DU-145 PC-3	Antineoplastic effect of β-elemene on prostate cancer cells and other types of solid tumor cells.	Li, Q.D.Q. et al.	*Journal of Pharmacy and Pharmacology*, 2010, 62, 8, 1018–1027.

Abstract No.	Species	Prostate Cancer Cells	Title of Research	First Named Author	Journal Reference
3074301	*Picrorhiza kurroa* Royle ex Benth (Scrophulariaceae)	PC-3	Antioxidant and antineoplastic activities of *Picrorhiza kurroa* extracts.	Rajkumar, V. et al.	*Food and Chemical Toxicology*, 2011, 49, 2, 363–369.
3064161	*Cayaponia tayuya* (root) (23, 24 dihydrocucurbitacin and cucurbitacin R)		Search for a novel antioxidant, anti-inflammatory/analgesic or antiproliferative drug: cucurbitacins hold the ace.	Bernard, S.A.	*Journal of Medicinal Plants Research*, 2010, 4, 25, 2821–2826.
3052586	Gossypol	PC-3	Radiosensitization of hormone-refractory prostate cancer cells by gossypol treatment.	Akagunduz, O. et al.	*Journal of B.U.ON.*, 2010, 15, 4, 763–767.
3053215	*Excoecaria agallocha* (3 flavonoid glycosides including 2 new compounds)	DU-145	New Hedgehog/GLI-signaling inhibitors from *Excoecaria agallocha*.	Rifai, Y. et al.	*Bioorganic & Medicinal Chemistry Letters*, 2011, 21, 2, 718–722.
3038542	Olive (leave extract) (oleurupein)	PC-3	Determination of the antitumor effects of oleurupein in prostate (PC-3), breast (MCF-7), and hepatoma (Hep3B) cells.	Köçkar, F. et al.	*BIBAD, Biyoloji Bilimleri Araştırma Dergisi*, 2010, 3, 2, 185–190.
3015979	Isoflavones: daidzein, puerarin, ipriflavone, genistein, neobavaisoflavone, and biochanin-A	LNCaP	Isoflavones augment the effect of tumor necrosis factor-related apoptosis-inducing ligand (TRAIL) on prostate cancer cells.	Szliszka, E. et al.	*Journal of Urology*, 2010, 63, 4, 182–186.
3007048	12 species of ethnomedically utilized plants (fruit and vegetables)		Induction of murine embryonic stem cell differentiation by medicinal plant extracts.	Reynertson, K.A. et al.	*Experimental Cell Research*, 2011, 317, 1, 82–93.
3004344	Triptolide (effects of mitogen activated protein kinases [MAPKs] on the activity of triptolide)	LNCaP PC-3	MAPKs are not involved in triptolide-induced cell growth inhibition and apoptosis in prostate cancer cell lines with different p53 status.	Li Wei et al.	*Planta Medica*, 2011, 77, 1, 27–31.
		2010 (Year published in Cabi Citations)			
3383686	Cisplatin with β-elemene	DU145 PC-3	Evaluation of cisplatin in combination with β-elemene as a regimen for prostate cancer chemotherapy.	Li, Q.D.Q. et al.	*Basic and Clinical Pharmacology and Toxicology*, 2010, 107, 5, 868–876.

Abstract No.	Species	Prostate Cancer Cells	Title of Research	First Named Author	Journal Reference
3369013	Retigeric acid B (naturally occurring pentacyclic triterpenic acid)	PC-3 LNCaP	A novel anticancer agent, retigeric acid B, displays proliferation inhibition, S phase arrest and apoptosis activation in human prostate cancer cells.	Liu Han et al.	Chemico-Biological Interactions, 2010, 188, 3, 598–606.
3351377	Salvia miltiorrhiza Bunge (roots) Tanshinone IIA (Tan IIA; 14,16-epoxy-20-nor-5(10),6,8,13,15-abietapentaene-11,12-dione)	PC-3 LNCaP	Tanshinone IIA induces mitochondria dependent apoptosis in prostate cancer cells in association with an inhibition of phosphoinositide 3-kinase/AKT pathway.	Won SukHyun et al.	Biological & Pharmaceutical Bulletin, 2010, 33, 11, 1828–1834.
3352221	Hops xanthohumol, a prenylated chalone		Growth inhibitory and apoptosis-inducing effects of xanthohumol, a prenylated chalone present in hops, in human prostate cancer cells.	Deeb, D. et al.	Anticancer Research, 2010, 30, 9, 3333–3339.
3352228	Gardenia obtusifolia (5,3'-dihydroxy-3,6,7,8,4'-pentamethoxyflavone)		A dihydroxy-pentamethoxyflavone from Gardenia obtusifolia suppresses proliferation and promotes apoptosis of tumor cells through modulation of multiple cell signaling pathways.	Phromnoi, K. et al.	Anticancer Research, 2010, 30, 9, 3599–3610.
3356476	Phyllanthus spp. (P. amarus, P. niruri, P. urinaria and P. watsonii) (Polyphenols e.g. ellagitannins, gallotannins, flavonoids, and phenolic acids)	PC-3	Phyllanthus spp. induces selective growth inhibition of PC-3 and MeWo human cancer cells through modulation of cell cycle and induction of apoptosis.	Tang YinQuan et al.	PLoS ONE, 2010, September, e12644.
3339736	Cannabis sativa (leaf ethanolic extract and its n-hexane fraction)	PC-3	Mitochondrial membrane depolarization and caspase dependent apoptosis induced by Cannabis sativa.	Irum Sehar et al.	Journal of Pharmacy Research, 2010, 3, 10, 2475–2479.
3339995	Docetaxel, oleic acid-coated hydroxyapatite nanoparticles	PC-3 DU-145	Docetaxel loaded oleic acid-coated hydroxyapatite nanoparticles enhance the docetaxel-induced apoptosis through activation of caspase-2 in androgen independent prostate cancer cells.	Luo Yun et al.	Journal of Controlled Release, 2010, 147, 2, 278–288.

Abstract No.	Species	Prostate Cancer Cells	Title of Research	First Named Author	Journal Reference
3340057	Phosphatidylinositol 3-kinase	DU-145	Inhibition of phosphatidylinositol 3-kinase promotes tumor cell resistance to chemotherapeutic agents via a mechanism involving delay in cell cycle progression.	McDonald, G.T. et al.	*Experimental Cell Research*, 2010, 316, 19, 3197–3206.
3341893	Corni fructus, ursolic acid	RC–58T/h/S A#4, Primary human cells	Apoptotic action of ursolic acid isolated from Corni fructus in RC-58T/h/SA#4 primary human prostate cancer cells.	Kwon SeongHyuk et al.	*Bioorganic & Medicinal Chemistry Letters*, 2010, 20, 22, 6435–6438.
3323069	Kava, Flavokawain B, a chalcone	DU-145 PC-3 LAPC-4 LNCaP	Flavokawain B, a kava chalcone, induces apoptosis via up-regulation of death-receptor 5 and Bim expression in androgen receptor negative, hormonal refractory prostate cancer cell lines and reduces tumor growth.	Tang, Y.X. et al.	*International Journal of Cancer*, 2010, 127, 8, 1758–1768.
3324742	*Tinospora crispa* (aerial parts) (15 *cis*-clerodane-type furanoditerpenoids)	PC-3	*cis*-clerodane-type furanoditerpenoids from *Tinospora crispa*.	Choudhary, M.I. et al.	*Journal of Natural Products*, 2010, 73, 4, 541–547.
3324743	*Pleuranthodium racemigerum*, (Zingiberaceae) (rhizome) (Diarylheptanoid)	PC-3	Diarylheptanoid from *Pleuranthodium racemigerum* with *in vitro* prostaglandin E_2 inhibitory and cytotoxic activity.	Wohlmuth, H. et al.	*Journal of Natural Products*, 2010, 73, 4, 743–746.
3324984	*Tacca chantrieri* (roots and rhizomes) (Evelynin, a cytotoxic benzoquinone-type retro-dihydrochalcone)	PC-3	Evelynin, a cytotoxic benzoquinone-type *retro*-dihydrochalcone from *Tacca chantrieri*.	Peng, J.N. et al.	*Journal of Natural Products*, 2010, 73, 9, 1590–1592.
3325114	*Pongamiopsis pervilleana* (roots) (3 new: (2'R)-4'-hydroxyemoroidocarpan, pongavilleanine and epipervilline; 2 known: emoroidocarpan and rotenolone)	DU-145, NSCLC N CI-H460	Antiproliferative compounds from *Pongamiopsis pervilleana* from the Madagascar dry forest.	Harinantenaina, L. et al.	*Journal of Natural Products*, 2010, 73, 9, 1559–1562.
3325122	From 450 flavonoids (*silico screening*): 3,6-dihydroxyflavone was found potent		Cytotoxic flavonoids as agonists of peroxisome proliferator-activated receptor γ on human cervical and prostate cancer cells.	Lee JeeYoung et al.	*Journal of Natural Products*, 2010, 73, 7, 1261–1265.

Abstract No.	Species	Prostate Cancer Cells	Title of Research	First Named Author	Journal Reference
3325305	Acacia pennata (leaves) Terpenoids and a flavonoid glycoside	DU-145	Terpenoids and a flavonoid glycoside from Acacia pennata leaves as Hedgehog/GLI-mediated transcriptional inhibitors.	Rifai, Y. et al.	Journal of Natural Products, 2010, 73, 5, 995–997.
3293978	Allium sativum Diallyl disulfide	LNCaP	Anti-invasive activity of diallyl disulfide through tightening of tight junctions and inhibition of matrix metalloproteinase activities in LNCaP prostate cancer cells.	Shin DongYeok et al.	Toxicology in Vitro, 2010, 24, 6, 1569–1576.
3293980	Inula racemosa. caspase-3 such as poly (ADP-ribose) polymerase (apoptosis)		Activation of caspases and poly (ADP-ribose) polymerase cleavage to induce apoptosis in leukemia HL-60 cells by Inula racemosa.	Pal, H.C. et al.	Toxicology in Vitro, 2010, 24, 6, 1599–1609.
3269323	Achyranthes aspera (Amaranthacea) (Leaves)		Anti-proliferative and anticancer properties of Achyranthes aspera: specific inhibitory activity against pancreatic cancer cells.	Subbarayan, P.R. et al.	Journal of Ethnopharmacology, 2010, 131, 1, 78–82.
3273404	Marchantin M (compound)	PC-3 LNCaP, DU-145 (K562, HepG2, MCF-7)	Marchantin M displays growth inhibitory effects on human prostate cancer cells.	Xu AiHui et al.	Journal of Shandong University (Health Sciences), 2010, 48, 5, 18–22.
3274108	Cruciferous vegetables such as watercress (phenethyl isothiocyanate)	LNCaP PC-3	Phenethyl isothiocyanate inhibits oxidative phosphorylation to trigger reactive oxygen species-mediated death of human prostate cancer cells.	Xiao, D. et al.	Journal of Biological Chemistry, 2010, 285, 34, 26558–26569.
3261491	Licorice compounds, Isoliquiritigenin	C4-2 LNCaP	Isoliquiritigenin, a natural antioxidant, selectively inhibits the proliferation of prostate cancer cells.	Zhang XiaoYu et al.	Clinical and Experimental Pharmacology and Physiology, 2010, 37, 8, 841–847.
3262635	Strobilanthes crispus A dichloromethane sub-fraction	PC-3 DU-145	Anticancer activity of a sub-fraction of dichloromethane extract of Strobilanthes crispus on human breast and prostate cancer cells in vitro.	Nik Soriani Yaacob et al.	BMC Complementary and Alternative Medicine, 2010, 10, 42.

Abstract No.	Species	Prostate Cancer Cells	Title of Research	First Named Author	Journal Reference
3262884	*Gardenia fructus* (extract) Genipin a metabolite of geniposide	PC-3	Genipin induced apoptosis associated with activation of the c-Jun NH_2-terminal kinase and p53 protein in HeLa cells.	Cao HouLi et al.	*Biological & Pharmaceutical Bulletin*, 2010, 33, 8, 1343–1348.
3247523	Genus *Aglaia* Flavaglines – silvestrol cyclopenta[b]benzofuran	Prostate cancer xenograft models	Antitumor activity and mechanism of action of the cyclopenta[b] benzofuran, silvestrol.	Cencic, R. et al.	*PLoS ONE*, 2009, April, e5223.
3247964	Streptavidin-saporin	LNCaP CWR22-Rv1 PC-3	Saporin toxin-conjugated monoclonal antibody targeting prostate-specific membrane antigen has potent anticancer activity.	Kuroda, K. et al.	*Prostate*, 2010, 70, 12, 1286–1294.
3251056	*Mentha arvensis, M. piperita, M. longifolia,* and *M. spicata* Essential oils	LNCaP	Seasonal variation in content, chemical composition and antimicrobial and cytotoxic activities of essential oils from four *Mentha* species.	Hussain, A.I. et al.	*Journal of the Science of Food and Agriculture*, 2010, 90, 11, 1827–1836.
3244049	*Rosmarinus officinalis* (leaves)	DU-145 PC-3	Inhibitory effects of rosemary extracts, carnosic acid and rosmarinic acid on the growth of various human cancer cell lines.	Yesil-Celiktas, O. et al.	*Plant Foods for Human Nutrition*, 2010, 65, 2, 158–163.
3232951	ProstaCaid: blend of vitamins, minerals, multiherb extracts, and derivatives	Human and mouse: LNCaP and CASP 2.1), (PC-3 and CASP 1.1)	ProstaCaid induces G2/M cell cycle arrest and apoptosis in human and mouse androgen–dependent and –independent prostate cancer cells.	Yan, J.	*Integrative Cancer Therapies*, 2010, 9, 2, 186–196.
3207619	Willow bark (phytopharmacon extract) Salicin (Apoptosis)		*In vitro* anti-antiproliferative effects of the willow bark extract STW 33-I.	Bonaterra, G.A. et al.	*Arzneimittel Forschung*, 2010, 60, 6, 330–335.
3219127	*Tremella aurantia* (fruiting bodies) (polysaccharides and 70% ethanol extracts)	LNCaP PC-3	Effect of polysaccharides and 70% ethanol extracts from medicinal mushrooms on growth of human prostate cancer LNCaP and PC-3 cells.	Kiho, T. et al.	*International Journal of Medicinal Mushrooms*, 2010, 12, 2, 205–211.
3185914	*Nigella sativa* Thymoquinone seed oil	C4-2B PC-3	Studies on molecular mechanisms of growth inhibitory effects of thymoquinone against prostate cancer cells: role of reactive oxygen species.	Koka, P.S. et al.	*Experimental Biology and Medicine*, 2010, 235, 6, 751–760.

Abstract No.	Species	Prostate Cancer Cells	Title of Research	First Named Author	Journal Reference
3200198	*Silybum marianum* (milk thistle) major flavonolignan diastereoisomers		Large-scale isolation of flavonolignans from *Silybum marianum* extract affords new minor constituents and preliminary structure-activity relationships.	Sy-Cordero, A. et al.	*Planta Medica*, 2010, 76, 6, 644–647.
3195146	Cyclic bisbibenzyls: Riccardin C, Pakyonol, Marchantin M, and Plagiochin E (apoptosis)	PC-3	Cyclic bisbibenzyls induce growth arrest and apoptosis of human prostate cancer PC3 cells.	Xu AiHui et al.	*Acta Pharmacologica Sinica*, 2010, 31, 5, 609–615.
3195337	*Costus specious* (root)	DU-145	The root part of *Costus specious* possesses *in vitro* cytotoxic potential against human cancer cell lines from colon, liver and prostate origin.	Vikas Sharma et al.	*Asian Journal of Experimental Chemistry*, 2009, 4, 1/2, 43–45.
3189833	*Pterocarpus marsupium* (Pterostilbene-dimethyl ester derivative of resveratrol) (apoptosis)	PC-3	In vitro evaluation of the cytotoxic, antiproliferative and antioxidant properties of pterostilbene isolated from *Pterocarpus marsupium*.	Ajanta Chakraborty et al.	*Toxicology in Vitro*, 2010, 24, 4, 1215–1228.
3190944	Mint (*Mentha spicata* L., Lamiaceae), ginger (*Zingiber officinale* Rosc., Zingiberaceae), lemon (*Citrus limon* Burm. F., Rutaceae), grapefruit (*Citrus paradisi* Macf., Rutaceae), jasmine (*Jasminum grandiflora* L., Oleaceae), lavender (Mill.,Lamiaceae), chamomile (*Matricaria chamomilla* L., Compositae), thyme (*Thymus vulgaris* L., Lamiaceae), rose (*Rosa damascena* Mill., Rosaceae) and cinnamon (*Cinnamomum zeylanicum* N. Lauraceae)	PC-3	Activities of ten essential oils towards *Propionibacterium acnes* and PC-3, A-549 and MCF-7 cancer cells.	Zu YuanGang et al.	*Molecules*, 2010, 15, 5, 3200–3210.
3176463	Cryptocaryone, (dihydrochalcone)	PC-3	Cryptocaryone, a natural dihydrochalcone, induces apoptosis in human androgen independent prostate cancer cells by death receptor clustering in lipid raft and nonraft compartments.	Chen YiCheng et al.	*Journal of Urology*, 2010, 183, 6, 2409–2418.

Abstract No.	Species	Prostate Cancer Cells	Title of Research	First Named Author	Journal Reference
3153093	*Calotropis gigantea* R.Br.	DU-145	*In vitro* cytotoxic potential of *Calotropis gigantea* R.Br. against human cancer cell lines.	Madhulika Bhagat; Vikas Sharma.	*International Journal of Medical Sciences (India)*, 2009, 2, 1, 46–49.
3172845	*Nigella sativa* (black cumin) Thymoquinone		Thymoquinone poly (lactide-co-glycolide) nanoparticles exhibit enhanced antiproliferative, anti-inflammatory, and chemosensitization potential.	Ravindran, J. et al.	*Biochemical Pharmacology*, 2010, 79, 11, 1640–1647.
3161050	Avicin G and avicin D Also Saponin	PC-3	Red blood cell permeabilization by hypotonic treatments, saponin, and anticancer avicins.	Arias, M. et al.	*Biochimica et Biophysica Acta, Biomembranes*, 2010, 1798, 6, 1189–1196.
3141812	Apigenin, baicalein, curcumin, epigallocatechin 3-gallate, genistein, quercetin, and resveratrol	human and mouse	Common botanical compounds inhibit the hedgehog signaling pathway in prostate cancer.	Slusarz, A. et al.	*Cancer Research*, 2010, 70, 8, 3382–3390.
3134683	Camptothecin, a Topoisomerase I inhibitor	LNCaP and PC-3/AR	Camptothecin disrupts androgen receptor signaling and suppresses prostate cancer cell growth.	Liu ShiCheng et al.	*Biochemical and Biophysical Research Communications*, 2010, 394, 2, 297–302.
3131851	*Strychnos usambarensis* (tree, East Africa) Isostrychnopentamine, an indolomonoterpenic alkaloid	PC-3	Isostrychnopentamine, an indolomonoterpenic alkaloid from *Strychnos usambarensis*, with potential antitumor activity against apoptosis-resistant cancer cells.	Balde, E.S. et al.	*International Journal of Oncology*, 2010, 36, 4, 961–965.
3117374	*Rheedia brasiliensis*, 2 prenylated benzophenones: triprenylated garciniaphenone and tetraprenylated benzophenone 7-epiclusianone Garciniaphenone and 7-epiclusianone	PC-03	Antiproliferative effect of benzophenones and their influence on cathepsin activity.	Murata, R.M. et al.	*Phytotherapy Research*, 2010, 24, 3, 379–383.
3119674	*Trichosanthes japonica* agglutinin-II (TJA-II) column, Fucα1-2Gal and βGalNAc (PSA) Implying elevated expression of α1,2-fucosylation and β-N-acetylgalactosaminylation of PSA during carcinogenesis.	LNCaP	α1,2-Fucosylated and β-N-acetylgalactosaminylated prostate-specific antigen as an efficient marker of prostatic cancer.	Fukushima, K. et al.	*Glycobiology*, 2010, 20, 4, 452–460.

Abstract No.	Species	Prostate Cancer Cells	Title of Research	First Named Author	Journal Reference
3121779	Ganodermataceae Donk and two reference species: European *Ganoderma lucidum* and Asian *G. lucidum*, *Ganoderma* aff. *tuberculosum*	PC-3	Antiproliferative activities of methanolic extracts from a neotropical *Ganoderma* species (Aphyllophoromycetideae): identification and characterization of a novel ganoderic acid.	Welti, S. et al.	*International Journal of Medicinal Mushrooms*, 2010, 12, 1, 17–31.
3098542	Taxol (paclitaxel and its semisynthetic analogue docetaxel)	CRPC-castration-resistant prostate cancer. PTEN-deficient C4-2 CRPC cells	Targeting the androgen receptor by taxol in castration-resistant prostate cancer.	Jiang JingTing et al.	*Molecular and Cellular Pharmacology*, 2010, 2, 1, 1–5.
3095648	Ginsenoside Rg3 with docetaxel	LNCaP PC-3 DU145	Combination of ginsenoside Rg3 with docetaxel enhances the susceptibility of prostate cancer cells via inhibition of NF-κB.	Kim SunMi et al.	*European Journal of Pharmacology*, 2010, 631, 1/3, 1–9.
3088598	Sun ginseng (SG) – Rg3, Rk1, and Rg5 ginsenosides KG-135, the ginsenoside-rich fraction of SG	DU-145 PC-3	KG-135, enriched with selected ginsenosides, inhibits the proliferation of human prostate cancer cells in culture and inhibits xenograft growth in athymic mice.	Yoo JiHye et al.	*Cancer Letters*, 2010, 289, 1, 99–110.
3077364	Endophytic fungi (marine-derived mangrove): SZ-685C, a marine anthraquinone, an anthracycline analogue (apoptosis)		SZ-685C, a marine anthraquinone, is a potent inducer of apoptosis with anticancer activity by suppression of the Akt/FOXO pathway.	Xie Gui'e et al.	*British Journal of Pharmacology*, 2010, 159, 3, 689–697.
3082611	*Omphalotus illudens* (basidiomycete): Illudin S and M (1, 2) (sesquiterpenes) Acylfulvene (4), irofulven (5)	Metastatic hormone-refractory PC failed prior treatment: 2 different standard chemotherapeutic regimens. Solid tumor cells *in vitro*, nontarget B-cell derived cell line	Structure-activity studies of urea, carbamate, and sulfonamide derivatives of acylfulvene.	McMorris, T.C. et al.	*Journal of Medicinal Chemistry*, 2010, 53, 3, 1109–1116.

Abstract No.	Species	Prostate Cancer Cells	Title of Research	First Named Author	Journal Reference
3043194	Epigallocatechin gallate, Cd^{2+} and EGCG+Cd^{2+} (Apotosis)	PC-3	Inhibitory effects of epigallocatechin gallate (EGCG) and Cd^{2+} on the growth of prostate cancer PC-3 cell.	Sun ShiLi et al.	Journal of Agricultural Biotechnology, 2009, 17, 5, 902–907.
3069080	Oleanane triterpenoid CDDO-Me (synthesized from oleanolic acid)	LNCaP PC-3	Oleanane triterpenoid CDDO-Me inhibits growth and induces apoptosis in prostate cancer cells through a ROS-dependent mechanism.	Deeb, D. et al.	Biochemical Pharmacology, 2010, 79, 3, 350–360.
3069512	Merremia emerginata Hexane, ethyl acetate and methanol	DU-145	Anticancer and anti-inflammatory activities of extracts of Merremia emerginata.	Babu, A.V. et al.	Biosciences, Biotechnology Research Asia, 2009, 6, 2, 835–838.
3065892	Fisetin (3,3',4',7-tetrahydroxyflavone)	PC-3	Antimetastatic potential of fisetin involves inactivation of the PI3K/Akt and JNK signaling pathways with downregulation of MMP-2/9 expressions in prostate cancer PC-3 cells.	Chien ChiSheng et al.	Molecular and Cellular Biochemistry, 2010, 333, 1/2, 169–180.
3065963	Acacetin (5,7-dihydroxy-4'-methoxyflavone)	DU-145	Acacetin, a flavonoid, inhibits the invasion and migration of human prostate cancer DU145 cells via inactivation of the p38 MAPK signaling pathway.	Shen KunHung et al.	Molecular and Cellular Biochemistry, 2010, 333, 1/2, 279–291.
3048265	Baihuasheshecao (Hedyotis diffusa), H. corymbosa	PC-3 LNCaP	Authentication of the antitumor herb baihuasheshecao with bioactive marker compounds and molecular sequences.	Li Ming et al.	Food Chemistry, 2010, 119, 3, 1239–1245.
3037737	Mentha spicata L. (Lamiaceae) lipophilic and hydrophilic fractions	PC-3	Antioxidant and cytotoxic activities of lipophilic and hydrophilic fractions of Mentha spicata L. (Lamiaceae).	Arumugam, P. et al.	International Journal of Food Properties, 2010, 13, 1, 23–31.
3039295	Alnus glutinosa (stem bark), Carpinus betulus (leaves and stem bark), Castanea sativa (stem bark), Fagus sylvatica (leaves), Ilex aquifolium (leaves), Larix decidua (leaves), Quercus petraea (stem bark), and Quercus robur (leaves), Robinia pseudoacacia (root)	PC-3	In vitro anticancer potential of tree extracts from the Walloon Region forest.	Frédérich, M. et al.	Planta Medica, 2009, 75, 15, 1634–1637.

Abstract No.	Species	Prostate Cancer Cells	Title of Research	First Named Author	Journal Reference
3016353	Banana (peel)	LNCaP & mouse	Banana peel extract suppressed prostate gland enlargement in testosterone-treated mice.	Akamine, K. et al.	*Bioscience, Biotechnology and Biochemistry*, 2009, 73, 9, 1911–1914.
3016402	*Senecio stabianus* Lacaita (Asteraceae) pyrrolizidine alkaloids	LNCaP	*In vitro* cytotoxic effects of *Senecio stabianus* Lacaita (Asteraceae) on human cancer cell lines.	Tundis, R. et al.	*Natural Product Research*, 2009, 23, 18, 1707–1718.
3012142	*Cinnamomum tenuifolium.* (stems) 3 new butanolides, tenuifolide A, isotenuifolide A, and tenuifolide B, a new secobutanolide, secotenuifolide A, and 1 new sesquiterpenoid, tenuifolin, along with 16 known compounds	DU-145	Cytotoxic compounds from the stems of *Cinnamomum tenuifolium*.	Lin RongJyh et al.	*Journal of Natural Products*, 2009, 72, 10, 1816–1824.
3000148	Gossypol with zoledronic acid	DU-145	Targeting apoptosis in the hormone- and drug-resistant prostate cancer cell line, DU-145, by gossypol/ zoledronic acid combination.	Sanli, U.A. et al.	*Cell Biology International*, 2009, 33, 11, 1165–1172.

CHAPTER 4

Triterpenoids and Sesquiterpenoids for Prostate Cancer Therapy

Muthu K. Shanmugam, Frank Arfuso, Alan Prem Kumar, and Gautam Sethi

CONTENTS

4.1   INTRODUCTION

Several classes of natural products and their derivatives play a pivotal role as anticancer agents. One important class of natural compounds, terpenoids, can be broadly classified into monoterpenoid

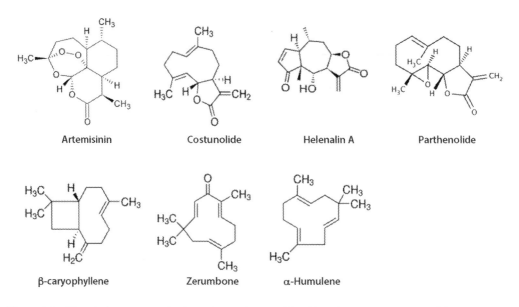

Figure 4.1 Chemical structures of selected sesquiterpenoids with anti-prostate cancer activity.

(10 carbon atoms), e.g., limonene, a-pinene, perillyl alcohol; sesquiterpenoid (15 carbon atoms) (Figure 4.1), e.g., parthenolide, zerumbone, artemisinin, costunolide, helenalin A; diterpenoid (20 carbon atoms), e.g., triptolide, acanthoic acid, tashinone IIA; triterpenoids/steroids (30 carbon atoms) (Figure 4.2), e.g., ursolic acid, oleanolic acid, betulinic acid, celastrol; and tetraterpenoids/carotenoids (40 carbon atoms), e.g., lycopene, astaxanthin. Sesquiterpenoids are naturally occurring 15-carbon compounds containing 3 isoprenoid units and are commonly found in a wide variety of plants, microorganisms, and marine life (Connolly and Hill, 2010; Shanmugam, et al., 2011a; Shanmugam, et al., 2012a). Sesquiterpenoids are classified according to the ring numbering system and the functional groups in the core structures such as acyclic, monocyclic, bicyclic, or tricyclic sesquiterpenoids (Chen, et al., 2011). These terpenoids have been shown to exhibit anti-inflammatory, anti-microbial, and anti-cancer activities (Bishayee, et al., 2011; Chen, et al., 2011; Petronelli, et al., 2009; Yadav, et al., 2010). In general, sesquiterpenoids have been shown to have cytotoxic activity against leukemia, breast, colon, lung, and liver cancer cells. However, sesquiterpenoids have shown exceptional prostate cancer specificity, and some of these compounds have been tested in human clinical trials (Chen, et al., 2011).

Moreover, in a randomized phase IIB clinical trial in patients with metastatic, hormone-refractory prostate cancer, the sesquiterpenoid compound hydroxymethylacylfulvene (HMAF, MGI 114) or irofulven, derived from the sesquiterpene *Illudin S*, was found to significantly improve the overall survival of patients who were non-responsive to docetaxel therapy (Chen, et al., 2011; Leggas, et al., 2002). Chen et al. (2011), reported the anti-prostate cancer activity of eremophilane sesquiterpenoids isolated from the rhizomes of *Ligularia fischeri*, which is commonly found in the Henan province of China. Numerous sesquiterpenoids have been isolated from the species *Inula*, and these compounds exhibit diverse biological activities – especially anti-inflammatory, cytotoxicity, and anti-tumor activity against LNCaP and PC3 prostate cancer cell lines, with IC50 values below 3 mM. *Inula* sesquiterpenoids induce apoptosis in these cell lines through the downregulation of nuclear factor kB (NF-kB) transcriptional activity (Cheng, et al., 2012; Huo, et al., 2008; Park and Kim, 1998; Wang, et al., 2014). In another study, sesquiterpenoids ST1 and ST2 isolated from myrrh, a resinous substance obtained from the *Commiphora* trees, inhibited prostate cancer

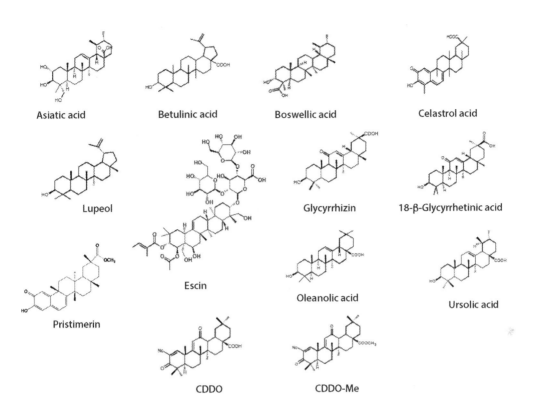

Figure 4.2 Chemical structures of selected triterpenoids with anti-prostate cancer activity.

cell proliferation and repressed androgen receptor (AR) transcriptional activity in LNCaP and PC3 cancer cell lines (Wang, et al., 2011). A new bisaboladiene sesquiterpenoid endoperoxide, 3, 6-epidioxy-1,10-bisaboladiene, isolated from *Cacalia delphiniifolia*, inhibited cell proliferation and induced apoptosis in the LNCaP cell line [IC50 = 23.4 mM] (Nishikawa, et al., 2008).

Interestingly, Deng et al. (2011) reported the isolation of a new sesquiterpenoid Linerenone from the plant *Lindera communis*, which exhibited significant cytotoxic activity against the androgen-independent prostate cancer cell line DU145. In another study, germacrane-type sesquiterpenoids myrrhanolide D and myrrhasin A, bearing an epoxy ring, were isolated from resinous exudates of the plant *Commiphora opobalsamum*. The isolated compound exhibited cytotoxic activity against DU145 and PC3 cells (Shen, et al., 2007). Rekha et al. (2013) reported that the two new sesqui-terpenoids isolated from the rhizome *Nardostachys jatamansi* were cytotoxic against different types of cancer cells, including the prostate cancer cell line DU145. Several cytotoxic sesquiter-penoids were isolated from the leaves and flowers of *Ratibida columnifera*. The sesquiterpenoid 9R-hydroxy-secoratiferolide-5R-O-(2-methylbutyrate) was found to be the most potent, and signifi-cantly inhibited LNCaP cell line proliferation and induced cell cycle arrest (Cui, et al., 1999). The sesquiterpene lactone vernolide, isolated from the leaves of *Vernonia amygdalina*, inhibited cell proliferation, induced cell S-phase cell cycle arrest, and blocked NF-kB and signal transducer and activator of transcription (STAT) 3 transcription activity in DU145 cells (Sinisi, et al., 2015).

A dose-dependent inhibition of prostate adenocarcinoma PC3 cell proliferation was observed when treated with Avarone, a sesquiterpene quinone isolated from the Mediterranean sponge *Dysidea avara* (Pejin, et al., 2014). a-santalol, a sesquiterpene alcohol, is a key constituent of sandal-wood essential oil extracted from the mature East Indian sandalwood tree, *Santalum album* L, and induces apoptosis in PC3 (androgen-independent and p53 null) and LNCaP (androgen-dependent and p53 wild-type) human prostate cancer cells by causing caspase-3 activation (Bommareddy, et al., 2012). In another study, a-santalol significantly inhibited the growth of a PC3 xenograft in nude mice and tumor associated angiogenesis by targeting the vascular endothelial growth factor receptor (VEGFR) 2 regulated AKT/mTOR/P70S6K signaling pathway (Saraswati, et al., 2013).

Marine organisms are also an important source of sesquiterpenoids. In a recent study, the total synthesis of sesquiterpene phenol dictyoceratin-C previously identified from the Indonesian marine sponge *Dactylospongia elegans* and its closely related compound dictyoceratin-A was reported. These two compounds exhibited potent hypoxia-selective cytotoxicity against DU145 cells (Sumii, et al., 2015).

4.2   SESQUITERPENOID LACTONE

4.2.1   Artemisinin

Artemisinin is a potent anti-malarial compound isolated from the herb *Artemisia annua* (Klayman, 1985). It is a sesquiterpenoid lactone that has recently been shown to have significant anti-proliferative effect against a variety of cancer cell lines (Efferth, 2007). A recent report by Willoughby et al. (2009) showed that artemisinin inhibited lymph node carcinoma of prostate (LNCaP) cell proliferation by inducing G1 phase cell cycle arrest associated with rapid downregulation of CDK2 and CDK4 protein levels. Interestingly, another study by Nakase et al. (2009) showed that an artemisinin-transferrin conjugate inhibited DU145 cell proliferation and induced mitochondrial pathway mediated apoptosis. *In vitro* treatment with a synthetic artemisinin dimer caused cell cycle arrest and induced apoptosis in prostate cancer cell lines at a low concentration compared to its parent compound artemisinin (Morrissey, et al., 2010). Similar to artemisinin, dihydroartemisinin (DHA) was cytotoxic to prostate cancer cells. However, DHA did not have any effect on normal prostate epithelial cells. He et al. (2010) showed that DHA upregulated death receptor 5 (DR5) and suppressed PI3K/AKT and ERK cell survival pathways in prostate cancer DU145, PC3, and LNCaP cells. Furthermore, DHA in combination with TRAIL, a natural ligand for death receptors, synergistically induced apoptosis in these cell lines. DHA also has an inhibitory effect on tumor angiogenesis. Zhuang et al. (2013) observed that DHA significantly suppressed VEGF mRNA and protein expression and induced apoptosis in the PC3M prostate cancer cell line.

4.2.2   Costunolide

Costunolide is a sesquiterpene lactone that has been demonstrated to inhibit cellular proliferation and induce apoptosis in hormone dependent (LNCaP) and independent (PC-3 and DU-145) prostate cancer cells in a dose-dependent manner (Hsu, et al., 2011).

4.2.3   Helenalin A

Helenalin A is a sesquiterpene lactone isolated from *Arnica montana*. It is a potent anti-inflammatory and anti-cancer compound specifically inhibiting the NF-kB transcription factor in a variety of cancer cell lines including prostate; however, its use is limited due to its high level of hepatic and lymphatic toxicity (Farhana, et al., 2005; Jin, et al., 2005).

4.2.4 Parthenolide

Parthenolide, a sesquiterpene lactone, is the most abundant molecule in the medicinal herb *Tanacetum parthenium*. Parthenolide has been shown to be a potent inhibitor of transcription factor NF-kB and its associated downstream targets in prostate cancer cells (Sweeney, et al., 2004). In another study, parthenolide inhibited proliferation of the androgen-independent cell line CWR22Rv1 *in vitro* and induced apoptosis at micro-molar concentrations. In a CWR22Rv1 xenograft mouse model, parthenolide inhibited tumor growth and augmented the efficacy of cancer chemotherapy compound docetaxel and anti-androgen bicalutamide, and restored sensitivity to anti-androgen therapy (Shanmugam, et al., 2006). In an androgen deprivation-resistant prostate cancer (ADRPC) xenograft mouse model, oral administration of parthenolide inhibited AR expression, prostate-specific antigen secretion, and tumor growth *in vivo* (Zhang, et al., 2009). Parthenolide also radiosensitized the androgen-independent DU145 cells that constitutively overexpress the tumor suppressor gene PTEN. Abrogation of PTEN expression by siRNA rendered DU145 cells more resistant to the combined effect of parthenolide and radiation (Sun, et al., 2007). Kawasaki et al. (2009) reported that parthenolide was cytotoxic to tumor initiating cells obtained from prostate cancer cells such as DU145, PC3, VCaP, and LAPC4, and from primary prostate tumor initiating cells. In addition, parthenolide inhibited tumor initiating cell-derived tumor formation in a xenograft mouse model (Kawasaki, et al., 2009). Remarkably, parthenolide inhibited X-ray induced NF-kB activation and completely suppressed split-dose repair in p53 null PC3 prostate cancer cells (Watson, et al., 2009). A novel water soluble analogue of parthenolide, dimethylaminoparthenolide, was shown to be a potent inhibitor of prostate cancer growth *in vitro* and *in vivo* (Shanmugam, et al., 2010). In PC3 cells, parthenolide selectively exhibits radiosensitization effects and activates NADPH oxidase, thereby inducing oxidative stress by increasing reactive oxygen species (ROS) production and decreasing antioxidant capacity. In contrast, there was no redox status change in normal cells, indicating redox as a selective target for cancer cell death (Sun, et al., 2010). In another similar study by Xu et al. (2013), parthenolide was shown to activate NADPH oxidase and induced ROS production. In this study they identified KEAP1 as the downstream redox target. Remarkably, parthenolide acts as a tumor cell-specific radiosensitizer and as a radioprotector on normal prostate cells (Xu, et al., 2013). The NF-kB transcription factor plays a major role in prostate tumor development. In addition to its radiosensitization effects, parthenolide also produced thermosensitization effects on androgen-independent prostate cancer cells. Parthenolide in combination with hyperthermia produced potent inhibition of prostate cancer cell proliferation, which was mediated by potent inhibition of NF-kB (Hayashi, et al., 2011). Parthenolide can reduce both hypoxic pro-inflammatory gene expression and hypoxia inducible factor (HIF) 1a in androgen-independent cells, thereby inhibiting tumor progression (Ravenna, et al., 2014).

4.2.5 β-Caryophyllene

β-Caryophyllene oxide, a sesquiterpene lactone, significantly inhibits constitutive and inducible STAT3 phosphorylation in a dose- and time-dependent manner in prostate cancer cells (Kim, et al., 2014a; Kim, et al., 2014b). Another similar study by the same group indicated that β-caryophylline oxide interferes with multiple signaling pathways such as PI3K/AKT/mTOR/S6K1 and mitogen-activated protein kinase (MAPK) pathways, thereby attenuating the growth of prostate cancer (Park, et al., 2011).

4.2.6 Zerumbone

Zerumbone (2,6,9,9-tetramethyl-[2E,6E,10E]-cycloundeca-2,6,10-trien-1-one) is a cyclic, eleven-membered sesquiterpene isolated from the rhizomes of *Zingiber zerumbet* Smith. Zerumbone has been shown to modulate an array of important molecular targets for both prevention and treatment of a variety of cancer types (Prasannan, et al., 2012). In a recent study, zerumbone in combination with paclitaxel was observed to inhibit prostate cancer growth synergistically through the negative regulation of Jak-2/STAT3 pathway in DU145 and PC3 cells (Jorvig and Chakraborty, 2015). In another study, zerumbone inhibited multiple targets in hormone refractive prostate cancer cells by targeting tubulin assembly, thereby inducing endoplasmic reticulum and mitochondrial stress, which resulted in autophagy and apoptosis of tumor cells (Chan, et al., 2015).

4.2.7 α-Humulene

α-Humulene is a monocyclic sesqiterpenoid and an analogue of zerumbone, which lacks the carbonyl group. α-Humulene is isolated from *Senecio ambiguus* subsp. *ambiguus* (Biv.) DC. The hexane extract inhibited hormone dependent prostate carcinoma LNCaP cell growth (Loizzo, et al., 2007; Tundis, et al., 2009).

4.3 TRITERPENOIDS AND PROSTATE CANCER

Research on natural products has provided a multitude of evidence on the nature and composition of bioactive phytochemicals present in seeds, fruits, cruciferous vegetables, and spices that are prospective entities to prevent inflammation-driven diseases (Aggarwal, et al., 2008; Aggarwal, et al., 2009; Gautam and Jachak, 2009; Kannaiyan, et al., 2011). In particular, triterpenoids isolated from various medicinal herbs have been shown to be potential therapeutic compounds for the treatment of a variety of malignancies (Aggarwal, et al., 2006; Aggarwal and Shishodia, 2006; Rabi and Gupta, 2008; Shanmugam, et al., 2011a). Among the triterpenoids, pentacyclic triterpenoids are the most extensively studied compounds, showing wide ranging anticancer activities (Shanmugam, et al., 2012a). Some of the naturally occurring pentacyclic triterpenoids are acetyl-11-keto-β-bosewellic acid (AKBA), asiatic acid (AA), α-amyrin, avicin, betulinic acid (BetA), bosewellic acid (BA), celastrol, escin, glycyrrhizin, 18-β-glycyrrhetinic acid, lupeol, madecassic acid, momordin I, oleanolic acid (OA), pristimerin, platycodon D, saikosaponins, soyasapogenol B, and ursolic acid (Connolly and Hill, 2010; Petronelli, et al., 2009). Furthermore, recent reports suggest that semisynthetic derivatives of oleanolic pentacyclic triterpenoids such as cyano-3,12-dioxooleana-1,9 (11)-dien-28-oic acid (CDDO), its methyl ester (CDDO-Me), and imidazolide (CDDO-Im) are more potent than natural triterpenoids in inducing apoptosis and inhibiting tumor growth *in vivo* (Deeb, et al., 2008; Liby, et al., 2007; Sporn, et al., 2011).

4.3.1 Acetyl-11-keto-β-boswellic Acid

Acetyl-11-keto-β-boswellic acid (AKBA) is the main bioactive pentacyclic triterpenoid molecule derived from *Boswellia serrata* and has been shown to suppress *in vitro* and *in vivo* growth of PC3 tumor (Syrovets, et al., 2005a; Syrovets, et al., 2005b). In both androgen-independent and -dependent PC3 and LNCaP cells respectively, AKBA-induced apoptosis was through upregulation of the death receptor 5 (DR5) mediated pathway and CAAT/enhancer binding protein homologous protein (CHOP) (Lu, et al., 2008). The specificity protein (Sp) family of transcription factors comprises critical molecules that play important roles in various cellular processes and are actively involved in the development and progress of cancers including prostate. Sp1 is upregulated in numerous cancers and indicates poor prognosis (Sankpal, et al., 2011). AKBA can abrogate AR expression in prostate cancer by suppressing Sp1 binding activity in the nucleus (Yuan, et al., 2008). In another study, AKBA was shown to inhibit prostate tumor growth by suppressing VEGFR2-induced angiogenesis (Pang, et al., 2009). Interestingly, VEGF and VEGFR2 have Sp1 binding sites and are regulated by Sp1 (Higgins, et al., 2006). In addition to AKBA, 3α-acetyl-11-keto-α-boswellic acid suppressed PC3 cell proliferation and inhibited tumor growth in a xenograft mouse model (Buchele, et al., 2006). Another semi-synthetic derivative of AKBA, propionyloxy derivative of 11-keto-β-boswellic acid, was found to inhibit PC3 cell proliferation *in vitro* (Chashoo, et al., 2011). Furthermore, a novel semisynthetic triterpenoid derivative, 3-cinnamoyl-11-keto-β-boswellic acid, inhibited PC3 prostate tumor growth *in vitro* and *in vivo* by targeting the mTOR pathway (Morad, et al., 2013).

4.3.2 Celastrol (Tripterine)

Celastrol (tripterine), a pentacyclic triterpenoid compound isolated from the Chinese herb Thunder God Vine, has been demonstrated to suppress almost all types of tumor cell proliferation (Kannaiyan, et al., 2011), including human prostate tumor growth in nude mice, by predominantly inhibiting the 26S proteasome pathway (Yang, et al., 2006). AR signaling is central to the progression of prostate cancer. Celastrol significantly inhibited AR signaling in a dose-dependent manner and also abrogated anchorage-independent cell growth and LNCaP cell colony formation in soft agar (Hieronymus, et al., 2006). Earlier studies have indicated that celastrol-mediated proteasome pathway inhibition is associated with AR suppression and immuno-reactivity to calpain, suggesting that AR degradation is intrinsic to the induction of apoptosis in prostate cancer cells (Yang, et al., 2008b). Interestingly, celastrol also sensitizes PC3 cells to radiation by inducing irreversible DNA damage to PC3 cells *in vitro* and *in vivo*, and is a potential candidate for novel adjuvant therapy in hormone refractive prostate cancer (Dai, et al., 2009). In another study by the same group, they observed that celastrol inhibited NF-kB and its downstream gene products in prostate cancer cells both *in vitro* and *in vivo* (Dai, et al., 2010). TRAIL receptors DR4 and DR5 are upregulated upon celastrol treatment in association with the induction of CHOP, thereby accelerating TRAIL-mediated apoptosis of PC3 cells (Sung, et al., 2010). In PC3 cells, celastrol was found to suppress VEGF-induced activation of the AKT/mTOR/ribosomal protein S6 kinase (P70S6K) pro-survival pathway, thereby inhibiting tumor growth in a xenograft mouse model (Pang, et al., 2010). Triptolide, which is a diterpenoid epoxide, is another active component extracted from the Chinese herb *Tripterygium wilfordii* Hook F, and inhibits PC3 and LNCaP growth by downregulating SENP1, AR, and cJUN expression both *in vitro* and *in vivo* (Chen, et al., 2012). The TMPRSS2/ERG (T/E) fusion gene is present in the majority of prostate cancers and is associated with constitutive activation of NF-kB signaling, and also can directly phosphorylate NF-kB p65 at Ser 536 residue. When VCaP cells were treated with celastrol, a dose- and time-dependent inhibition of AR, ERG, and NF-kB was reported, and a similar effect was observed in a xenograft mice study (Shao, et al., 2013). Recently, liposome-encapsulated celastrol displayed efficient serum stability, cellular internalization, and anti-prostate tumor activity, which was comparable to that of the free drug reconstituted in dimethyl sulfoxide (Wolfram, et al., 2014). In another study, cell-penetrating peptide-coated tripterine-loaded nanostructured lipid carriers (CT-NLC) exhibited potent anti-cancer activity against PC3 prostate tumor cells *in vitro* and *in vivo* (Yuan, et al., 2013). Moreover, celastrol was found to abrogate IL-6 gene expression by downregulation of NF-kB in prostate cancer cells (Chiang, et al., 2014). Interestingly, celastrol can also inhibit the hERG (human ether-à-go-go-related gene) channel in androgen-independent DU145 cells, thereby abrogating cell cycle progression (Ji, et al., 2015).

4.3.3 Asiatic Acid

Asiatic acid (AA) is a member of the ursane type of triterpenoid. It has been reported to induce apoptosis of PPC-1 prostate cancer cells, which was mediated by an increase in intracellular calcium and caspase-3 activation (Gurfinkel, et al., 2006). Although AA has anti-cancer activity against a variety of tumor cell lines, its application is limited by poor bioavailability and thereby limited cytotoxicity. In a recent report, a semi-synthetic derivative of AA was found to be more cytotoxic than the parent compound, and the cytotoxicity was associated with anti-angiogenic activity (Jing, et al., 2015).

4.3.4 Betulinic Acid

Betulinic acid (BetA) is a pentacyclic triterpenoid isolated from the bark of white birch that exhibits cytotoxic activity against a variety of cancer cells (Kessler, et al., 2007). Papineni et al. (2008) showed that BetA inhibited transcription factor specificity protein 1 (sp1), sp3, and sp4, thereby preventing the expression of the tumor survival angiogenic factor VEGF and survivin in LNCaP prostate cancer cells. BetA itself, being a catalytic inhibitor of topoisomerases, inhibits the formation of apoptotic topoisomerase I-DNA cleavable complexes induced by drugs such as camptothecin, staurosporin, and etoposide in DU145 cells (Ganguly, et al., 2007). In another study, BetA was found to inhibit both constitutive and TNFa-induced NF-kB activation in PC3 cells (Rabi and Gupta, 2008; Rabi, et al., 2008). However, in addition to its anti-cancer activity, the semi-synthetic derivative dimethyl succinyl betulinic acid (bevirimat) is now in phase IIb clinical trials as a "maturation inhibitor" (Lee, 2010). In a drug combination experiment with docetaxel and 2-methoxyestradiol, BetA induced synergistic apoptotic cell death in LNCaP cells and non-apoptotic cell death in DU145 and PC3 cells (Parrondo, et al., 2010). In another study using hypoxic PC3 cells, BetA inhibited binding of HIF-1a and STAT3 to the VEGF promoter, thereby inhibiting tumor-associated angiogenesis (Shin, et al., 2011). In prostate cancer cells, BetA suppressed multiple deubiquitinases, leading to accumulation of polyubiquitinated proteins, reduced oncoprotein production, and induction of apoptotic cell death (Reiner, et al., 2013). BetA (10 mg/kg) produced a similar effect in transgenic adenocarcinoma of prostate (TRAMP) mice tumors but had no effect on normal mouse tissue (Reiner, et al., 2013).

4.3.5 Escin

Escin, the main bioactive compound isolated from the plant *Aesculus hippocastanum* (horse chestnut), inhibited cell proliferation of castration-resistant prostate cancer (CRPC) cells, PC3 and DU145, and induced G2/M cell cycle arrest, downregulated cyclin B1, and induced p21 expression *in vitro*. *In vivo*, escin was shown to significantly reduce CRPC growth (Piao, et al., 2014).

4.3.6 Glycyrrhizin and 18-β-glycyrrhetinic Acid

Glycyrrhetinic acid (GA) is the active metabolite of glycyrrhizic acid, one of the components of licorice extract. GA significantly suppressed the rate of proliferation of LNCaP cells, but it had no effect on the proliferation of PC3 and DU145 cells (Hawthorne and Gallagher, 2008). In another study, GA was observed to inhibit LNCaP and DU145 cells in a dose-dependent manner and induce caspase-independent apoptosis in those cell lines (Thirugnanam, et al., 2008). GA inhibited DU145 growth and proliferation, inhibited HUVEC tube formation, and downregulated NF-kB, VEGF, and MMP9 expression. GA also suppressed nonsteroidal anti-inflammatory gene-1 (NSD-1) expression in DU145 cells (Shetty, et al., 2011).

4.3.7 Lupeol

Lupeol is a triterpenoid compound present in fruits and vegetables. It has been demonstrated to dose-dependently inhibit cell proliferation and induce apoptotic cell death. In a CWR22Rnu1 prostate tumor xenograft mice model, lupeol produced a significant inhibition of tumor growth with concomitant reduction in prostate-specific antigen secretion (Saleem, et al., 2005; Siddiqui, et al., 2008; Syed, et al., 2008). Prasad et al. showed that lupeol inhibited the expression of cyclin B, cdc25C, and plk1, while no change was observed in the expression of gadd45, p21(waf1/cip1), and cdc2 genes. In addition, lupeol induced the expression of 14-3-3 sigma genes with potent induction of apoptosis in PC3 cells (Prasad, et al., 2008a; Prasad, et al., 2008b). Saleem et al. (2009) reported that lupeol treatment significantly reduced levels of beta-catenin in the cytoplasmic and nuclear fractions, glycogen synthase kinase 3 beta (GSK3beta)-axin complex (regulator of beta-catenin stability), MMP-2, and T-cell factor (TCF)-responsive element in prostate cancer cells. In another study by the same group, it was demonstrated that lupeol dose-dependently inhibited cyclin A, B1, D1, D2, E2, CDK2, increased CDK inhibitor p21, arrested cell proliferation, and downregulated the anti-apoptotic protein cFLIP (Khan, et al., 2010; Saleem, et al., 2009). Interestingly, lupeol also suppressed androgen analog (1881)-induced AR transcriptional activity, reduced prostate-specific antigen levels, competitively inhibited binding to the AR receptor, and sensitized androgen-independent cells to anti-hormone therapy (Siddique, et al., 2011; Siddique and Saleem, 2011).

4.3.8 Pristimerin

Pristimerin is a quinonemethide triterpenoid derived from the plant *Triterpygium wilfordii* Hook with the potential of being a promising anticancer agent. In AR-negative PC3 cells and AR-positive LNCaP cells, pristimerin induced apoptosis by inhibiting proteasome function (Yang, et al., 2008a). It has been reported that pristimerin-induced apoptosis of LNCaP and PC3 cells was mediated through the mitochondrial apoptotic pathway, inhibiting Bcl-2 and survivin though a ROS-dependent ubiquitin proteasomal degradation pathway (Liu, et al., 2013; Liu, et al., 2014). Pristimerin reversed the hypoxia-induced metastatic phenotype such as invasiveness, cancer stem cell characteristics, and epithelial-mesenchymal transition in hypoxia-induced PC3 cells (Zuo, et al., 2015). Pristimerin was also shown to inhibit human telomerase reverse transcriptase (hTERT) in prostate cancer cells by suppressing transcription factors STAT3, SP1, cMYC, and protein kinase B/AKT that regulate hTERT transcriptionally and post-translationally (Liu, et al., 2015).

4.3.9 Saikosaponin

Saikosaponin-d (SSd), a triterpene saponin compound derived from *Bupleurum radix*, has been shown to have a cytotoxic effect on various cancer cell lines. Saikosaponin inhibited DU145 cell proliferation in a dose-dependent manner, induced cell cycle arrest at G0/G1 phase, upregulated p53 and p21 levels, and induced mitochondrial-dependent apoptosis (Yao, et al., 2014).

4.3.10 Oleanolic Acid

Oleanolic acid (OA; 3b-hydroxyolean-12-en-28-oic acid) is a bioactive pentacyclic triterpenoid belonging to the family Oleaceae. It has been isolated from more than 1600 plant species, the majority of which are edible plants and medicinal herbs (Liby and Sporn, 2012; Shanmugam, et al., 2014). Major advancements in triterpenoid research during the current decade have been made in the synthesis of synthetic triterpenoids. For example, the OA derivative, 2-cyano-3, 12-dioxoole-ana-1,9 (11)-dien-28-oic acid (CDDO) and its C-28 methyl ester (CDDO-ME, or bardoxolone methyl) and C28 imidazole (CDDO-IM) demonstrated potent anti-inflammatory and anti-tumor activities (Honda, et al., 2000a; Honda, et al., 2000b; Liby and Sporn, 2012; Suh, et al., 1999). CDDO-ME- and CDDO-IM-induced inhibition of growth of LNCaP, ALVA31, DU145, PC3, and PPC1 prostate cancer cells lines was associated with increased expression of TRAIL receptors DR4 and DR5 (Hyer, et al., 2008). Treatment with CDDO-ME inhibited LNCaP and PC3 prostate cancer cell proliferation and induced apoptosis, which was associated with suppression of hTERT gene expression and inhibition of the AKT/NF-kB/mTOR pathway (Liu, et al., 2012a; Liu, et al., 2012b). Hao et al. (2013) described the anti-tumor activity of 12 derivatives of OA that exhibited the most potent cytotoxicity against PC3 cancer cells. Deeb et al. (2008), showed that CDDO-ME inhibited hormone-refractory PC3 (AR^-) and C4-2 (AR^+) prostate cancer growth and progression by modulating pAKT-, pmTOR-, and NF-kB-signaling proteins and their downstream targets, such as pBad and pFoxo3a (for AKT), pS6K1, peIF-4E and p4E-BP1 (for mTOR), and COX-2, VEGF, and cyclin D1 (for NF-kappaB), both *in vitro* and *in vivo*. In another study, CDDO-ME induced ROS in LNCaP and PC3 cells from both non-mitochondrial and mitochondrial sources and induced apoptosis in these cells (Deeb, et al., 2010). CDDO and CDDO-ME prevented the progression of prostate cancer in the TRAMP mice model (Gao, et al., 2011). In addition, inhibition of development of pre-neoplastic lesions by CDDO-ME in TRAMP mice was associated with a significant decrease in TERT and its associated regulatory molecules in the prostate gland. Thus TERT is a likely target of CDDO-Me for both the prevention and treatment of prostate cancer (Liu, et al., 2012a; Liu, et al., 2012b).

4.3.11   Ursolic Acid

Ursolic acid (3b-hydroxy-urs-12-en-28-oic-acid), an ursane-type pentacyclic triterpenoid, belongs to the cyclosqualenoid family. It is abundantly present in medicinal plants such as *Rosemarinus officinalis, Eriobotrya japonica, Calluna vulgaris, Ocimum sanctum*, and *Eugenia jambolana* (Ngo, et al., 2011; Shanmugam, et al., 2013). Ursolic acid was previously reported to be cytotoxic to a variety of tumor cells, to induce apoptosis (Shanmugam, et al., 2011c), and to inhibit tumor promotion, metastasis, and angiogenesis in nude mice xenograft and in transgenic tumor models (Kiran, et al., 2008). Our group has investigated the potential effect of ursolic acid on the NF-kB- and STAT3-signaling pathways in both DU145 and LNCaP cells. We found that ursolic acid inhibited both constitutive and TNF-a-induced activation of NF-kB in DU145 and LNCaP cells in a dose-dependent manner. Ursolic acid also downregulated the expression of various NF-kB- and STAT3-regulated gene products involved in proliferation, survival, and angiogenesis, and induced apoptosis in both cell lines (Shanmugam, et al., 2011c). Activation of CXCR4/CXCL12-signaling pathway has been implicated in tumor cell ability to metastasize to organs such as liver and lungs (Teicher and Fricker, 2010). Moreover, we found that ursolic acid downregulated the CXCR4 expression irrespective of the HER2 status in a dose- and time-dependent manner, and this downregulation was also mediated by inhibition of NF-kB activation (Shanmugam, et al., 2011b). Limami et al. (2012) showed that puriergic receptors P2Y(2)/src/p38/COX2-signaling pathway was integral to the development of resistance to ursolic acid-induced apoptosis in DU145 cells. Ursolic acid is known to chemosensitize tumor cells to a number of chemotherapeutic agents (Pathak, et al., 2007; Prasad, et al., 2012). In another study, ursolic acid was shown to radiosensitize DU145, CT26, and B16F10 cells and accelerated cell death in these cell lines (Koh, et al., 2012). Shin et al. (2012), demonstrated that autophagy inhibitors in combination with ursolic acid synergistically induce autophagy in PC3 cells and induced apoptosis, increased the expression of LC3-II (an autophagosome marker in mammals), and triggered monodansyl-cadaverine integration into autolysosomes (Shin, et al., 2012; Zhang, et al., 2010). Wang et al. (2011) showed that ursolic acid and its cis- and trans-3-O-p-hydroxycinnamoyl esters derivatives inhibited the growth of MMP activity associated with tumor invasion and metastasis in DU145 cells. Intraperitoneal administration of ursolic acid

(200 mg/kg b.w.) for 6 weeks inhibited the growth of DU145 cells in nude mice without any significant effect on body weight (Shanmugam, et al., 2013; Shanmugam, et al., 2011c). In addition, ursolic acid–enriched diet (1% w/w) produced chemopreventive effects in the TRAMP (Shanmugam, et al., 2012b). In this model, ursolic acid demonstrated significantly reduced tumor growth without any effects on total body weight and prolonged overall survival (days) of mice compared to untreated control mice. It was also observed that ursolic acid downregulated the activation of NF-kB, STAT3, AKT, and IKKa/b phosphorylation in the dorsolateral prostate (DLP) tissues, which correlated with the decrease in circulating TNF-a and IL-6 in mouse serum (Shanmugam, et al., 2012b).

4.4 CONCLUSION AND PERSPECTIVES

Several terpenoids are found in nature and are structurally diverse, in particular the sesquiterpenoids and triterpenoids. These different classes of terpenoids have been shown to inhibit cancer cell proliferation, survival, metastasis, and angiogenesis, and induce apoptosis. In addition, when combined with standard chemotherapeutic agents or targeted agents, a synergistic effect is produced. This is probably attributed to their effects on multiple oncogenic signaling cascades in a wide variety of tumor models. It is becoming very clear that cancer is a complex disease, and many intrinsic as well as extrinsic factors play key roles in its development and progression. In particular, prostate cancer contains phenotypically and functionally distinct cells that pose clear clinical challenges to various available therapies. These include prostate cancer stem cells, AR status, tumor-associated macrophages, and castration-resistant prostate cancer. Considering the complexity that drives prostate cancer, simultaneously targeting multiple cancer-related proteins by the above discussed terpenoids would provide critical clues for anticancer drug development. Several clinical studies with oleanolic acid semisynthetic derivatives such as CDDO, CDDO-ME, and CDDO-IM have provided novel insights on their potency and efficacy in humans. All these studies support the potential use of terpenoids for therapy, and additional clinical trials are needed to bring these exciting molecules to clinical practice for the benefit of society.

REFERENCES

Aggarwal, B. B. Ichikawa, H. Garodia, P. et al. 2006. From traditional Ayurvedic medicine to modern medicine: identification of therapeutic targets for suppression of inflammation and cancer. *Expert opinion on therapeutic targets*, 10, 87–118.

Aggarwal, B. B. Kunnumakkara, A. B. Harikumar, K. B. et al. 2008. Potential of spice-derived phytochemicals for cancer prevention. *Planta Med*, 74, 1560–1569.

Aggarwal, B. B. Shishodia, S. 2006. Molecular targets of dietary agents for prevention and therapy of cancer. *Biochem Pharmacol*, 71, 1397–1421.

Aggarwal, B. B. Vijayalekshmi, R. V. Sung, B. 2009. Targeting inflammatory pathways for prevention and therapy of cancer: short-term friend, long-term foe. *Clinical cancer research : an official journal of the American Association for Cancer Research*, 15, 425–430.

Bishayee, A. Ahmed, S. Brankov, N. et al. 2011. Triterpenoids as potential agents for the chemoprevention and therapy of breast cancer. *Frontiers in bioscience : a journal and virtual library*, 16, 980–996.

Bommareddy, A. Rule, B. VanWert, A. L. et al. 2012. alpha-Santalol, a derivative of sandalwood oil, induces apoptosis in human prostate cancer cells by causing caspase-3 activation. *Phytomedicine*, 19, 804–811.

Buchele, B. Zugmaier, W. Estrada, A. et al. 2006. Characterization of 3alpha-acetyl-11-keto-alpha-boswellic acid, a pentacyclic triterpenoid inducing apoptosis in vitro and in vivo. *Planta Med*, 72, 1285–1289.

Chan, M. L. Liang, J. W. Hsu, L. C. et al. 2015. Zerumbone, a ginger sesquiterpene, induces apoptosis and autophagy in human hormone-refractory prostate cancers through tubulin binding and crosstalk between endoplasmic reticulum stress and mitochondrial insult. *Naunyn Schmiedebergs Arch Pharmacol*, 388, 1223–1236.

Chashoo, G. Singh, S. K. Sharma, P. R. et al. 2011. A propionyloxy derivative of 11-keto-beta-boswellic acid induces apoptosis in HL-60 cells mediated through topoisomerase I & II inhibition. *Chem Biol Interact*, 189, 60–71.

Chen, Q. F. Liu, Z. P. Wang, F. P. 2011. Natural sesquiterpenoids as cytotoxic anticancer agents. *Mini Rev Med Chem*, 11, 1153–1164.

Chen, Y. N. Huang, T. F. Chang, C. H. et al. 2012. Antirestenosis effect of butein in the neointima formation progression. *J Agric Food Chem*, 60, 6832–6838.

Cheng, X. R. Li, W. W. Ren, J. et al. 2012. Sesquiterpene lactones from Inula hookeri. *Planta Med*, 78, 465–471.

Chiang, K. C. Tsui, K. H. Chung, L. C. et al. 2014. Celastrol blocks interleukin-6 gene expression via down-regulation of NF-kappaB in prostate carcinoma cells. *PLoS One*, 9, e93151.

Connolly, J. D. Hill, R. A. 2010. Triterpenoids. *Nat Prod Rep*, 27, 79–132.

Cui, B. Lee, Y. H. Chai, H. et al. 1999. Cytotoxic sesquiterpenoids from Ratibida columnifera. *J Nat Prod*, 62, 1545–1550.

Dai, Y. Desano, J. Tang, W. et al. 2010. Natural proteasome inhibitor celastrol suppresses androgen-independent prostate cancer progression by modulating apoptotic proteins and NF-kappaB. *PLoS One*, 5, e14153.

Dai, Y. DeSano, J. T. Meng, Y. et al. 2009. Celastrol potentiates radiotherapy by impairment of DNA damage processing in human prostate cancer. *Int J Radiat Oncol Biol Phys*, 74, 1217–1225.

Deeb, D. Gao, X. Dulchavsky, S. A. et al. 2008. CDDO-Me inhibits proliferation, induces apoptosis, down-regulates Akt, mTOR, NF-kappaB and NF-kappaB-regulated antiapoptotic and proangiogenic proteins in TRAMP prostate cancer cells. *J Exp Ther Oncol*, 7, 31–39.

Deeb, D. Gao, X. Jiang, H. et al. 2010. Oleanane triterpenoid CDDO-Me inhibits growth and induces apoptosis in prostate cancer cells through a ROS-dependent mechanism. *Biochem Pharmacol*, 79, 350–360.

Efferth, T. 2007. Willmar Schwabe Award 2006: antiplasmodial and antitumor activity of artemisinin – from bench to bedside. *Planta Med*, 73, 299–309.

Farhana, L. Dawson, M. I. Fontana, J. A. 2005. Apoptosis induction by a novel retinoid-related molecule requires nuclear factor-kappaB activation. *Cancer Res*, 65, 4909–4917.

Ganguly, A. Das, B. Roy, A. et al. 2007. Betulinic acid, a catalytic inhibitor of topoisomerase I, inhibits reactive oxygen species-mediated apoptotic topoisomerase I-DNA cleavable complex formation in prostate cancer cells but does not affect the process of cell death. *Cancer Res*, 67, 11848–11858.

Gao, X. Deeb, D. Liu, Y. et al. 2011. Prevention of prostate cancer with oleanane synthetic triterpenoid CDDO-Me in the TRAMP mouse model of prostate cancer. *Cancers (Basel)*, 3, 3353–3369.

Gautam, R. Jachak, S. M. 2009. Recent developments in anti-inflammatory natural products. *Med Res Rev*, 29, 767–820.

Gurfinkel, D. M. Chow, S. Hurren, R. et al. 2006. Disruption of the endoplasmic reticulum and increases in cytoplasmic calcium are early events in cell death induced by the natural triterpenoid Asiatic acid. *Apoptosis*, 11, 1463–1471.

Hao, J. Liu, J. Wen, X. et al 2013. Synthesis and cytotoxicity evaluation of oleanolic acid derivatives. *Bioorg Med Chem Lett*, 23(7), 2074–2077.

Hawthorne, S. Gallagher, S. 2008. Effects of glycyrrhetinic acid and liquorice extract on cell proliferation and prostate-specific antigen secretion in LNCaP prostate cancer cells. *J Pharm Pharmacol*, 60, 661–666.

Hayashi, S. Koshiba, K. Hatashita, M. et al. 2011. Thermosensitization and induction of apoptosis or cell-cycle arrest via the MAPK cascade by parthenolide, an NF-kappaB inhibitor, in human prostate cancer androgen-independent cell lines. *Int J Mol Med*, 28, 1033–1042.

He, Q. Shi, J. Shen, X.L. et al. 2010. Dihydroartemisinin upregulates death receptor 5 expression and cooperates with TRAIL to induce apoptosis in human prostate cancer cells. *Cancer Biol Ther*, 9(10), 819–824.

Hieronymus, H. Lamb, J. Ross, K. N. et al. 2006. Gene expression signature-based chemical genomic prediction identifies a novel class of HSP90 pathway modulators. *Cancer Cell*, 10, 321–330.

Higgins, K. J. Liu, S. Abdelrahim, M. et al. 2006. Vascular endothelial growth factor receptor-2 expression is induced by 17beta-estradiol in ZR-75 breast cancer cells by estrogen receptor alpha/Sp proteins. *Endocrinology*, 147, 3285–3295.

Honda, T. Gribble, G. W. Suh, N. et al. 2000a. Novel synthetic oleanane and ursane triterpenoids with various enone functionalities in ring A as inhibitors of nitric oxide production in mouse macrophages. *J Med Chem*, 43, 1866–1877.

Honda, T. Rounds, B. V. Bore, L. et al. 2000b. Synthetic oleanane and ursane triterpenoids with modified rings A and C: a series of highly active inhibitors of nitric oxide production in mouse macrophages. *J Med Chem*, 43, 4233–4246.

Hsu, J. L. Pan, S. L. Ho, Y. F. et al. 2011. Costunolide induces apoptosis through nuclear calcium2+ overload and DNA damage response in human prostate cancer. *J Urol*, 185, 1967–1974.

Huo, Y. Shi, H. Wang, M. et al. 2008. Complete assignments of 1H and 13C NMR spectral data for three sesquiterpenoids from Inula helenium. *Magn Reson Chem*, 46, 1208–1211.

Hyer, M. L. Shi, R. Krajewska, M. et al. 2008. Apoptotic activity and mechanism of 2-cyano-3,12-dioxoolean -1,9-dien-28-oic-acid and related synthetic triterpenoids in prostate cancer. *Cancer Res*, 68, 2927–2933.

Ji, N. Li, J. Wei, Z. et al. 2015. Effect of celastrol on growth inhibition of prostate cancer cells through the regulation of hERG channel in vitro. *Biomed Res Int*, 2015, 308475.

Jin, F. Liu, X. Zhou, Z. et al. 2005. Activation of nuclear factor-kappaB contributes to induction of death receptors and apoptosis by the synthetic retinoid CD437 in DU145 human prostate cancer cells. *Cancer Res*, 65, 6354–6363.

Jing, Y. Wang, G. Ge, Y. et al. 2015. Synthesis, anti-tumor and anti-angiogenic activity evaluations of asiatic Acid amino Acid derivatives. *Molecules*, 20, 7309–7324.

Jorvig, J. E. Chakraborty, A. 2015. Zerumbone inhibits growth of hormone refractory prostate cancer cells by inhibiting JAK2/STAT3 pathway and increases paclitaxel sensitivity. *Anticancer Drugs*, 26, 160–166.

Kannaiyan, R. Shanmugam, M. K. Sethi, G. 2011. Molecular targets of celastrol derived from Thunder of God Vine: potential role in the treatment of inflammatory disorders and cancer. *Cancer letters*, 303, 9–20.

Kawasaki, B. T. Hurt, E. M. Kalathur, M. et al. 2009. Effects of the sesquiterpene lactone parthenolide on prostate tumor-initiating cells: An integrated molecular profiling approach. *Prostate*, 69, 827–837.

Kessler, J. H. Mullauer, F. B. de Roo, G. M. et al. 2007. Broad in vitro efficacy of plant-derived betulinic acid against cell lines derived from the most prevalent human cancer types. *Cancer Lett*, 251, 132–145.

Khan, N. Adhami, V. M. Mukhtar, H. 2010. Apoptosis by dietary agents for prevention and treatment of prostate cancer. *Endocr Relat Cancer*, 17, R39–52.

Kim, C. Cho, S. K. Kapoor, S. et al. 2014a. beta-Caryophyllene oxide inhibits constitutive and inducible STAT3 signaling pathway through induction of the SHP-1 protein tyrosine phosphatase. *Mol Carcinog*, 53, 793–806.

Kim, C. Cho, S. K. Kim, K. D. et al. 2014b. beta-Caryophyllene oxide potentiates TNFalpha-induced apoptosis and inhibits invasion through down-modulation of NF-kappaB-regulated gene products. *Apoptosis*, 19, 708–718.

Kiran, M. S. Viji, R. I. Sameer Kumar, V. B. et al. 2008. Modulation of angiogenic factors by ursolic acid. *Biochem Biophys Res Commun*, 371, 556–560.

Klayman, D. L. 1985. Qinghaosu (artemisinin): an antimalarial drug from China. *Science*, 228, 1049–1055.

Koh, S. J. Tak, J. K. Kim, S. T. et al. 2012. Sensitization of ionizing radiation-induced apoptosis by ursolic acid. *Free Radic Res*, 46, 339–345.

Lee, K. H. 2010. Discovery and development of natural product-derived chemotherapeutic agents based on a medicinal chemistry approach. *J Nat Prod*, 73, 500–516.

Leggas, M. Stewart, C. F. Woo, M. H. et al. 2002. Relation between Irofulven (MGI-114) systemic exposure and tumor response in human solid tumor xenografts. *Clin Cancer Res*, 8, 3000–3007.

Liby, K. T. Sporn, M. B. 2012. Synthetic oleanane triterpenoids: multifunctional drugs with a broad range of applications for prevention and treatment of chronic disease. *Pharmacol Rev*, 64, 972–1003.

Liby, K. T. Yore, M. M. Sporn, M. B. 2007. Triterpenoids and rexinoids as multifunctional agents for the prevention and treatment of cancer. *Nat Rev Cancer*, 7, 357–369.

Limami, Y. Pinon, A. Leger, DY. et al. 2012. The P2Y2/Src/p38/COX-2 pathway is involved in the resistance to ursolic acid-induced apoptosis in colorectal and prostate cancer cells. *Biochimie*, 94(8), 1754–1763.

Liu, Y. Gao, X. Deeb, D. et al. 2012a. Telomerase reverse transcriptase (TERT) is a therapeutic target of oleanane triterpenoid CDDO-Me in prostate cancer. *Molecules*, 17, 14795–14809.

Liu, Y. Gao, X. Deeb, D. et al. 2012b. Oleanane triterpenoid CDDO-Me inhibits Akt activity without affecting PDK1 kinase or PP2A phosphatase activity in cancer cells. *Biochem Biophys Res Commun*, 417, 570–575.

Liu, Y. B. Gao, X. Deeb, D. et al. 2013. Pristimerin induces apoptosis in prostate cancer cells by downregulating Bcl-2 through ROS-dependent ubiquitin-proteasomal degradation pathway. *J Carcinog Mutagen*, Suppl 6, 005.

Liu, Y. B. Gao, X. Deeb, D. et al. 2014. Ubiquitin-proteasomal degradation of antiapoptotic survivin facilitates induction of apoptosis in prostate cancer cells by pristimerin. *Int J Oncol*, 45, 1735–1741.

Liu, Y. B. Gao, X. Deeb, D. et al. 2015. Role of telomerase in anticancer activity of pristimerin in prostate cancer cells. *J Exp Ther Oncol*, 11, 41–49.

Loizzo, M. R. Tundis, R. Statti, G. A. et al. 2007. Jacaranone: a cytotoxic constituent from Senecio ambiguus subsp. ambiguus (biv.) DC. against renal adenocarcinoma ACHN and prostate carcinoma LNCaP cells. *Arch Pharm Res*, 30, 701–707.

Lu, M. Xia, L. Hua, H. et al. 2008. Acetyl-keto-beta-boswellic acid induces apoptosis through a death receptor 5-mediated pathway in prostate cancer cells. *Cancer Res*, 68, 1180–1186.

Morad, S. A. Schmid, M. Buchele, B. et al. 2013. A novel semisynthetic inhibitor of the FRB domain of mammalian target of rapamycin blocks proliferation and triggers apoptosis in chemoresistant prostate cancer cells. *Mol Pharmacol*, 83, 531–541.

Morrissey, C. Gallis, B. Solazzi, J. W. et al. 2010. Effect of artemisinin derivatives on apoptosis and cell cycle in prostate cancer cells. *Anticancer Drugs*, 21, 423–432.

Nakase, I. Gallis, B. Takatani-Nakase, T. et al. 2009. Transferrin receptor-dependent cytotoxicity of artemisinin-transferrin conjugates on prostate cancer cells and induction of apoptosis. *Cancer Lett*, 274(2), 290–298.

Ngo, S. N. Williams, D. B. Head, R. J. 2011. Rosemary and cancer prevention: preclinical perspectives. *Crit Rev Food Sci Nutr*, 51, 946–954.

Nishikawa, K. Aburai, N. Yamada, K. et al. 2008. The bisabolane sesquiterpenoid endoperoxide, 3,6-epidioxy-1,10-bisaboladiene, isolated from Cacalia delphiniifolia inhibits the growth of human cancer cells and induces apoptosis. *Biosci Biotechnol Biochem*, 72, 2463–2466.

Pang, X. Yi, Z. Zhang, J. et al. 2010. Celastrol suppresses angiogenesis-mediated tumor growth through inhibition of AKT/mammalian target of rapamycin pathway. *Cancer Res*, 70, 1951–1959.

Pang, X. Yi, Z. Zhang, X. et al. 2009. Acetyl-11-keto-beta-boswellic acid inhibits prostate tumor growth by suppressing vascular endothelial growth factor receptor 2-mediated angiogenesis. *Cancer Res*, 69, 5893–5900.

Papineni, S. Chintharlapalli, S. Safe, S. 2008. Methyl 2-cyano-3,11-dioxo-18 beta-olean-1,12-dien-30-oate is a peroxisome proliferator-activated receptor-gamma agonist that induces receptor-independent apoptosis in LNCaP prostate cancer cells. *Mol Pharmacol*, 73(2), 553–565.

Park, E. J. Kim, J. 1998. Cytotoxic sesquiterpene lactones from Inula britannica. *Planta Med*, 64, 752–754.

Park, K. R. Nam, D. Yun, H. M. et al. 2011. beta-Caryophyllene oxide inhibits growth and induces apoptosis through the suppression of PI3K/AKT/mTOR/S6K1 pathways and ROS-mediated MAPKs activation. *Cancer Lett*, 312, 178–188.

Parrondo, R. de las Pozas, A. Reiner, T. et al. 2010. NF-kappaB activation enhances cell death by antimitotic drugs in human prostate cancer cells. *Mol Cancer*, 9, 182.

Pathak, A. K. Bhutani, M. Nair, A. S. et al. 2007. Ursolic acid inhibits STAT3 activation pathway leading to suppression of proliferation and chemosensitization of human multiple myeloma cells. *Mol Cancer Res*, 5, 943–955.

Pejin, B. Iodice, C. Tommonaro, G. et al. 2014. Further in vitro evaluation of cytotoxicity of the marine natural product derivative 4'-leucine-avarone. *Nat Prod Res*, 28, 347–350.

Petronelli, A. Pannitteri, G. Testa, U. 2009. Triterpenoids as new promising anticancer drugs. *Anti-cancer drugs*, 20, 880–892.

Piao, S. Kang, M. Lee, Y. J. et al. 2014. Cytotoxic effects of escin on human castration-resistant prostate cancer cells through the induction of apoptosis and G2/M cell cycle arrest. *Urology*, 84, 982 e981–987.

Prasad, S. Kalra, N. Shukla, Y. 2008a. Induction of apoptosis by lupeol and mango extract in mouse prostate and LNCaP cells. *Nutr Cancer*, 60, 120–130.

Prasad, S. Nigam, N. Kalra, N. et al. 2008b. Regulation of signaling pathways involved in lupeol induced inhibition of proliferation and induction of apoptosis in human prostate cancer cells. *Mol Carcinog*, 47, 916–924.

Prasad, S. Yadav, V. R. Sung, B. et al. 2012. Ursolic acid inhibits growth and metastasis of human colorectal cancer in an orthotopic nude mouse model by targeting multiple cell signaling pathways: chemosensitization with capecitabine. *Clin Cancer Res*, 18, 4942–4953.

Prasannan, R. Kalesh, K. A. Shanmugam, M. K. et al. 2012. Key cell signaling pathways modulated by zerumbone: role in the prevention and treatment of cancer. *Biochem Pharmacol*, 84, 1268–1276.

Rabi, T. Gupta, S. 2008. Dietary terpenoids and prostate cancer chemoprevention. *Frontiers in bioscience : a journal and virtual library*, 13, 3457–3469.

Rabi, T. Shukla, S. Gupta, S. 2008. Betulinic acid suppresses constitutive and TNFalpha-induced NF-kappaB activation and induces apoptosis in human prostate carcinoma PC-3 cells. *Mol Carcinog*, 47, 964–973.

Ravenna, L. Principessa, L. Verdina, A. et al. 2014. Distinct phenotypes of human prostate cancer cells associate with different adaptation to hypoxia and pro-inflammatory gene expression. *PLoS One*, 9, e96250.

Reiner, T. Parrondo, R. de Las Pozas, A. et al. 2013. Betulinic acid selectively increases protein degradation and enhances prostate cancer-specific apoptosis: possible role for inhibition of deubiquitinase activity. *PLoS One*, 8, e56234.

Rekha, K. Rao, R.R. Pandey, R. et al. 2013. Two new sesquiterpenoids from the rhizomes of Nardostachys jatamansi. *J Asian Nat Prods Res*, 15, 111–116.

Saleem, M. Kweon, M. H. Yun, J. M. et al. 2005. A novel dietary triterpene Lupeol induces fas-mediated apoptotic death of androgen-sensitive prostate cancer cells and inhibits tumor growth in a xenograft model. *Cancer Res*, 65, 11203–11213.

Saleem, M. Murtaza, I. Witkowsky, O. et al. 2009. Lupeol triterpene, a novel diet-based microtubule targeting agent: disrupts survivin/cFLIP activation in prostate cancer cells. *Biochem Biophys Res Commun*, 388, 576–582.

Sankpal, U. T. Goodison, S. Abdelrahim, M. et al. 2011. Targeting Sp1 transcription factors in prostate cancer therapy. *Med Chem*, 7, 518–525.

Saraswati, S. Kumar, S. Alhaider, A. A. 2013. alpha-santalol inhibits the angiogenesis and growth of human prostate tumor growth by targeting vascular endothelial growth factor receptor 2-mediated AKT/mTOR/P70S6K signaling pathway. *Mol Cancer*, 12, 147.

Shanmugam, M. K. Dai, X. Kumar, A. P. et al. 2013. Ursolic acid in cancer prevention and treatment: molecular targets, pharmacokinetics and clinical studies. *Biochem Pharmacol*, 85, 1579–1587.

Shanmugam, M. K. Dai, X. Kumar, A. P. et al. 2014. Oleanolic acid and its synthetic derivatives for the prevention and therapy of cancer: preclinical and clinical evidence. *Cancer Lett*, 346, 206–216.

Shanmugam, M. K. Kannaiyan, R. Sethi, G. 2011a. Targeting cell signaling and apoptotic pathways by dietary agents: role in the prevention and treatment of cancer. *Nutr Cancer*, 63, 161–173.

Shanmugam, M. K. Manu, K. A. Ong, T. H. et al. 2011b. Inhibition of CXCR4/CXCL12 signaling axis by ursolic acid leads to suppression of metastasis in transgenic adenocarcinoma of mouse prostate model. *Int J Cancer*, 129, 1552–1563.

Shanmugam, M. K. Nguyen, A. H. Kumar, A. P. et al. 2012a. Targeted inhibition of tumor proliferation, survival, and metastasis by pentacyclic triterpenoids: potential role in prevention and therapy of cancer. *Cancer Lett*, 320, 158–170.

Shanmugam, M. K. Ong, T. H. Kumar, A. P. et al. 2012b. Ursolic acid inhibits the initiation, progression of prostate cancer and prolongs the survival of TRAMP mice by modulating pro-inflammatory pathways. *PLoS One*, 7, e32476.

Shanmugam, M. K. Rajendran, P. Li, F. et al. 2011c. Ursolic acid inhibits multiple cell survival pathways leading to suppression of growth of prostate cancer xenograft in nude mice. *J Mol Med (Berl)*, 89, 713–727.

Shanmugam, R. Jayaprakasan, V. Gokmen-Polar, Y. et al. 2006. Restoring chemotherapy and hormone therapy sensitivity by parthenolide in a xenograft hormone refractory prostate cancer model. *Prostate*, 66, 1498–1511.

Shanmugam, R. Kusumanchi, P. Cheng, L. et al. 2010. A water-soluble parthenolide analogue suppresses in vivo prostate cancer growth by targeting NFkappaB and generating reactive oxygen species. *Prostate*, 70, 1074–1086.

Shao, L. Zhou, Z. Cai, Y. et al. 2013. Celastrol suppresses tumor cell growth through targeting an AR-ERG-NF-kappaB pathway in TMPRSS2/ERG fusion gene expressing prostate cancer. *PLoS One*, 8, e58391.

Shen, T. Wan, W. Yuan, H. et al. 2007. Secondary metabolites from Commiphora opobalsamum and their antiproliferative effect on human prostate cancer cells. *Phytochemistry*, 68, 1331–1337.

Shetty, A. V. Thirugnanam, S. Dakshinamoorthy, G. et al. 2011. 18alpha-glycyrrhetinic acid targets prostate cancer cells by down-regulating inflammation-related genes. *Int J Oncol*, 39, 635–640.

Shin, J. Lee, H. J. Jung, D. B. et al. 2011. Suppression of STAT3 and HIF-1 alpha mediates anti-angiogenic activity of betulinic acid in hypoxic PC-3 prostate cancer cells. *PLoS One*, 6, e21492.

Shin, S. W. Kim, S. Y. Park, J. W. 2012. Autophagy inhibition enhances ursolic acid-induced apoptosis in PC3 cells. *Biochim Biophys Acta*, 1823, 451–457.

Siddique, H. R. Mishra, S. K. Karnes, R. J. et al. 2011. Lupeol, a novel androgen receptor inhibitor: implications in prostate cancer therapy. *Clin Cancer Res*, 17, 5379–5391.

Siddique, H. R. Saleem, M. 2011. Beneficial health effects of lupeol triterpene: a review of preclinical studies. *Life Sci*, 88, 285–293.

Siddiqui, I. A. Afaq, F. Adhami, V. M. et al. 2008. Prevention of prostate cancer through custom tailoring of chemopreventive regimen. *Chem Biol Interact*, 171, 122–132.

Sinisi, A. Millan, E. Abay, S. M. et al. 2015. Poly-electrophilic sesquiterpene lactones from Vernonia amygdalina: new members and differences in their mechanism of thiol trapping and in bioactivity. *J Nat Prod*, 78, 1618–1623.

Sporn, M. B. Liby, K. T. Yore, M. M. et al. 2011. New synthetic triterpenoids: potent agents for prevention and treatment of tissue injury caused by inflammatory and oxidative stress. *J Nat Prod*, 74, 537–545.

Suh, N. Wang, Y. Honda, T. et al. 1999. A novel synthetic oleanane triterpenoid, 2-cyano-3,12-dioxoolean-1,9-dien-28-oic acid, with potent differentiating, antiproliferative, and anti-inflammatory activity. *Cancer Res*, 59, 336–341.

Sumii, Y. Kotoku, N. Fukuda, A. et al. 2015. Enantioselective synthesis of dictyoceratin-A (smenospondiol) and -C, hypoxia-selective growth inhibitors from marine sponge. *Bioorg Med Chem*, 23, 966–975.

Sun, Y. St Clair, D. K. Fang, F. et al. 2007. The radiosensitization effect of parthenolide in prostate cancer cells is mediated by nuclear factor-kappaB inhibition and enhanced by the presence of PTEN. *Mol Cancer Ther*, 6, 2477–2486.

Sun, Y. St Clair, D. K. Xu, Y. et al. 2010. A NADPH oxidase-dependent redox signaling pathway mediates the selective radiosensitization effect of parthenolide in prostate cancer cells. *Cancer Res*, 70, 2880–2890.

Sung, B. Park, B. Yadav, V. R. et al. 2010. Celastrol, a triterpene, enhances TRAIL-induced apoptosis through the down-regulation of cell survival proteins and up-regulation of death receptors. *J Biol Chem*, 285, 11498–11507.

Sweeney, C. Li, L. Shanmugam, R. et al. 2004. Nuclear factor-kappaB is constitutively activated in prostate cancer in vitro and is overexpressed in prostatic intraepithelial neoplasia and adenocarcinoma of the prostate. *Clin Cancer Res*, 10, 5501–5507.

Syed, D. N. Suh, Y. Afaq, F. et al. 2008. Dietary agents for chemoprevention of prostate cancer. *Cancer Lett*, 265, 167–176.

Syrovets, T. Buchele, B. Krauss, C. et al. 2005a. Acetyl-boswellic acids inhibit lipopolysaccharide-mediated TNF-alpha induction in monocytes by direct interaction with IkappaB kinases. *Journal of immunology*, 174, 498–506.

Syrovets, T. Gschwend, J. E. Buchele, B. et al. 2005b. Inhibition of IkappaB kinase activity by acetyl-boswellic acids promotes apoptosis in androgen-independent PC-3 prostate cancer cells in vitro and in vivo. *J Biol Chem*, 280, 6170–6180.

Teicher, B. A. Fricker, S. P. 2010. CXCL12 (SDF-1)/CXCR4 pathway in cancer. *Clin Cancer Res*, 16, 2927–2931.

Thirugnanam, S. Xu, L. Ramaswamy, K. et al. 2008. Glycyrrhizin induces apoptosis in prostate cancer cell lines DU-145 and LNCaP. *Oncol Rep*, 20, 1387–1392.

Tundis, R. Loizzo, M. R. Bonesi, M. et al. 2009. In vitro cytotoxic effects of Senecio stabianus Lacaita (Asteraceae) on human cancer cell lines. *Nat Prod Res*, 23, 1707–1718.

Wang, G. W. Qin, J. J. Cheng, X. R. et al. 2014. Inula sesquiterpenoids: structural diversity, cytotoxicity and anti-tumor activity. *Expert Opin Investig Drugs*, 23, 317–345.

Wang, X. L. Kong, F. Shen, T. et al. 2011. Sesquiterpenoids from myrrh inhibit androgen receptor expression and function in human prostate cancer cells. *Acta Pharmacol Sin*, 32, 338–344.

Watson, C. Miller, D. A. Chin-Sinex, H. et al. 2009. Suppression of NF-kappaB activity by parthenolide induces X-ray sensitivity through inhibition of split-dose repair in TP53 null prostate cancer cells. *Radiat Res*, 171, 389–396.

Willoughby, J.A. Sr. Sundar, S.N. Cheung, M. et al. 2009. Artemisinin blocks prostate cancer growth and cell cycle progression by disrupting Sp1 interactions with the cyclin-dependent kinase-4 (CDK4) promoter and inhibiting CDK4 gene expression. *J Biol Chem*, 284(4), 2203–2213.

Wolfram, J. Suri, K. Huang, Y. et al. 2014. Evaluation of anticancer activity of celastrol liposomes in prostate cancer cells. *J Microencapsul*, 31, 501–507.

Xu, Y. Fang, F. Miriyala, S. et al. 2013. KEAP1 is a redox sensitive target that arbitrates the opposing radiosensitive effects of parthenolide in normal and cancer cells. *Cancer Res*, 73, 4406–4417.

Yadav, V. R. Prasad, S. Sung, B. et al. 2010. Targeting inflammatory pathways by triterpenoids for prevention and treatment of cancer. *Toxins*, 2, 2428–2466.

Yang, H. Chen, D. Cui, Q. C. et al. 2006. Celastrol, a triterpene extracted from the Chinese "Thunder of God Vine," is a potent proteasome inhibitor and suppresses human prostate cancer growth in nude mice. *Cancer Res*, 66, 4758–4765.

Yang, H. Landis-Piwowar, K. R. Lu, D. et al. 2008a. Pristimerin induces apoptosis by targeting the proteasome in prostate cancer cells. *J Cell Biochem*, 103, 234–244.

Yang, H. Murthy, S. Sarkar, F. H. et al. 2008b. Calpain-mediated androgen receptor breakdown in apoptotic prostate cancer cells. *J Cell Physiol*, 217, 569–576.

Yao, M. Yang, J. Cao, L. et al. 2014. Saikosaponind inhibits proliferation of DU145 human prostate cancer cells by inducing apoptosis and arresting the cell cycle at G0/G1 phase. *Mol Med Rep*, 10, 365–372.

Yuan, H. Q. Kong, F. Wang, X. L. et al. 2008. Inhibitory effect of acetyl-11-keto-beta-boswellic acid on androgen receptor by interference of Sp1 binding activity in prostate cancer cells. *Biochem Pharmacol*, 75, 2112–2121.

Yuan, L. Liu, C. Chen, Y. et al. 2013. Antitumor activity of tripterine via cell-penetrating peptide-coated nanostructured lipid carriers in a prostate cancer model. *Int J Nanomedicine*, 8, 4339–4350.

Zhang, L. Altuwaijri, S. Deng, F. et al. 2009. NF-kappaB regulates androgen receptor expression and prostate cancer growth. *Am J Pathol*, 175, 489–499.

Zhang, Y. Kong, C. Zeng, Y. et al. 2010. Ursolic acid induces PC-3 cell apoptosis via activation of JNK and inhibition of Akt pathways in vitro. *Mol Carcinog*, 49, 374–385.

Zhuang, W. Wang, G. Li, L. et al. 2013. Omega-3 polyunsaturated fatty acids reduce vascular endothelial growth factor production and suppress endothelial wound repair. *J Cardiovasc Transl Res*, 6(2), 287–293.

Zuo, J. Guo, Y. Peng, X. et al. 2015. Inhibitory action of pristimerin on hypoxiamediated metastasis involves stem cell characteristics and EMT in PC-3 prostate cancer cells. *Oncol Rep*, 33, 1388–1394.

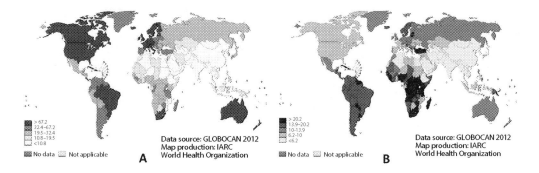

Figure 2.1 (A) Worldwide incidence of prostate cancer as estimated in 2012. (B) Worldwide mortality due to prostate cancer as estimated in 2012. (GLOBOCAN Data, 2012. Map provided by IARC, WHO.)

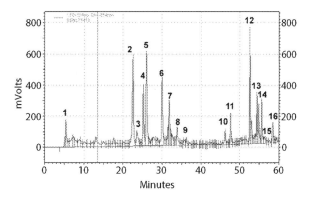

Figure 7.2 Fractionation of SENL was performed using a Kinetex C18 column on a Shimadzu HPLC system. Column temperature was maintained at 40°C. The autosampler injected 20 μL of sample. Mobile phase A was 100% water and phase B was 100% methanol. A flow rate of 1.0 mL/min, starting with a 50-minute linear gradient from 50% to 100% B, 50 to 56 minutes with 100% B, and 56 to 58 minutes to 10% B, and a total run time of 60 minutes, was used with UV detection at 254 nm.

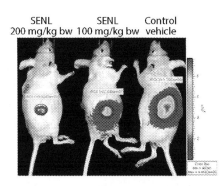

Figure 7.3 SENL inhibited the growth of LNCaP-luc2 prostate cancer xenografts in nude mice. Bioluminescence imaging of mice implanted with LNCaP-luc2 tumors. Group 1 (n=8) animals received vehicle control (olive oil) orally. Group 2 (n=8) and 3 (n=8) animals were administered SENL, 100 or 200 mg/kg body weight, by gavage 6 days a week. A representative image of the mice from each group at the end of 9 weeks of treatment is shown.

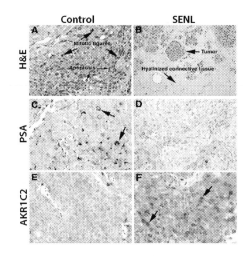

Figure 7.4 Histologic changes of LNCaP-luc2 tumor tissues of mice treated with SENL, 200mg/kg body weight. At the end of 9 weeks, xenograft tumor tissues were collected and stained with hematoxylin and eosin. Two sections of tumor tissue from each of eight mice in a group were examined for histologic changes. (A) Tumor tissue of vehicle-treated mouse showing mitotic figures (thick arrows), and apoptosis (thin arrows). (B) Tumor tissue of SENL-treated mice shows nests of tumor cells separated by hyalinization. (C–D) Immunohistochemistry analysis for *PSA* expression in the tumor tissues of vehicle-treated and SENL-treated mice. (E–F) Immunohistochemistry analysis for *AKR1C2* expression in the tumor tissues of vehicle-treated and SENL-treated mice. Brown staining represents positive staining for *PSA* and *AKR1C2* expression. Original magnification, ·400.

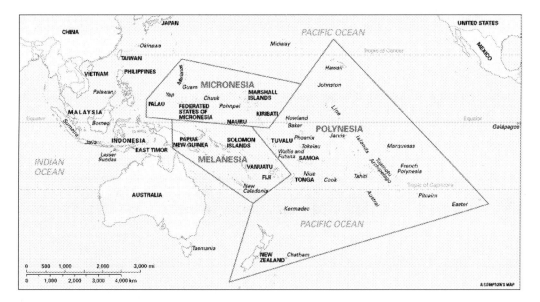

Figure 8.1   Kava consumption areas (Melanesia) in the South Pacific Islands.

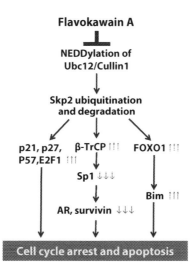

Flavokawain A

⊣

NEDDylation of Ubc12/Cullin1

↓

Skp2 ubiquitination and degradation

p21, p27, P57,E2F1 ⇑⇑⇑ **β-TrCP** ⇑⇑⇑ **FOXO1** ⇑⇑⇑

Sp1 ⇓⇓⇓

AR, survivin ⇓⇓⇓ **Bim** ⇑⇑⇑

Cell cycle arrest and apoptosis

Figure 8.3   Schematic presentation of mechanisms of flavokawain's anticancer action.

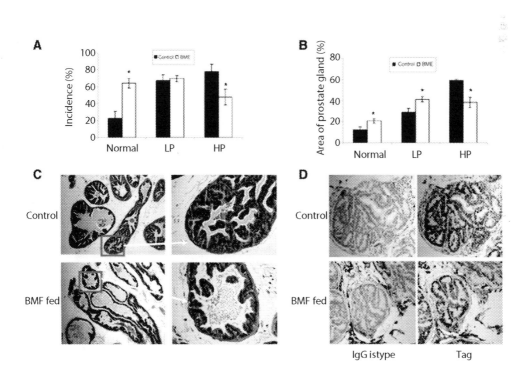

Figure 9.3   Oral BME administration in TRAMP mice delays prostate tumor progression. (A) The incidence of histologic grades classified as normal prostate (N), low-grade PIN (LP), and high-grade PIN (HP) in the DLP from control and BME-fed mice. Ten representative fields of each section of each mouse were scored for incidence of each histologic grade. The error bars represent variability of results in histologic grading between the two researchers (*, P < 0.0002, 0.5 and 0.003, respectively). (B) The percentage of the area corresponding to the normal prostate, LP and HP in the DLP of control and BME-treated mice was scored by two researchers (*, P < 0.002, 0.001, and 0.0001, respectively). (C) H&E staining of the DLP from control and BME-fed mice sacrificed at 21 weeks of age (magnification 100× left panels and 400× right panels). (D) SV40 T-antigen expression in a representative DLP of a control and BME-fed TRAMP mouse (magnification, 200×). (Reprinted with permission from Ru et al., *Cancer Prev Res* 2011; 4: 2122–2130).

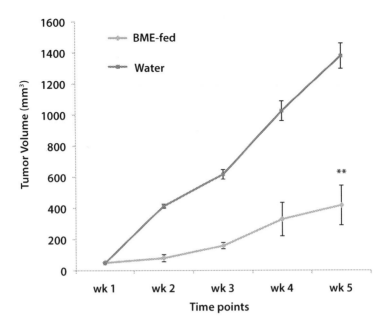

Figure 9.4 BME feeding halts prostate cancer growth in xenograft model.

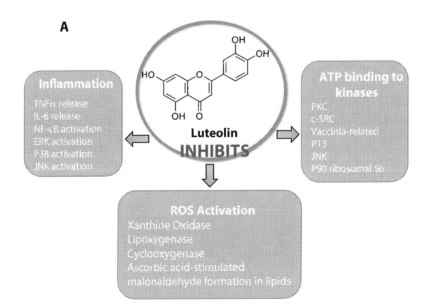

Figure 10.3 Activities of luteolin, ellagic acid, and punicic acid. (A) Luteolin attenuates ROS damage, inflammation, and proliferation. ROS is attenuated through downregulation of xanthine oxidase, lipoxygenase, cyclooxygenase, and ascorbic acid-stimulated malonaldehyde formation in lipids. Inflammation is attenuated through inhibition of LSP-stimulated TNFα release, IL-6 release, NF-κB activation, ERK, P38, and JNK. Proliferation is attenuated through inhibition of ATP binding to PKC, c-SRC, vaccinia-related kinase, PI3K, JNK, and P90 ribosomal S6 kinase. (B) Ellagic acid attenuates inflammation through upregulation of IL-10, and GSH, and downregulates NF-kB. These regulations lead to the downregulation of IL-1β, TNF-α, iNOS, COX-2, and PGE-2. (C) Punicic acid inhibits testosterone to DHT conversion through the inhibition of the enzyme, 5α-reductase type 1, which reduces the androgen receptor nuclear translocation.

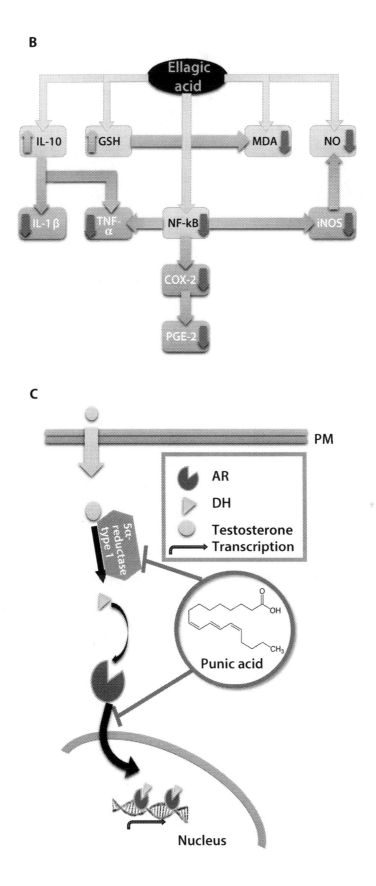

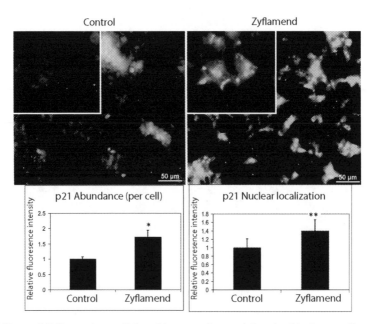

Figure 11.5 Effects of Zyflamend on cellular p21 expression as determined by immunofluorescent imaging using castrate-resistant CWR22Rv1 cells (Huang E-C et al., 2014). Cells pretreated with 200 µg/ml Zyflamend for 24 h (right) were compared with control cells (left). Nuclei are shown in blue. Mean p21 abundance per cell (green) was calculated [(total p21 fluorescence)/(nuclei count)]. To assess nuclear accumulation, p21 fluorescence was also measured within discrete nuclear regions (defined using a DAPI intensity threshold). A summary of the data is presented as the mean ± SD in relative fluorescence units. *p<0.01; **p<0.001.

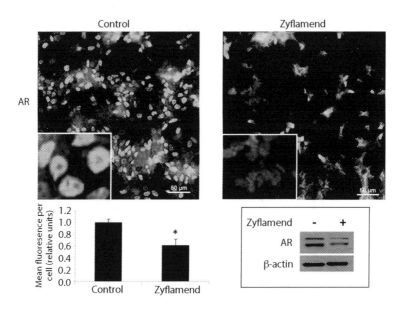

Figure 11.6 Effects of Zyflamend on cellular androgen receptor (AR) expression as determined by immunofluorescent imaging using castrate-resistant CWR22Rv1 cells (Huang E-C et al., 2011). Cells pretreated with 200 µg/ml Zyflamend for 24 h (right) were compared with control cells (left). Nuclei are shown in blue. Mean AR abundance per cell (green) was calculated [(total AR fluorescence)/(nuclei count)]. A summary of the data is presented as the mean ± SD in relative fluorescence units, *p<0.05, along with a representative western blot (protein levels).

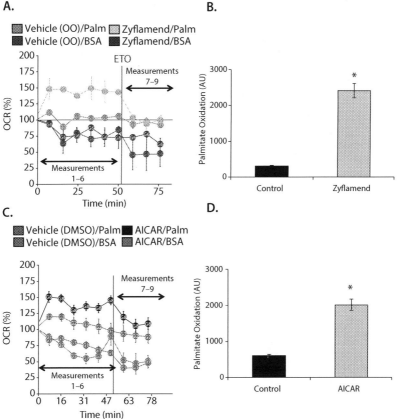

Figure 11.9 The effect of Zyflamend and AICAR on fatty acid (palmitate) oxidation in castrate-resistant CWR22Rv1 cells (Zhao et al., 2015). Percent change in oxygen consumption rate (%OCR) in CWR22Rv1 cells treated with vehicle (olive oil or DMSO), Zyflamend or AICAR for 1 h. Then, BSA or palmitate was injected and the %OCR was measured over six cycles. At the end of the six cycles, etomoxir (50 µM), a fatty acid oxidation inhibitor, was injected and %OCR was measured over three additional cycles. The total contribution of palmitate oxidation toward %OCR is observed after injection of etomoxir (A, C). The relative palmitate oxidation was determined by determining the difference before and after etomoxir injection in vehicle groups compared to Zyflamend or AICAR treatment groups. Data points for panels (B) and (D) represent the average OCR (%) over 3–5 replicates per experimental condition. Error bars represent +/- the SEM. [Abbreviations: AU, arbitrary units; ETO, etomoxir (carnitine palmitoyl transferase-1 inhibitor)] AU, Arbitrary units – area under the curve after injection of palmitate for each treatment and normalized to etomoxir treatment.

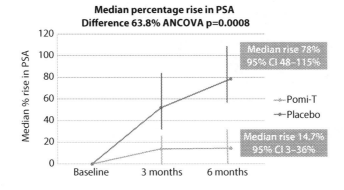

Figure 12.3 Graph demonstrating the medium change in PSA between men taking Pomi-T or placebo.

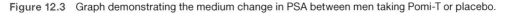

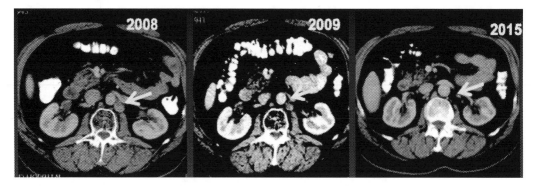

Figure 12.6 CT scan showing reduced size of paraortic lymphadenopathy after broccoli soup and Pomi-T intake.

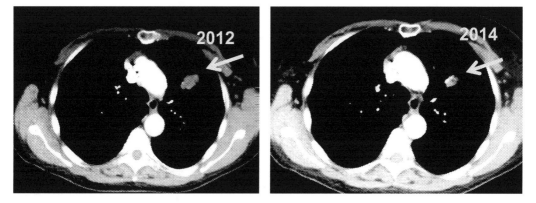

Figure 12.7 CT scan showing reduced size of a proven lung metastasis following lifestyle interventions.

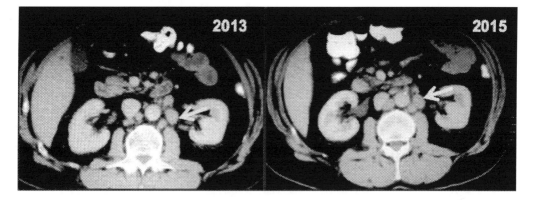

Figure 12.8 CT showing reduced size of PET positive paraortic lymphadenopathy following intense lifestyle interventions.

CHAPTER 5

Green Tea Polyphenols in the Prevention and Therapy of Prostate Cancer

Eswar Shankar, Jeniece Montellano, and Sanjay Gupta

CONTENTS

ABBREVIATIONS

8-OHdG: 8-hydroxy-2'–deoxyguanosine
ASAP: atypical small acinar proliferation
Cdk: cyclin-dependent kinases
CI: confidence interval
COX-2: cyclooxygenase-2
CYP: cytochrome P450
DNA: deoxyribonucleic acid
DNMT: DNA methyltransferases
EC: (-)-epicatechin
ECG: (-)-epicatechin-3-gallate
EGC: (-)-epigallocatechin

EGCG: (-)-epigallocatechin-3-gallate
ERK: extracellular-regulated kinases
GI: gastrointestinal
GTP: green tea polyphenols
HDAC: histone deacetylases
HGF: hepatocyte growth factor
HGPIN: high-grade prostatic intraepithelial neoplasia
hK2:   human kallikrein 2
HR: hazard ratio
IGF: insulin-like growth factor
IGFBP: insulin growth factor binding protein
IKK: IκB kinase
Lys: lysine
MBD: methyl-binding domain protein
MCM-7:   minichromosome maintenance protein-7
MMP: matrix metalloproteinases
NF-κB: nuclear factor-κappaB
NIK: NF-κB inducing kinase
NOAEL: no-observed-adverse-effect-level
ODC: ornithine decarboxylase
OR: odds ratio
PCNA: proliferating cell nuclear antigen
PI3K: phosphatidylinositol-3-kinases
PSA: prostate-specific antigen
RANK: receptor activator of nuclear factor-κB
ROS: reactive oxygen species
Sp1:   specificity protein 1
STAT3:   signal transducer and activator of transcription 3
TGF: transforming growth factor
VEGF: vascular endothelial growth factor

5.1 INTRODUCTION

Prostate cancer is the most commonly diagnosed cancer in men in the United States and other Western nations. According to the American Cancer Society, approximately 220,800 new cases and 27,540 deaths from prostate cancer are projected to occur in the United States in 2015 (ACS 2015, Siegal et al., 2014). Despite widespread screening efforts and advancement in therapeutic regimens, incidence of prostate cancer is still on the rise and continues to be the second-leading cause of cancer-related deaths among men in the United States. The occurrence of prostate cancer seems mostly sporadic, with <10% inherited, although several genetic and environmental factors are attributed in controlling the development of this disease (Syed et al., 2007). The incidence of prostate cancer in the United States is highest among African Americans, followed by Caucasian and Hispanic men, while Asian-American men exhibit the lowest risk (Shavers et al., 2009). Geographic variations attributed to the incidence of prostate cancer exhibit higher rates in North America and northern Europe, intermediate levels in the Mediterranean region, and relatively low in many parts of Asia (Shavers et al., 2009; Zlotta et al. 2013). Although racial background and family history are the most common risk factors for prostate cancer, the other major risk factors that contribute to the development of prostate cancer are age, environmental factors, and lifestyle. Aging remains a critical factor that seems to be responsible for the progression of prostate cancer (Moyad and Carroll 2004 a,b). The strong correlation between aging and the onset of prostate cancer is evident from pathological examination of prostate tissue in aging men (Hankey et al., 1999). There is a characteristic age-related decrease in the ratio of androgens to estrogen in men which may contribute to prostate cancer initiation. An additional strong risk factor for prostate cancer is a positive family history of the disease. There is evidence for both autosomal dominant and X-linked inheritance in families with a history of prostate cancer. Consequently, there is considerable scientific interest in identifying highly penetrant alleles in genes associated with hereditary prostate cancer (Kommu et al., 2004). Environmental factors also play an important role in the risk of prostate cancer; variations in dietary patterns have shown to be related to an increase in prostate cancer incidence among Asian immigrants who adopt a Western diet (Lee et al., 2007; Zhu et al., 2015). Lifestyle factors have also been implicated in the development of prostate cancer. Diet is an important part of lifestyle; ecological studies have implicated a "Western-style" diet in the development of prostate cancer (Lin et al., 2015). In fact, high incidence of prostate cancer is observed in American men consuming Western stereotypical diets, which are quite different from Asian diets. The typical Western diet contains high amounts of fats and meats, both of which have been implicated as candidate risk factors for prostate cancer. In comparison, Asian diets are low-fat, plant-based diets rich in fruits and vegetables having high fiber content and certain beverages with high polyphenolic content.

There is considerable interest in ascertaining whether plant-based diets offer protection against prostate cancer. A number of macronutrients, micronutrients, and other dietary constituents have been or are currently being evaluated as potential preventive/therapeutic agents for prostate cancer. Dietary agents have gained considerable attention as anticancer agents since they possess low intrinsic toxicity, high abundance, and the potential to target various signaling pathways that have relevance to cancer development and progression. This approach has practical implications in reducing the risk and incidence of prostate cancer. Although several carcinogenic environmental factors that are beyond anyone's control also play a role, individuals are free to modify their dietary and lifestyle habits. Several studies have focused on the antioxidant and non-antioxidant effects of various dietary substances in the prevention of prostate cancer. Among all, one such agent is green tea polyphenols, consumed as a beverage for nearly 5,000 years by the Chinese and Asian populations, making it the most consumable and popular beverage in the world, next to water. This chapter highlights review of the literature and studies thus far conducted with green tea polyphenols on various aspects including epidemiologic, case control studies, and preclinical and clinical findings on prostate cancer.

5.2   GREEN TEA POLYPHENOLS

Tea is a universal beverage that provides health benefits and reduces the risk of several human cancers. Its consumption in the world is second only to water, with a per capita worldwide consumption of approximately 0.12 liters per day (Graham, 1992). Produced from the leaves of the plant *Camellia sinensis*, the manufacturing process used for tea preparation is available in four different forms, as green, black, oolong, and white tea. Green tea is prepared by preventing the oxidation of green leaf polyphenols; in black tea, most of these substances are oxidized; in oolong tea, they are partially oxidized. White tea is made from new-growth buds and young leaves by inactivating polyphenol oxidation through the process of steaming and drying. During tea production, only 20% is green tea and less than 2% is oolong tea (McKay and Blumberg 2002). The polyphenolic composition of green tea includes catechins (30–42%), flavonols (5–10%), other flavonoids such as theogallin (2–3%), gallic acid (0.5%), quinic acid (2%), theanine (4–6%), and methylxanthins (7–9%). The major polyphenols present in black tea are catechins (3–10%), flavanols (6–8%), methylxanthines

(8–11%), theaflavins (3–6%) and thearubigens (12–18%). The major catechins present in green tea are (-)-epigallocatechin-3-gallate (EGCG), (-)-epigallocatechin (EGC), (-)-epicatechin-3-gallate (ECG), and (-)-epicatechin (EC). EGCG contributes more than two-fifths the total amount of phenols present in green tea and has been widely reported for its health benefits. A typical cup of green tea, brewed with 2.5 mg of tea leaves in 250 mL hot water, contains 620 to 880 mg of water-extractable solids, of which about one-third are catechins. The presumed beneficial effects of tea in the prevention of cancer as well as cardiovascular, neurodegenerative, obesity, and other diseases have been extensively studied (Graham 1992; McKay and Blumberg 2002; Legeay et al., 2015).

5.2.1   Pharmacokinetics, Distribution and Metabolism of Green Tea Polyphenols

The beneficial health effects of tea catechins are fundamentally related to their bioavailability, absorption, and distribution in various organs, as well as metabolism and excretion from the body. Green tea catechins (EGCG, ECG, EGC, and EC) are relatively high molecular weight compounds (300–450 Da) comprised of more than 5 hydroxyl groups (Zhang et al., 2004). They have low bioavailability due to their large size. The level of catechins in plasma does not exceed 1 μM when consumed in typical amounts (1–2 cups, 100–200 mg of catechins). The low bioavailability of tea catechins is attributed to its low solubility in the gastrointestinal (GI) fluid, poor membrane permeability, degradation/metabolism in the GI tract, transporter-mediated intestinal secretion/efflux, and pre-systemic hepatic elimination. The degradation of tea catechins in the GI tract is considered a prime cause for its low bioavailability (Chow et al., 2003; 2005; Johnson et al., 2010). Pharmacokinetic studies with green tea catechins exhibit low oral bioavailability, with estimates ranging from 1 to 2%, and are stable at pH <6.5; however, EGC and EGCG are rapidly degraded at a pH >7.4. Pharmacokinetic studies performed using Polyphenon E, a standardized pharmaceutical grade preparation of green tea polyphenols (200 mg of EGCG, 37 mg of EGC, 31 mg of EC per capsule), on healthy volunteers exhibit the presence of EGC and EC in the body after Polyphenon E administration, predominantly in conjugated forms. A greater oral bioavailability of free catechins can be achieved by taking Polyphenon E capsules on an empty stomach after an overnight fast. In another human study, 5 days of continuous green tea intake resulted in the presence of EGC (100 pmol/g), EC (43 pmol/g), EGCG (40 pmol/g), and ECG (21 pmol/g) in prostate tissues (Henning et al., 2006; Johnson et al., 2010). Catechin metabolites – namely EGCG, ECG, EGC, and EC – determined in humans after oral intake of green tea demonstrate a higher portion of the methylated EGC than that of ECG and EGCG in the human plasma. A greater amount of EGCG is present in the free form than EGC and EC, which are mostly in the conjugated form. One hour after drinking tea, 77% of EGCG remains in the free form in human plasma, and 31% EGC and 21% EC are present. After consuming a tea supplement and pure catechin, over 80% of catechin found in plasma was in the bound form. EGC has not been detected at all, whereas 57 to 71% of ECG was present in the glucuronidated form, 23 to 36% in the sulfonated form, and 3 to 13% in the free form. In urine, over 90% of EGC remains in the sulfonated form. It is suggested that food may delay gastric emptying as well as raise the pH of the stomach, which decreases the stability of green tea catechins (Johnson et al., 2010).

5.2.2   Epidemiologic Studies with Green Tea Polyphenols

Initial evidence from epidemiologic studies suggested that the risk of many cancers was significantly reduced in a region of the world where green tea is consumed as a part of the daily diet. A detailed review of clinical studies critically assessed the association between green tea consumption and the risk of cancer incidence and mortality (Yuan et al., 2011). There were 51 prospective controlled interventional and observational studies of 1.6 million participants conducted, which either assessed the associations between green tea consumption and risk of cancer incidence or reported cancer mortality (Thakur et al., 2012a). The results from studies assessing associations between green tea and risk of digestive tract cancer incidence were highly contradictory. There was limited evidence that green tea could reduce the incidence of liver cancer. There was conflicting evidence for esophageal, gastric, colon, rectum, and pancreatic cancers. In prostate cancer, observational studies with higher methodological quality and the one randomized controlled trial suggested a decreased risk in men consuming higher quantities of green tea or green tea extracts (Boehm et al., 2009). However, there was limited to moderate evidence that the consumption of green tea reduced the risk of lung cancer, especially in men, and urinary bladder cancer. There was also evidence that green tea consumption could increase the risk of the latter. There was moderate to strong evidence that green tea consumption does not decrease the risk of participants dying from gastric cancer. Similarly, limited moderate to strong evidence for lung, pancreatic, and colorectal cancer was observed in the green tea consumption group (Boehm et al., 2009).

A number of epidemiologic studies have examined the association between green tea intake and the risk of prostate cancer. All studies were conducted in Japanese or Chinese populations (Adhami and Mukthar, 2013). Two case-control studies in the Chinese population examined and found an inverse relation between green tea intake and prostate cancer risk. One study in southeast China included 130 patients with prostate cancer and 274 hospital inpatients as controls. It found an inverse relation between green tea intake and prostate cancer; the odds ratio (OR) was 0.28 (95% CI: 0.17, 0.47) for drinkers relative to nondrinkers, with a dose-response relation (P-trend <0.001) (Jian et al., 2004). Another study performed in 140 prostate cancer cases and an equal number of hospital patients as controls found an inverse but non-significant association (Yuan et al., 2011). Four prospective cohort studies conducted in Japanese populations examined the association between green tea consumption and the risk of prostate cancer. An early study in men of Japanese ancestry in Hawaii found that green tea consumption was associated with a non-significant increased risk of prostate cancer (HR: 1.47; 95% CI: 0.99, 1.13) (Severson et al., 1989). The other three studies found no association between green tea intake and prostate cancer risk (Allen et al., 2004, Sonoda et al., 2004; Kikuchi et al., 2006). Only one prospective cohort study examined the association between green tea consumption and risk of prostate cancer stratified by disease stage. A dose-dependent inverse relation was observed for risk of advanced prostate cancer (P-trend = 0.01): the HR was 0.52 (95% CI: 0.28, 0.96) for men who consumed ≥5 cups green tea/day compared with <1 cup/day. On the other hand, there was no association between green tea consumption and risk of localized prostate cancer (Kurahashi et al., 2008). These results suggest that green tea constituents may have an effect in reducing the growth of prostate tumors (Adhami and Mukthar, 2013).

5.2.3 Meta-Analysis of Cohort and Case-Control Studies on Green Tea Polyphenols

In a meta-analysis Lin et al. (2014) evaluated 21 published studies on green tea and prostate cancer. These articles were mostly case-control studies that observed the relationship between tea consumption and prostate cancer risk. When the results were population-stratified for Asian and non-Asian, there appeared to be no relationship; stratification by tea type yielded no benefit for green or black tea; when stratified by case-control study, there was a borderline inverse association between tea intake and the overall risk of prostate cancer. The lack of association could be due to the unknown tea concentrations in many of the studies as well as an overall lower quantity of tea consumption. This lower concentration can affect the anticancer potential of green tea. Fei et al. (2014) conducted a meta-analysis in which 21 studies were examined as well. The case-control studies exhibited a protective effect of tea consumption against prostate cancer, but a summary of the cohort studies showed no significant association. A significant association was observed between tea consumption and risk of prostate cancer, with the highest level of tea consumption protecting against low-grade cancer. No statistical effect was noted on high-grade or advanced prostate cancer. The authors concluded that more relevant randomized controlled trials were needed, with cohort studies to be conducted on larger populations.

5.3 GREEN TEA POLYPHENOLS AND PROSTATE CANCER

5.3.1 Cell Culture Studies

Earlier studies using green tea polyphenols in cell cultures have shown they exert their anticancer effects by a number of different mechanisms, including reduction of cellular proliferation by inhibition of oxidative stress, angiogenesis, invasion, and metastasis, and induction of cell cycle arrest and apoptosis. In addition to these studies, green tea polyphenols have been shown to inhibit the activity of 5α-reductase, which converts testosterone into the active metabolite 5α-dihydroxytestosterone and is overexpressed in prostate cancer (Liao and Hjipakka, 1995). EGCG also inhibits the expression of androgen-regulated prostate-specific antigen (PSA) and hK2 genes in androgen-responsive human prostate cancer LNCaP cells. Furthermore, EGCG has been shown to decrease expression of Sp1 and its DNA binding to the androgen receptor gene, which possesses Sp1 binding sites (Ren et al., 2000). Another study demonstrated that EGCG physically interacts with the ligand-binding domain of the androgen receptor, restricting the growth of androgen-responsive prostate cancer cells (Siddiqui et al., 2011). Studies from our laboratory have demonstrated that EGCG causes apoptosis in human prostate cancer cells by both intrinsic and extrinsic pathways, independent of their p53 or androgen status. Another study from our group demonstrated that EGCG is capable of repressing class I histone deacetylases (HDACs), which are overexpressed in prostate cancer (Thakur et al., 2012b). Treatment of LNCaP cells with GTPs or EGCG resulted in dose- and time-dependent inhibition of class I HDACs (HDAC1, 2, 3, and 8), albeit at varying levels. EGCG-mediated downregulation of class I HDACs led to p53 activation through acetylation at the Lys373 and Lys382 residues in prostate cancer cells (Thakur et al., 2012c). The increased GTP/EGCG-mediated p53 acetylation enhanced its binding on the promoters of p21/waf1 and Bax, which was associated with increased accumulation of cells in the G0/G1 phase of the cell cycle and induction of apoptosis. Discontinuation of treatment with GTP/EGCG resulted in the loss of p53 acetylation at both the sites in these cells (Gupta et al., 2012). Brusselsmans et al. (2003) have shown that EGCG dose-dependently inhibited fatty acid synthase activity in LNCaP cells, resulting in a decrease in endogenous lipid synthesis, inhibition of cell growth, and induction of apoptosis. GTP has been found to reduce oxidation in prostate cancer cells, preventing further mutations and metastasis. Henning et al. (2011) have shown that EGCG indirectly assist in stimulating the antioxidant response through upregulation of Nrf2 transcription factor. Nrf2 stimulation increases the expression of multiple antioxidant enzymes through the antioxidant-response element. In human prostate cancer cell lines, Nrf2 is suppressed by hypermethylation in the promoter region, resulting in the inhibition of the levels of antioxidant enzymes and thereby elevating ROS levels. Kanwal et al. (2014) further demonstrated that treatment with GTP/EGCG resulted in reduced ROS and 8-OHdG production, causing reduced DNA damage in prostate epithelial cells. Chung et al. (2001) demonstrated that EGCG treatment to highly aggressive human prostate cancer DU145 cells led to induction of apoptosis and growth suppression associated with mitochondrial depolarization. EGCG treatment in prostate cancer cells causes a delay in metastatic growth through suppression of insulin-like growth factor (IGF-1 and IGF-2), which controls cell survival and proliferation and often leads to transformation and metastasis (Henning et al., 2006; 2011). EGCG is an inhibitor of IGF-1 receptor, with an

IC_{50} of 14 μM, resulting in the prevention of malignant cell growth (Li et al., 2007). In a study conducted by Siddiqui et al. (2004), EGCG inhibited the levels of phosphatidylinositol-3-kinases (PI3K) and p-Akt as well as increased the transcription of extracellular-signal-regulated kinases (ERK1/2) in prostate cancer DU145 and LNCaP cells. A study by Adhami et al. (2003) demonstrated that EGCG treatment of LNCaP cells resulted in a decrease of NF-κB DNA binding activity, affecting the downstream targets regulating inflammatory responses, cell proliferation, angiogenesis, and metastasis. Inhibition of transcription factors NF-κB as well as inhibition of the phosphorylation of ERK1/2 facilitates the inhibition of matrix metalloprotease (MMP)-2 and MMP-9 in DU145 cells, preventing metastasis (Vayalil and Katiyar, 2004). In another study, EGCG inhibited Shc activation via transforming growth factor (TGF) α-induced activation of ErbB1, induced WAF1/p21 and KIP1/p27, and decreased cell cycle regulatory molecules viz. cdk4 cdk2, cyclins D1 and E (Bhatia and Agarwal, 2001).

Recent studies on green tea polyphenols in prostate cancer have focused on the mechanism(s) by which green tea may contribute its role in the reversal of epigenetically silenced genes that occurs during the transformation of normal prostate epithelial to neoplastic stage and its progression towards malignancy. EGCG has been shown to inhibit DNA methyltransferase 1 (DNMT1), a major enzyme involved in the hypermethylation of CpG islands that are present in the promoter region and exons of several genes (Fang et al., 2003; 2007). Studies from our laboratory have demonstrated the dual potential of green tea polyphenols to alter DNA methylation and chromatin remodeling of glutathione-S transferase pi (GSTP1) gene promoter, without causing toxicity in prostate cancer cells. Exposure of human prostate cancer LNCaP cells to GTP for up to 7 days resulted in dose- and time-dependent re-expression of GSTP1, which correlated with DNMT1 inhibition. GTP treatment further resulted in extensive demethylation in the proximal GSTP1 promoter and regions distal to the transcription factor binding sites. GTP exposure in a time-dependent fashion diminished the mRNA and protein levels of methyl-binding domain proteins, including MBD1, MBD4, and MeCP2, HDAC 1-3, and increased the levels of acetylated histone H3 (LysH9/18) and H4. In addition, GTP treatment reduced MBD2 association with accessible Sp1 binding sites leading to increased binding and transcriptional activation of the *GSTP1* gene. GTP treatment did not result in global hypomethylation, rather it promoted maintenance of genomic integrity (Pandey et al., 2010).

5.3.2 Animal Studies

Earlier *in vivo* studies on green tea polyphenols by Liao et al. (1995) demonstrated that EGCG causes growth-inhibitory activity when injected into mice with human prostate cancer xenografts. We earlier reported that oral feeding of GTP in drinking water for 7 days before testosterone administration resulted in a decrease in testosterone-caused induction of ornithine decarboxylase (ODC) activity in sham-operated and castrated rats (Gupta et al., 1999). Similar results were obtained with C57BL/6 mice in which testosterone treatment at similar dosage resulted in a twofold increase in ODC activity in the ventral prostate, and prior oral feeding with GTP resulted in inhibition of this induction. Gupta et al. (2001) administered a GTP infusion at a human achievable dose (equivalent to 6 cups of green tea/day) to transgenic adenocarcinoma of mouse prostate (TRAMP) for 24 weeks, starting from 8 weeks of age. The mice exhibited inhibition of prostate cancer development and complete inhibition of distant-site metastasis. GTP intake also increased tumor-free and overall survival of these mice. Sequential MRI analysis demonstrated a significant decrease in prostate and genitourinary weight; inhibition of serum IGF-1, and restoration of IGFBP-3 levels and reduction in the protein expression of proliferating cell nuclear antigen (PCNA) in the prostate compared with water-fed TRAMP mice. Further extension of this work demonstrated a significant decrease in the levels of angiogenic and metastatic markers viz. VEGFA, MMP2, and MMP9, along with abrogation of PI3K pathway. McCarthy et al. (2007) have shown that treatment of TRAMP mice with green tea polyphenols resulted in inhibition of minichromosome maintenance protein (MCM)-7, which has been implicated in prostate cancer progression, growth, and invasion. Siddiqui et al. (2008) demonstrated that continuous GTP infusion for 28 weeks resulted in marked reduction in expression of NF-κB, IKKα, IKKβ, RANK, NIK, and STAT-3 in dorsolateral prostate of TRAMP mice. The level of transcription factor osteopontin was also downregulated, and there was shift in balance between Bax and Bcl2 favoring apoptosis in the dorsolateral prostate of GTP fed TRAMP mice. Siddiqui et al. (2008) used mice to determine the effective GTP doses, and found that 0.05% GTP in drinking water was effective, while 0.01% was not. This indicates a need to find the ideal dose for humans as well, as concentration affects efficacy. The 0.05% concentration was associated with a significant decrease in PSA levels, an increase in apoptosis, and a decrease in VEGF (Siddiqui et al., 2008). Similarly, Harper et al. (2007) found that a concentration of 0.06% ECGC allowed for significant red cell proliferation, induced apoptosis and a decrease in the androgen receptor, IGF-1, IGF-1R, phospho-ERK1/2, COX-2, and inducible nitric oxide synthase. In an experiment conducted by Roomi et al. (2005), athymic nude mice implanted with PC-3 cells and maintained on a diet consisting of lysine, proline, arginine, ascorbic acid, and green tea extract resulted in inhibition of tumor growth and MMP-9, VEGF secretion, and mitosis in tissues. Loss of E-cadherin has been associated with prostate cancer progression. Saleem et al. (2005) demonstrated that GTP feeding to TRAMP mice restores E-cadherin to normal levels. These results are promising in revealing the therapeutic potential of green tea.

Some *in vivo* studies with green tea polyphenols have not shown encouraging results in suppressing prostate cancer. Zhou et al. (2003) conducted a study in which black tea was capable of reducing PSA levels and tumor sizes, but not green tea. However, this could be due to application of high dosage and the quality of tea leaves used. The study used 15 g of tea leaves per liter of water, which is a much higher intake than humans normally ingest. Green tea may lose its efficacy at very high dose, or the procedure in which the leaves were brewed could have decreased its polyphenol concentration.

5.3.3 Human Studies

The efficacy of green tea polyphenols in prostate cancer suppression in humans has largely varied. The timing of treatment and dosage have been demonstrated as vital to maximizing treatment potential. Adhami and Mukhtar (2013) reviewed several clinical studies and found that patients with advanced or hormone-refractory prostate cancer did not respond well to treatment, but subjects with high-grade prostatic intraepithelial neoplasia (HGPIN) lesions and patients scheduled for prostatectomies both responded well to green tea polyphenol treatment. This suggests that the chemopreventive potential of green tea is maximized when interception is done at earlier stages of cancer, and it decreases with more advanced stage. Bettuzzi et al. (2006) demonstrated an 80% reduction in prostate cancer diagnosis when subjects with HGPIN were subjected to 200 mg of green tea catechins three times a day. This inhibition was long-lasting, as a follow-up study 2 years later exhibited that the incidence of prostate cancer was lower in the patients who took green tea supplements (Bettuzzi et al., 2007). The results also showed a lower incidence of urinary tract symptoms in patients pretreated with green tea polyphenols (Bettuzzi et al., 2006). This could suggest a lower incidence of BPH and therefore a lower incidence of development of prostate cancer. McLarty et al. (2009) used Polyphenon E treatment on patients who were scheduled for prostatectomy and found a significant reduction in the serum PSA levels. In addition, a significant decrease was noted in the levels of HGF, VEGF, IGF-1, and IGFBP3, biomarkers relevant for prostate cancer development.

Some clinical studies of green tea polyphenols on prostate cancer demonstrated conflicting results or lack of efficacy. Jatoi et al. (2003) reported a phase II trial with GTP and prostate cancer; however, it was found that this report was poorly planned and executed, as critiqued (Adhami and

Mukhtar, 2013). The results of this report stated that green tea lacks the ability to prevent prostate cancer, which initiated criticism for green tea therapy. Henning et al. (2015) conducted a study on the effects of drinking 6 cups of green tea per day for patients scheduled for radical prostatectomy, although not all of their results were significant. Serum PSA values underwent a small but statistically significant decrease and there was a significant decrease in urinary 8-OHdG in men in the green tea group, indicating a decrease in systemic antioxidant activity. However, there were no significant differences in the markers of proliferation, apoptosis, or oxidative DNA damage in green tea–supplemented group (Henning et al., 2015). This suggests that the lack of effects of green tea polyphenols might be due to poor bioavailability in the prostate tissue or may be due to pleotropic effects of green tea polyphenols. In a randomized, double-blind, placebo-controlled intervention trial conducted by Nguyen et al. (2012), lower levels of IGF-1, PSA, and a lower ratio of 8-OHdG to dG were noted in the green tea–treated group, but none were statistically significant. Overall, a trend among the systemic biomarkers suggested chemopreventive activity, but there was no statistical significance. This may be due to limited sample size and duration of the study (3–6 weeks). In another study, 19 patients with hormone-refractory prostate cancer were provided with green tea capsules (250 mg twice daily) for a minimum of 2 months (Choan et al., 2005). The study concluded that green tea had minimal clinical activity against hormone-refractory prostate cancer. A recent randomized, double-blind, placebo-controlled trial of Polyphenon E, containing 400 mg EGCG per day, in men with HGPIN and/or atypical small acinar proliferation (ASAP) was conducted. It was observed that daily intake of Polyphenon E for 1 year accumulated in plasma and was well tolerated but did not reduce the likelihood of prostate cancer in men with baseline HGPIN or ASAP (Kumar et al., 2015).

5.3.4   Safety and Toxicity Studies on Green Tea Polyphenols

There are few reports of adverse reactions with green tea, as some cultures consume greater than 10 cups of green tea per day. The most notable side effect observed to date in clinical trials is reports of "jitteriness" that has been suggested to be a result of caffeine intake. Pharmaceutical grade preparations used in research such as Polyphenon E have limited caffeine (~0.5% w/w) and are considered caffeine-free. Consumption of green tea polyphenols as dietary supplements significantly increases the amount of green tea catechins on a daily basis when compared to ingesting tea as a beverage inducing liver toxicity. The cytotoxicity studies of green tea extract on rat hepatocytes showed uncertainty on the toxic effect of EGCG (100–500 μg/mL medium), regardless of the fact that the concentrations used were significantly greater (i.e., >100X) than observed in human serum after green tea consumption. Evaluation of the EGCG-rich product Teavigo® suggested doses of 200 mg/kg/day of EGCG in animals is the no-observed-adverse-effect-level (NOAEL). Chow et al. (2003) observed that it is safe for healthy individuals to take green tea polyphenol products, 8–16 cups in amounts equivalent to the EGCG, once a day or in divided doses twice a day for 4 weeks. This increased systemic availability of free EGCG is greater than 60% after chronic green tea polyphenol administration at a high daily bolus dose of either 800 mg EGCG or Polyphenon E once daily. Results also suggest that green tea catechin administration does not cause clinically significant effects on the disposition of drugs metabolized by cytochromes P450 (CYP) enzymes.

5.3.5   Limitations of Green Tea Polyphenol Therapy

It is difficult to control the variety of variables in human clinical studies. The genetic variability in humans can often give negative results, and it is vital to find the proper at-risk population with the correct genetic viability in the GI tract in order for the green tea polyphenol treatment to maximize its effectiveness. This limits the treatment potential of green tea in regard to prostate cancer. Further studies will need to examine both larger populations and conduct more controlled experiments. Yang et al. (2009) observed that smoking and alcohol consumption interferes with the efficacy of GTPs, and the quantity as well as quality of tea can often determine whether the treatment reduces incidence of prostate cancer. Current studies are attempting to help offset these multiple variables. It has been found that the oral bioavailability of green tea catechins is low due to the harsh conditions of the GI tract (Khan et al., 2014). The concentrations of green tea catechins found in humans after consumption is often 5 to 50 times less than the concentrations shown to exert biological activities in *in vitro* models. Khan et al. (2014) demonstrated that encapsulated EGCG in chitosan, a natural linear polysaccharide, was capable of increasing the retention time of treatment for nude mice. This resulted in delayed tumor growth, decrease in tumor size in the expression of CD31 and VEGF-positive cells (which are responsible for angiogenesis), a dose-dependent decrease in serum PSA, and an increase in the activation of caspases and apoptosis. While this study was conducted in mice, it holds potential for chemoprevention in humans, and could help in resolving the issue of variability of green tea polyphenol metabolism.

5.4 CONCLUSIONS AND FUTURE DIRECTION

Intensive effort in the last three decades to evaluate the role of green tea polyphenols in prostate cancer prevention or treatment comprises of epidemiological, pre-clinical and early clinical investigations. Research in *in vitro* and *in vivo* models using EGCG, the major constituent of green tea, has shown it to downregulate pro-inflammatory pathways, multiple kinases, and insulin-like growth factor axis, as well as blunt the effects of androgens. Additional studies using xenograft tumor models and transgenic mice suggest that green tea polyphenols can suppress the tumorigenic potential of prostate cancer. Clinical investigations confirm the safe and tolerable use of defined green tea products. The main focus of clinical trials of green tea has been to reduce the incidence and proliferation of precancerous HGPIN lesions or suppress late-stage hormone-refractory prostate cancer progression; there is a significant disparity in the knowledge available for patients who are classified as having localized prostate cancer. This group of patients may signify an ideal population, as they often undergo "watchful waiting" without any pharmaceutical interventions and PSA testing as a routinely used biomarker. More recently, short-term supplementation with green tea polyphenols in patients undergoing radical prostatectomy was found to decrease serum biomarkers associated with prostate cancer. No appropriate biomarker of the various pathways that are influenced by green tea polyphenols has been developed. The current scenario requires development of new biomarkers and their validation, and may be integrated with the ongoing mechanistic *in vitro* and *in vivo* models in order to assess the efficacy of green tea in prostate cancer and later validate in clinical settings. To date PSA testing remains the gold standard for monitoring and detecting prostate cancer, but it fails to identify a small but significant proportion of aggressive cancers. Only about 30% of men with higher PSA values than "cutoff" have a positive biopsy. However, 25% of men treated for prostate cancer require additional treatment due to disease recurrence, while in some men prostate cancer growth remains sluggish. In these individuals, treatment is unnecessary and harmful, as these men do not benefit from treatment and are at a risk of treatment-related side effects and complications. The main challenge is to develop safe and cost-effective agents as well as improved diagnostic and prognostic biomarkers for prostate cancer that need to be validated in clinical trials.

Recent reports on the additive or synergistic effects of green tea polyphenols to increase the efficacy of chemo- or radiation therapy is a promising area of research and emphasis should be provided on more well-designed and well-planned studies (Hussain et al., 2005; Jang et al., 2005; Ping et al., 2010). This approach has the potential to enhance the efficacy of conventional therapies by adjustment of dose and time periods needed to achieve optimal results. In addition, development of new derivatives of tea polyphenols with improved bioavailability, low toxicity, and high effi-cacy is needed. Studies to develop techniques such as nanotechnology should be encouraged and could lead to sustained and precise delivery of polyphenols to the target site(s), thereby achieving improved efficacy and effective treatments to improve patient outcomes after treatment with green tea polyphenols.

ACKNOWLEDGEMENTS

The original work from authors' laboratory outlined in this review was supported by United States Public Health Service Grants RO1CA115491, R21CA193080, R03CA186179 and The Gateway for Cancer Research to SG. The authors would like to thank Albert Lee, undergraduate at Case Western Reserve University, for his contribution in compiling and summarizing some of the sources. We apologize to those investigators whose original work could not be cited owing to the space limitations.

REFERENCES

Adhami, V.M. Ahmad, N. Mukhtar, H. 2003. Molecular targets for green tea in prostate cancer prevention. *J Nutr* 133: 2417S–2424S.

Adhami, V.H. Mukthar, H. 2013. Human cancer chemoprevention: hurdles and challenges. In *Natural Products in Cancer Prevention and Therapy,* J.M. Pezzuto, N. Suh (Eds.). Berlin: Springer. *Top Curr Chem* 329: 203–220.

Allen, N.E. Sauvaget, C. Roddam, A.W. et al. 2004. A prospective study of diet and prostate cancer in Japanese men. *Cancer Causes Control* 15(9): 911–920.

American Cancer Society (ACS). 2015. Prostate cancer. Available at: http://www.cancer.org/cancer/prostatecancer/detailedguide/prostate-cancer-key-statistics.

Bettuzzi, S. Brausi, M. Rizzi, F. et al. 2006. Chemoprevention of human prostate cancer by oral administration of green tea catechins in volunteers with high-grade prostate intraepithelial neoplasia: a preliminary report from a one-year proof-of-principle study. *Cancer Res* 66(2): 1234–1240.

Bettuzzi, S. Rizzi, F. Belloni, L. 2007. Clinical relevance of the inhibitory effect of green tea catechins (GtCs) on prostate cancer progression in combination with molecular profiling of catechin-resistant tumors: an integrated view. *Pol J Vet Sci.* 10(1): 57–60.

Bhatia, N. Agarwal, R. 2001. Detrimental effect of cancer preventive phytochemicals silymarin, genistein and epigallocatechin 3-gallate on epigenetic events in human prostate carcinoma DU145 cells. *Prostate* 46(2): 98–107.

Boehm, K. Borrelli, F. Ernst, E. et al. 2009. Green tea (Camellia sinensis) for the prevention of cancer. *Cochrane Database Syst Rev* (3):CD005004.

Brusselmans, K. De Schrijver, E. Heyns, W. et al. 2003. Epigallocatechin-3-gallate is a potent natural inhibi-tor of fatty acid synthase in intact cells and selectively induces apoptosis in prostate cancer cells. *Int J Cancer* 106(6): 856–862.

Choan, E. Segal, R. Jonker, D. et al. 2005. A prospective clinical trial of green tea for hormone refractory prostate cancer: an evaluation of the complementary/alternative therapy approach. *Urol Oncol* 23(2): 108–113.

Chow, H.H. Cai, Y. Hakim, I.A. et al. 2003. Pharmacokinetics and safety of green tea polyphenols after multiple-dose administration of epigallocatechin gallate and polyphenon E in healthy individuals. *Clin Cancer Res* 9(9): 3312–3319.

Chow, H.H. Hakim, I.A. Vining, D.R. et al. 2005. Effects of dosing condition on the oral bioavailability of green tea catechins after single-dose administration of Polyphenon E in healthy individuals. *Clin Cancer Res* 11(12): 4627–4633.

Chung, L.Y. Cheung, T.C, Kong, S.K. et al. 2001. Induction of apoptosis by green tea catechins in human prostate cancer DU145 cells. *Life Sci* 68(10): 1207–1214.

Fang, M.Z. Wang, Y. Ai, N. et al. 2003. Tea polyphenol (-)-epigallocatechin-3-gallate inhibits DNA methyltransferase and reactivates methylation-silenced genes in cancer cell lines. *Cancer Res* 63(22): 7563–7570.

Fang, M. Chen, D. Yang, C.S. 2007. Dietary polyphenols may affect DNA methylation. *J Nutr* 137 (1 Suppl): 223S–228S.

Fei, X. Shen, Y. Li, X. et al. 2014. The association of tea consumption and the risk and progression of prostate cancer: a meta-analysis. *Int J Clin Exp Med* 7(11): 3881–3891.

Graham, H.N. 1992. Green tea composition, consumption, and polyphenol chemistry. *Prev Med* 21(3): 334–350.

Gupta, K. Thakur, V.S. Bhaskaran, N. et al. 2012. Green tea polyphenols induce p53-dependent and p53-independent apoptosis in prostate cancer cells through two distinct mechanisms. *PLoS One* 7(12): e52572.

Gupta, S. Ahmad, N. Mohan, R.R. et al. 1999. Prostate cancer chemoprevention by green tea: in vitro and in vivo inhibition of testosterone-mediated induction of ornithine decarboxylase. *Cancer Res* 59(9): 2115–2120.

Gupta, S. Hastak, K. Ahmad, N. et al. 2001. Inhibition of prostate carcinogenesis in TRAMP mice by oral infusion of green tea polyphenols. *Proc Natl Acad Sci U S A* 98(18): 10350–10355.

Hankey, B.F. Feuer, E.J. Clegg, L.X. et al. 1999. Cancer surveillance series: interpreting trends in prostate cancer – part I: evidence of the effects of screening in recent prostate cancer incidence, mortality, and survival rates. *J Natl Cancer Inst* 91(12): 1017–1024.

Harper, C.E. Patel, B.B. Wang, J. et al. 2007. Epigallocatechin-3-Gallate suppresses early stage, but not late stage prostate cancer in TRAMP mice: mechanisms of action. *Prostate* 67(14): 1576–1589.

Henning, S.M. Aronson, W. Niu, Y. et al. 2006. Tea polyphenols and theaflavins are present in prostate tissue of humans and mice after green and black tea consumption. *J Nutr* 136: 1839–1843.

Henning, S.M. Wang, P. Heber, D. 2011. Chemopreventive effects of tea in prostate cancer: green tea versus black tea. *Mol Nutr Food Res* 55(6): 905–920.

Henning, S.M. Wang, P. Said, J.W. et al. 2015. Randomized clinical trial of brewed green and black tea in men with prostate cancer prior to prostatectomy. *Prostate* 75(5): 550–559.

Hussain, T. Gupta, S. Adhami, V.M. et al. 2005. Green tea constituent epigallocatechin-3-gallate selectively inhibits COX-2 without affecting COX-1 expression in human prostate carcinoma cells. *Int J Cancer* 113 (4): 660–669.

Jang, E.H. Choi, J.Y. Park, C.S. et al. 2005. Effects of green tea extract administration on the pharmacokinetics of clozapine in rats. *J Pharm Pharmacol* 57 (3): 311–316.

Jatoi, A. Ellison, N. Burch, P.A. et al. 2003. A phase II trial of green tea in the treatment of patients with androgen independent metastatic prostate carcinoma. *Cancer* 97(6): 1442–1446.

Jian, L. Xie, L.P. Lee, A.H. et al. 2004. Protective effect of green tea against prostate cancer: a case-control study in southeast China. *Int J Cancer* 108(1): 130–135.

Johnson, J.J. Bailey, H.H. Mukhtar, H. 2010. Green tea polyphenols for prostate cancer chemoprevention: a translational perspective. *Phytomedicine* 7(1): 3–13.

Kanwal, R. Pandey, M. Bhaskaran, N. et al. 2014. Protection against oxidative DNA damage and stress in human prostate by glutathione S-transferase P1. *Mol Carcinog* 53(1): 8–18.

Khan, N. Bharali, D.J. Adhami, V.M. et al. 2014. Oral administration of naturally occurring chitosan-based nanoformulated green tea polyphenol EGCG effectively inhibits prostate cancer cell growth in a xenograft model. *Carcinogenesis* 35(2): 415–423.

Kikuchi, N. Ohmori, K. Shimazu, T. et al. 2006. No association between green tea and prostate cancer risk in Japanese men: the Ohsaki Cohort Study. *Br J Cancer* 95(3): 371–373.

Kommu, S. Edwards, S. and Eeles, R. 2004. The clinical genetics of prostate cancer. *Hered Cancer Clin Prac* 2(3): 111–121.

Kumar, N.B. Pow-Sang, J. Egan, K.M. et al. 2015. Randomized, placebo-controlled trial of green tea catechins for prostate cancer prevention. *Cancer Prev Res (Phila)* pii: canprevres.0324.2014. [Epub ahead of print].

Kurahashi, N. Sasazuki, S. Iwasaki, M. et al. 2008. Green tea consumption and prostate cancer risk in Japanese men: a prospective study. *Am J Epidemiol* 167(1): 71–77.

Lee, J. Demissie, K. Lu, S.E. Rhoads, G.G. 2007. Cancer incidence among Korean-American immigrants in the United States and native Koreans in South Korea. *Cancer Control* 14(1): 78–85.

Legeay, S. Rodier, M. Fillon, L. et al. 2015. Epigallocatechin gallate: a review of its beneficial properties to prevent metabolic syndrome. *Nutrients* 7(7): 5443–5468.

Li, M. He, Z. Ermakova, S. et al. 2007. Direct inhibition of insulin-like growth factor-I receptor kinase activity by (-)-epigallocatechin-3-gallate regulates cell transformation. *Cancer Epidemiol Biomarkers Prev* 16(3): 598–605.

Liao, S. Hiipakka, R.A. 1995. Selective inhibition of steroid 5 alpha-reductase isozymes by tea epicatechin-3-gallate and epigallocatechin-3-gallate. *Biochem Biophys Res Commun* 214(3): 833–838.

Liao, S. Umekita, Y. Guo, J. et al. 1995. Growth inhibition and regression of human prostate and breast tumors in athymic mice by tea epigallocatechin gallate. *Cancer Lett* 96 (2): 239–243.

Lin, P.H. Aronson, W. Freedland, S.J. 2015. Nutrition, dietary interventions and prostate cancer: the latest evidence. *BMC Med* 13: 3.

Lin, Y.W. Hu, Z.H. Wang, X. et al. 2014. Tea consumption and prostate cancer: an updated meta-analysis. *World J Surg Oncol* 12: 38–45.

McCarthy, S. Caporali, A. Enkemann, S. et al. 2007. Green tea catechins suppress the DNA synthesis marker MCM7 in the TRAMP model of prostate cancer. *Mol Oncol* 1(2): 196–204.

McKay, D.L., Blumberg J.B. 2002. The role of tea in human health: An update. *J. Am. Coll. Nutr* 21: 1–13.

McLarty, J. Bigelow, R.L. Smith, M. et al. 2009. Tea polyphenols decrease serum levels of prostate-specific antigen, hepatocyte growth factor, and vascular endothelial growth factor in prostate cancer patients and inhibit production of hepatocyte growth factor and vascular endothelial growth factor in vitro. *Cancer Prev Res*. 2(7): 673–682.

Moyad, M.A. Carroll, P.R. 2004a. Lifestyle recommendations to prevent prostate cancer, part I: time to redirect our attention? *Urol Clin North Am* 31(2): 289–300.

Moyad, M.A. Carroll, P.R. 2004b. Lifestyle recommendations to prevent prostate cancer, part I: time to redirect our attention? *Urol Clin North Am* 31(2): 301–311.

Nguyen, M.M. Ahmann, F.R. Nagle, R.B. et al. 2012. Randomized, double-blind, placebo-controlled trial of polyphenon E in prostate cancer patients before prostatectomy: evaluation of potential chemopreventive activities. *Cancer Prev Res* (Phila) 5(2): 290–298.

Pandey, M. Shukla, S. Gupta, S. 2010. Promoter demethylation and chromatin remodeling by green tea polyphenols leads to re-expression of GSTP1 in human prostate cancer cells. *Int J Cancer* 126(11): 2520–2533.

Ping, S.Y. Hour, T.C. Lin, S.R. et al. 2010. Taxol synergizes with antioxidants in inhibiting hormonal refractory prostate cancer cell growth. *Urol Oncol* 28(2): 170–179.

Ren, F. Zhang, S. Mitchell, S.H. et al. 2000. Tea polyphenols down-regulate the expression of the androgen receptor in LNCaP prostate cancer cells. *Oncogene* 19(15): 1924–1932.

Roomi, M.W. Ivanov, V. Kalinovsky, T. et al. 2005. In vivo antitumor effect of ascorbic acid, lysine, proline and green tea extract on human prostate cancer PC-3 xenografts in nude mice: evaluation of tumor growth and immunohistochemistry. *In Vivo* 19(1): 179–183.

Saleem, M. Adhami, V.M. Ahmad, N. et al. 2005. Prognostic significance of metastasis-associated protein S100A4 (Mts1) in prostate cancer progression and chemoprevention regimens in an autochthonous mouse model. *Clin Cancer Res* 11(1): 147–153.

Severson, R.K. Nomura, A.M. Grove, J.S. et al. 1989. A prospective study of demographics, diet, and prostate cancer among men of Japanese ancestry in Hawaii. *Cancer Res* 49(7): 1857–1860.

Shavers, V.L. Underwood, W. Moser, RP. 2009. Race/ethnicity and the perception of the risk of developing prostate cancer. *Am J Prev Med* 37(1): 64–7.

Siddiqui, I.A. Adhami, V.M. Afaq, F. et al. 2004. Modulation of phosphatidylinositol-3-kinase/protein kinase B- and mitogen-activated protein kinase-pathways by tea polyphenols in human prostate cancer cells. *J Cell Biochem* 91(2): 232–242.

Siddiqui, I.A. Asim, M. Hafeez, B.B. et al. 2011. Green tea polyphenol EGCG blunts androgen receptor function in prostate cancer. *FASEB J* 25(4): 1198–1207.

Siddiqui, I.A. Shukla, Y. Adhami, V.M. et al. 2008. Suppression of NFkappaB and its regulated gene products by oral administration of green tea polyphenols in an autochthonous mouse prostate cancer model. *Pharm Res* 25(9): 2135–2142.

Siegel, R. Ma, J. Zou, Z. Jemal, A. 2014. Cancer statistics, 2014. *CA: A Cancer J Clin* 64: 9–24.

Sonoda, T. Nagata, Y. Mori, M. et al. 2004. A case-control study of diet and prostate cancer in Japan: possible protective effect of traditional Japanese diet. *Cancer Sci* 95(3): 238–142.

Syed, D.N. Khan, N. Afaq, F. Mukhtar, H. 2007. Chemoprevention of prostate cancer through dietary agents: progress and promise. *Cancer Epidemiol Biomarkers Prev* 16(11): 2193–2203.

Thakur, V.S. Gupta, K. Gupta, S. 2012a. The chemopreventive and chemotherapeutic potentials of tea polyphenols. *Curr Pharm Biotechnol* 13(1): 191–199.

Thakur, V.S. Gupta, K. Gupta, S. 2012b. Green tea polyphenols causes cell cycle arrest and apoptosis in prostate cancer cells by suppressing class I histone deacetylases. *Carcinogenesis* 33(2): 377–384.

Thakur, V.S. Gupta, K. Gupta, S. 2012c. Green tea polyphenols increase p53 transcriptional activity and acetylation by suppressing class I histone deacetylases. *Int J Oncol* 41(1): 353–361.

Vayalil, P.K. Katiyar, S.K. 2004. Treatment of epigallocatechin-3-gallate inhibits matrix metalloproteinases-2 and -9 via inhibition of activation of mitogen-activated protein kinases, c-jun and NF-kappaB in human prostate carcinoma DU-145 cells. *Prostate* 59(1): 33–42.

Yang, C.S. Wang, X. Lu, G. et al. 2009. Cancer prevention by tea: animal studies, molecular mechanisms and human relevance. *Nat Rev Cancer* 9 (6): 429–439.

Yuan, J.M. Sun, C. Butler, L.M. 2011. Tea and cancer prevention: epidemiological studies. *Pharmacol Res* 64(2): 123–135.

Zhang, L. Zheng, Y. Chow, M.S. et al. 2004. Investigation of intestinal absorption and disposition of green tea catechins by Caco-2 monolayer model. *Int J Pharm* 287(1–2): 1–12.

Zhou, J.R. Yu, L. Zhong, Y. et al. 2003. Soy phytochemicals and tea bioactive components synergistically inhibit androgen-sensitive human prostate tumors in mice. *J Nutr* 133 (2): 516–521.

Zhu, Y. Wang, H. Qu, Y.Y. et al. 2015 Prostate cancer in East Asia: evolving trend over the last decade. *Asian J Androl* 17(1): 48–57.

Zlotta, A.R. Egawa, S. Pushkar, D. et al. 2013. Prevalence of prostate cancer on autopsy: cross-sectional study on unscreened Caucasian and Asian men. *J Natl Cancer Inst* 105(14): 1050–1058.

CHAPTER 6

Plumbagin and Prostate Cancer Therapy

R.S. Reshma, Revathy Nadhan, and Priya Srinivas

CONTENTS

6.1 INTRODUCTION

Prostate cancer is the fourth most common cancer, among the total cancers in both the sexes when analyzed together, and the second most common cancer in men (GLOBOCAN IARC 2012; (Ferlay et al. 2015)). In addition, cancer of the prostate is the fifth leading cause of cancer mortality in men. Unlike many other types of cancer, prostate cancer progresses very slowly (Schmid, McNeal, and Stamey 1993). At primary stages, the prostate cells involved in cancer progression are androgen dependent, wherein androgen binds to the androgen receptor (AR) and activates androgen-responsive elements (ARE) of the promoters of genes that are transactivated by AR. This type of prostate cancer is known as androgen-dependent prostate cancer, androgen-sensitive prostate cancer, or hormone-sensitive prostate cancer (HSPC). As the disease progresses, the prostate cancer cells do not require androgen for their growth and become androgen independent. This advanced cancer that progresses in spite of androgen deprivation therapy (ADT), via mutated AR or AR-independent pathways, is known as androgen-independent prostate cancer, androgen-insensitive prostate cancer, or hormone-refractory prostate cancer (HRPC) (Arnold and Isaacs 2002; Scher and Sawyers 2005; Silvestris et al. 2005; Karantanos, Corn, and Thompson 2013). These subtypes are also termed castration-sensitive prostate cancer (CSPC) for HSPC and castration-resistant prostate cancer (CRPC) for HRPC. The term CRPC was introduced possibly due to the insensitivity of the advanced prostate cancer to the castration methods of treatment such as reduction of available androgen, testosterone, or dihydrotestosterone or through inhibition of paracrine or intacrine androgen production by chemical or surgical means (Mostaghel et al. 2007; Saad and Hotte 2010).

6.2   PROSTATE CANCER: STANDARD THERAPY AND CURRENT DRUGS

Being a male reproductive organ, the prostate gland is influenced by the effect of many hormones either synthesized by itself or reaching the site by endocrine circulation. The major hormones which play a role in the prostate tumorigenesis include androgen, estrogen, progesterone, and luteinizing hormone-releasing hormone (LHRH). The overexpression of androgen receptors, estrogen receptors, progesterone receptors, and LHRH has paved the way to the use of their inhibitors for efficient therapy against prostate tumors.

The most commonly used therapy for the initial stage of prostate cancer is ADT, which is the blockage of the production or use of androgens. This therapy invariably fails once the disease progresses to metastatic CRPC (mCRPC) (Hotte and Saad 2010). Recently, a combination of chemotherapy and immunotherapy with hormone therapy has emerged as a standard approach for the treatment of mCRPC (Mitsiades et al. 2012). Although phase III clinical trials with many of these agents alone or in combination have helped in improving the survival benefits of prostate cancer patients, several criticisms and challenges still exist. Various treatment methods and current drugs used in prostate cancer therapy and their mode of action are described in Table 6.1.

6.3   USE OF ROS INDUCERS FOR CANCER TREATMENT

An elevated level of oxidative stress has been detected in almost all types of cancers, in which they upregulate many factors, leading to tumor development and progression (Liou and Storz 2010). Oxidative stress may be the result of either an increase in reactive oxygen species (ROS) generation or a loss of function of ROS scavengers (Khandrika et al. 2009). ROS, like hydroxyl radicals, peroxides, and superoxides, leads to damage of biomolecules including DNA, as well as stimulation of signaling pathways associated with cell proliferation, apoptosis, etc. (Sauer, Wartenberg, and Hescheler 2001). Intracellular antioxidants including enzymatic ones such as glutathione peroxidase, thioredoxine, catalase, superoxide dismutase, etc., and non-enzymatic ones such as glutathione, thiols, certain vitamins and metals, or phytochemicals such as isoflavones, polyphenols, and flavonoids, help the cells in scavenging ROS, thus preventing the biomolecules from oxidative damage (Seifried et al. 2007). ROS generated by various chemotherapeutic agents can also be used as an effective means for selectively eradicating malignant cells (Schumacker 2006).

Depending on the tumor type, various ROS inducers have been studied as effective therapeutics. For example, Sulindac, an FDA-approved drug, enhances intracellular ROS levels and increases

Table 6.1 Various Treatment Methods and Current Drugs Used in Prostate Cancer Therapy and Their Mode of Action

Method	Current Drug	Mode of Action	References
		CSPC	
Hormone Therapy			
Orchiectomy	–	Reduces production of testosterone by removal of one or both testicles	(Eisenberger et al. 1998)
Luteinizing hormone-releasing hormone (LHRH) agonists	Leuprolide Goserelin Buserelin	Reduces the level of testosterone by preventing secretion of LH by downregulating the LH receptors, rendering the pituitary gland irresponsive to further stimulation by LHRH	(Labrie et al. 1996; Schmitt et al. 2001)
LHRH antagonists	Abarelix Degarelix	Reduces the level of testosterone by binding to LHRH receptors, preventing LHRH binding on pituitary cells	(Weckermann and Harzmann 2004; Crawford and Hou 2009)
Estrogen	Diethyl-stilbestrol	Suppresses pituitary secretion of LH, then inhibits testicular testosterone production as antiandrogens Increases serum sex hormone–binding globulin, reducing free testosterone in circulation	(Oh 2002; Bosland 2005)
Antiandrogens	Flutamide Enzalutamide Bicalutamide Nilutamide MDV 3100	Competes with androgens for binding with AR	(Cookson et al. 2013; Scher et al. 2010)
Androgen synthesis inhibitor (17α-hydroxy /17,20-lyase (CYP17) inhibitor)	Ketoconazole Amino-gluthethimide	Prevents androgen production by adrenal gland, prostate cells, and testicles by blocking testosterone production from cholesterol	(Small et al. 2004)
		CRPC	
Prostatectomy	–	Surgical removal of the prostate gland	(Eschwege et al. 1995)
Hormone Therapy			
• Antiandrogen	ARN 509 BMS 641988	AR inhibitor, sensitive to prostate cancer with overexpressed AR	(Clegg et al. 2012; Attar et al. 2009)
• Androgen synthesis inhibitor	Abiraterone Orteronel TOK – 001	CYP 17 inhibitor, blocks testosterone synthesis AR and CYP inhibitors	(de Bono et al. 2011; Kaku et al. 2011; Bruno et al. 2011)
Immunotherapy	Sipuleucal T	Stimulates T-cell immune response targeted against PAP	(Beer et al. 2011; Madan et al. 2012)
	Ipilimumab	Blocks immune checkpoint molecule CTLA-4	
	Prostvac VF	Recombinant vaccine	
Chemotherapy	Mitoxanthrone Docetaxel Carbazitoxel Satraplatin	Topoisomerase II inhibitor Mitotic block; interrupts microtubule stabilization	(Tannock et al. 2004; Hurwitz 2015; Sternberg et al. 2005)
Radiotherapy	Radium 223 dichloride	Alpha emitter	(Parker et al. 2013)

the sensitivity of colon and lung cancer cells to H_2O_2-induced apoptosis (Marchetti et al. 2009). Aminoflavone, an intracellular ROS inducer, was reported to induce apoptosis via caspase 3 activation in breast cancer cells (McLean et al. 2008). Phytochemicals have also been reported to be potential cancer chemotherapeutic agents, as they can inhibit the proliferation of cancer cells by elevating intracellular ROS levels. Epigallocate-3-gallate, benzyl isothiocyanate, and capsaicin have been reported to elevate intracellular ROS levels and induce apoptosis in pancreatic cancer (Shankar, Suthakar, and Srivastava 2007; Srivastava and Singh 2004).

6.4 ROS INDUCTION AND PROSTATE CANCER TREATMENT

Oxidative stress, characterized by ROS generation, plays a vital role in the aggressive phenotypic behavior of prostate cancer (Paschos et al. 2013). Oxidative stress is correlated with prostate cancer progression and response to therapy by regulating molecules such as DNA, transcription factors, enhancers, cell cycle regulators, etc. (Gupta-Elera et al. 2012). Previous studies have shown that generation of ROS can be a cause of prostate cancer; thus strategies for lowering of ROS generation rather than neutralization of generated ROS could be an effective therapeutic measure (Kumar et al. 2008). Conversely, some studies state that accumulation of ROS leads to prostatic disorders that in turn cause more ROS generation; thus treatment strategies aiming at neutralization of ROS would be necessary to maintain homeostasis (Khandrika et al. 2009). A drop in the ROS level below the optimum may affect the cell proliferation and immune system, whereas a rise in ROS level along with lowering of antioxidants may interrupt the normal functioning of the prostate, causing cancerous phenotype (Waris and Ahsan 2006). Therefore, an optimal level of ROS is needed for cells for their normal functioning, depending on the physiological conditions, so both ROS scavengers and ROS inducers are effectively studied in treating cancers. An ROS inducer can become an ROS scavenger as well, depending on the ROS content or the substrate available in the system.

Green tea extract and green tea catechins have been reported to suppress cell growth and induce apoptosis in human prostate cancer cells through an increase in reactive oxygen species formation and mitochondrial depolarization (Chung et al. 2001). Similarly, sulforaphane and berberine were reported to induce apoptosis by disruption of the mitochondrial membrane potential, release of apoptogenic molecules from mitochondria, and cleavage of caspases and PARP proteins. The effect of these compounds on prostate cancer was shown to be initiated by ROS generation irrespective of their androgen responsiveness (Singh et al. 2005; Meeran, Katiyar, and Katiyar 2008). Naphthaquinone derivatives have also been reported to induce cytotoxicity in prostate cancer, and exhibits synergistic effects with radiation by accumulation of ROS and mitochondrial dysfunction (Ross et al. 1985). A number of 1,4-naphthoquinone derivatives have been reported to possess powerful pharmacological effects associated with antitumor activities in both androgen-dependent and androgen-independent prostate cancer cells (Habib, Bekhit, and Park 2003; Copeland et al. 2007). Plumbagin, a 1,4-naphthoquinone derivative, has been proved to be a potential anticancer agent by inhibiting cell invasion and inducing apoptosis in prostate cancer cells, but not in non-tumorigenic prostate cells (Nair et al. 2008; Ahmad et al. 2008; Aziz, Dreckschmidt, and Verma 2008).

6.5 PLUMBAGIN AND CANCER THERAPY

Naphthaquinones constitute a large group of plant secondary metabolites, possessing a wide variety of pharmacological activities such as antimicrobial, antioxidant, anti-inflammatory, and anticancerous properties. Plumbagin is a naphthaquinone derivative, isolated from the roots of the medicinal plant *Plumbago* species (known as Chitraka in the ancient Ayurvedic texts of Charaka).

Plumbagin is also present in *Juglans* sp. black walnut, butter walnut, butternut, etc. (Sandur et al. 2006). Apart from its antimicrobial (Jeyachandran et al. 2009) and anti-cancerous properties (Padhye et al. 2012), plumbagin has been shown to possess a broad range of potential health benefits including neuroprotection, contraception, immunosuppression, and cardiotonic potential (Son et al. 2010).

Plumbagin is chemically represented as 5-hyroxy-2-methyl-1,4-naphthaquinone (Figure 6.1: Plumbagin). The biological activity of plumbagin may be due to (i) the presence of two carbonyl groups that have the ability to accept one and/or two electrons to form radical anion/dianion species; (ii) asymmetry caused by the strong intramolecular hydrogen bonding of the carbonyl group with the adjacent hydroxyl function; (iii) contraction of the carbon-oxygen and carbon-carbon bonds due to the enhanced electron donating ability of the methyl group; (iv) chelating property of the hydroxyl group to form stable complexes with several trace metals of biological relevance; and/or (v) acid-base properties. It has been reported that redox cycling and bionucleophile reactions play a key role in quinone action; thus, plumbagin also acts as an inhibitor of the electron transport chain

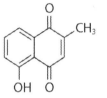

Figure 6.1   Plumbagin (5-hyroxy-2-methyl-1,4-naphthaquinone).

Table 6.2   Previous Studies Reporting the Anticancerous Role of Plumbagin in Various Cancer Cell Lines

Cancer Type	Cell Lines	References
Breast	MDA-MB-231, MCF 7	(Kuo, Hsu, and Cho 2006; Qiao et al. 2015; Lee et al. 2012; Yan et al. 2013; Ahmad et al. 2008)
Ovarian	BG1, PEO-1, PE0-4 OVCAR-5	(Srinivas, Annab, et al. 2004; Thasni et al. 2008; Sinha et al. 2013)
Lung	H460, H23, A549, H292, LLC	(Hsu et al. 2006; Li et al. 2014; Hwang et al. 2015; Gomathinayagam et al. 2008; Xu et al. 2013)
Colon	HCT116	(Chen et al. 2013; Eldhose et al. 2014; Raghu and Karunagaran 2014)
Melanoma	A375, SKMEL 28	(Wang et al. 2008; Anuf et al. 2014)
Tongue squamous cell	SCC25, Tca 8113	(Pan et al. 2015; Qiu et al. 2013)
Oral squamous cell	OSCC	(Ono et al. 2015)
Leukemia	NB4, U937	(Xu and Lu 2010; Gaascht et al. 2014)
Gastric	MKN 28 AGS, MKN45, SNU16, SGC-7901	(Manu et al. 2011; Joo et al. 2015; Li et al. 2012)
Myeloma	U266 MM.1S	(Sandur et al. 2010)
Pancreatic	PANC1, DXPC3, B2PC3	(Chen et al. 2009; Wang et al. 2015)
Cervical	SiHa	(Hwang et al. 2015)
Bone	U2OS	(Tian et al. 2012)
Liver	HepG2	(Shih et al. 2009)

by abstracting electrons and diverting the electron flow to dioxygen molecules to form superoxide radicals (Chesis et al. 1984).

Plumbagin has been shown to possess anticancer properties against various types of cancers (Padhye et al. 2012), while it is comparatively much less cytotoxic to normal cells (Aziz, Dreckschmidt, and Verma 2008; Nair et al. 2008; Ahmad et al. 2008). Previous studies reporting the anticancerous role of plumbagin against different cancer cell lines are summarized in Table 6.2.

6.6   PLUMBAGIN: MECHANISM OF ACTION

The anticancerous action of plumbagin relies on four major reactions: (i) ROS generation; (ii) topoisomerase II inhibition; (iii) microtubule stabilization; and/or (iv) DNA intercalation (Figure 6.2). These steps can subsequently lead to a cascade of reactions interrupting cell proliferation, cell cycle progression, angiogenesis, migration, and invasion and eventually resulting in inducing cell cycle arrest and apoptosis.

1. ROS generation: The quinone structure allows plumbagin to conduct electrons from two-electron donors to single-electron acceptors and transfer them to molecular oxygen, thus acting as a ROS generator (Srinivas, Gopinath, et al. 2004). Nazeem et al. (2009) showed that the endogenous copper ions bound to chromatin activate plumbagin via copper redox reaction, leading to the generation of ROS and a plumbagin semiquinone intermediate. ROS generated by plumbagin may act as signaling molecule either by cascading various pathways or directly, resulting in DNA damage.

2. Topoisomerase II inhibition: Plumbagin acts as a Topo II poison by stabilizing the Topoisomerase II-DNA cleavable complex (Fujii et al. 1992). This stabilization prevents the relegation step, leading to accumulation of double-strand DNA breaks and trigger apoptosis (Mizutani et al. 2002). Wang et al. (2001) reported that plumbagin causes topoisomerase II inactivation through thiol group modification of the topoisomerase enzyme through Michael addition. The topoisomerase II inactivation

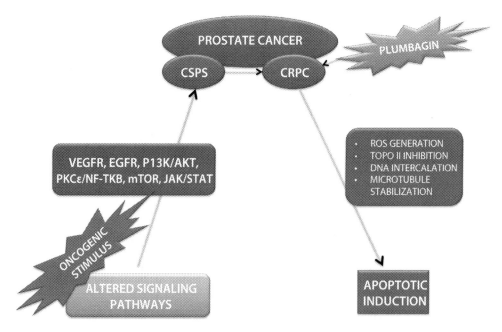

Figure 6.2   Representative figure of the action of plumbagin on prostate cancer.

inhibits the ability of cells to change DNA topology and thus blocks DNA synthesis. ROS generated by plumbagin at low concentration may also act as signaling molecules, mediating apoptosis through topoisomerase II inactivation. Li et al. (1999) reported that hydrogen peroxide generated by plumbagin inhibits topoisomerase II activity by oxidizing the thiol group of the enzyme.

3. Microtubule stabilization: Binding of plumbagin to tubulin alters the microtubule dynamics, leading to mitotic spindle dysfunction. Inhibition of microtubule dynamics blocks cell division through mitosis and activates the pathways leading to apoptosis. Thus, molecules that can stabilize microtubule-disturbing dynamics can be used as an anticancer drug for targeted therapies. Plumbagin perturbs the interphase microtubule network at the colchicine binding site and inhibits the polymerization of tubulin (Acharya, Bhattacharyya, and Chakrabarti 2008).

4. DNA intercalation: DNA is the critical target of the activity of many compounds, including phytochemicals. Plumbagin can intercalate into DNA to a lesser extent, but better than shikonin and lawsone (Fujii et al. 1992). Spectroscopic studies showed that some interactions take place between DNA and plumbagin, leading to some local denaturation changes and significant disruption of the hydrogen bonds between adenine and thymine. The non-obvious DNA intercalation may be due to the methyl group in the naphthalene skeleton (Vaverkova et al. 2014).

In addition to the above mechanisms, plumbagin can interact directly with some receptors triggering various signaling pathways, which are discussed later.

6.7 ANTICANCER ACTIVITY OF PLUMBAGIN IN PROSTATE CANCER

Plumbagin has been reported to possess antitumor activities in both androgen-sensitive and -insensitive cell lines. Several studies have been carried out which reported the selective anticancer potential of plumbagin on prostate cancer cells and animal models, without affecting the normal prostate cells. Previous reports showing the mode of action of plumbagin in prostate cancer cell lines/animals is described in Table 6.3.

Table 6.3 Anticancer Activity of Plumbagin in Prostate Cancer Cell Lines/Animals

Animals/Cells	Mode of Action of Plumbagin	References
PC-3, DU 145	Inhibits PI3K/Akt/mTOR pathway Downregulates sirtuin 1 in coordination with AMPK, p38MAPK, visfatin and ROS-associated pathway	(Zhou et al. 2015)
PC-3, DU 145	Modulates proteins regulating cell cycle, autophagy, apoptosis, EMT pathways	(Qiu et al. 2015)
LNCaP, C4-2	Downregulates AR transactivation, AR level, AR-targeted PSA; accelerates AR degradation Downregulates IL6 induced interaction of Stat3 with AR Blocks androgen and nonandrogen activation of AR signaling	(Hafeez, Colson, and Verma 2010)
PC-3, LNCaP, C4-2	Induces ROS generation leading to apoptosis Depletes GSH levels Alters the expression of genes such as MnSoD2	(Powolny and Singh 2008)
DU 145 cells, xenografts	Downregulates PKCε, PI3K, pAkt, pStat, pJAK2 Downregulates DNA binding activity of TFAP1, NFKβ, Stat3 Downregulates BclxL, cdc25A, COX-2	(Aziz, Dreckschmidt, and Verma 2008)
Pten KO mice	Downregulates PKCε, Akt, Stat3, COX-2 Inhibits EMT markers vimentin, slug	(Hafeez et al. 2015)
Xenograft mice	Inhibits expression of PKCε, Stat3, Stat3 downstream target genes, proliferative, metastatic, and angiogenesis markers	(Hafeez et al. 2013)
TRAMP mice	Downregulates PKCε, pStat3, PCNA, neuroendocrine markers	(Hafeez et al. 2012)

6.8 PLUMBAGIN AND CRPC THERAPY

Using both *in vitro* and *in vivo* preclinical models, Aziz, Dreckschmidt, and Verma (2008) reported that plumbagin can inhibit growth and invasion of CRPC cells. Intraperitonial administration of plumbagin is reported to reduce tumor weight and volume and thus growth of tumor in CRPC cell implants. This is the first report on the anticancer activity of plumbagin in CRPC. Subsequently, Powolny and Singh (2008) reported that irrespective of androgen responsiveness, plumbagin is reported to induce apoptosis in human prostate cancer cells. Plumbagin can modulate the expression of different proteins regulating the cell cycle, apoptosis, autophagy, and EMT in androgen-independent prostate cancer cells PC-3 and DU 145 (Zhou et al. 2015; Qiu et al. 2015).

Progression of CRPC from androgen-dependent prostate cancer is related to continuous AR activation, which leads to increased sensitivity of AR to low androgen levels and altered ligand specificity. Plumbagin is proven to inhibit prostate cancer cells blocking androgen and non-androgen–induced activation of AR signaling. Plumbagin can inhibit the AR protein level and increase AR degradation (Hafeez, Colson, and Verma 2010), thus proving effective in CRPC therapy.

PKCε can be considered as a predictive marker of prostate cancer aggressiveness. Stat3 activated by PKCε acts as a non-androgen activator of AR. Both of these molecules can lead to androgen-independent AR activation, prostate cancer cell survival, and CRPC progression (Hafeez et al. 2011). Plumbagin is reported to inhibit the progression of prostatic intraepithelial neoplasia to carcinoma via inhibition of PKCε, Stat3, and neuroendocrine markers (Hafeez et al. 2012). Plumbagin can also inhibit the growth and liver metastasis of prostate cancer cells in orthotopic xenograft tumors by inhibiting PKCε, Stat3, Stat3 downstream target genes, and proliferative, metastatic, and angiogenesis markers (Hafeez et al. 2013).

PTEN deletion can also lead to the progression of invasive carcinoma from prostatic intraepithelial neoplasia. Hafeez et al. (2015) reported that plumbagin can inhibit tumor development in castrated PTEN knockout mice, which again proved that plumbagin inhibits growth of both primary prostate cancer and CRPC.

6.9 CURRENT THERAPEUTIC TARGETS FOR PROSTATE CANCER

Various therapeutic targets for prostate cancer which are now in use are also found to be the targets of plumbagin. The molecules and signaling pathways reported to be specific targets of plumbagin are explained below.

6.9.1 Receptors

1. *Androgen receptor (AR):* AR-directed therapies targeting androgen synthesis and AR pathways are implemented in ongoing phase II and III trials for the treatment of CSPC. Several mechanisms responsible for the post-castration activation of AR in CRPC include partial inhibition of AR ligand signaling, AR amplification, expression of AR splice variants, malfunctioning of AR co-regulators, etc. (Scher and Sawyers 2005). Intracrine androgen metabolic enzymes also influence the development of CRPC. Thus, a combinatorial approach of anti-androgens and enzyme inhibitors could be effective in CRPC patients (Mitsiades et al. 2012). Abedinpour et al. (2013) proved that the combination of androgen ablation, which is the standard treatment for CSPC along with plumbagin, can provide significant prostate cancer regression *in vivo*. Microenvironmental factors might also play a significant role in increasing the therapeutic efficacy of the new strategy, combining plumbagin with castration.

2. *Estrogen receptor α (ERα):* Plumbagin has been reported to inhibit ER signaling by interfering with the binding of ERα to ERE by induction of truncated 46kDa ERα isoform and thus inhibiting nuclear translocation of ERα from cytoplasm (Thasni et al. 2008). Alterations in ERα and/or ERβ

expression can alter growth response of prostate cancer to ADT, thus leading to progression of prostate cancer (Linja et al. 2003). Hence, plumbagin might inhibit CRPC progression by inhibiting ERα translocation, which needs to be further examined.

3. *Death receptor TRAIL:* Death receptor TRAIL has been reported to be upregulated by plumbagin in melanoma (Li et al. 2014) and leukemia cells (Sun and McKallip 2011). K. Thasni et al. (2013) proved that plumbagin induced apoptosis by directly docking with death receptors TNFR-TRAIL as agonists. TRAIL-based therapies show selective antitumor activity in prostate cancer by inducing apoptosis in cancer cells but not in normal cells, thus suggesting them as potential anti-prostate cancer agents (Li et al. 2010). Plumbagin may thus act as a potent apoptosis inducer via targeting TRAIL receptor in CRPC cells, which has to be further verified experimentally.

4. *Nuclear receptor CRM1:* The nuclear export receptor CRM1 (XPO1), the active transporter of tumor suppressors, has been proven to be a direct cellular target of plumbagin (Liu et al. 2014). Gravina et al. (2014) showed that selective inhibition of CRM1-dependent nuclear export represents a novel advance for the treatment of CRPC. This inhibitory potential could impart the therapeutic properties of plumbagin to prostate cancer.

6.9.2 Neuroendocrine Markers

Previous reports proved that neuroendocrine cells were responsible for the transition of CSPC cells to CRPC cells (Dutt and Gao 2009). Neuropeptides transmitted signals through G-coupled receptors and subsequently activated AR in the absence of androgen (Chuu et al. 2005). Plumbagin could downregulate the expression of neuromarkers, synaptophysin, and chromogranin A (Hafeez et al. 2012) and could thus be effective in inhibiting the process of CRPC in the hormone refractory stage.

6.9.3 AR-Independent Pathways

Many alternative growth and survival signaling cascades bypassing the AR pathways play a major role in the development of CRPC. The key signaling cascades include VEGFR, EGFR, PI3K/AKT, PKCε/NFKB, mTOR, JAK/STAT, Wnt signaling pathways, etc. Novel therapeutic targets in prostate cancer – EGFR, VEGFR, PI3K/AKT/mTOR pathways targeting angiogenesis, PKCε/NFKB, IL6/JAK/STAT targeting proliferation, survivin targeting apoptosis, PARP targeting DNA repair, etc. – are now undergoing phase II and III trials, all of which are proved to be the targets of plumbagin.

Plumbagin has been reported to induce cell cycle arrest and apoptosis through multiple pathways by modulating several pro-apoptotic and pro-survival factors. Plumbagin can activate apoptotic factors like Bax, Bak, BclX5, caspase 3, caspase 9, etc. and downregulate anti-apoptotic proteins like IAPI, XIAP, Bcl2, BclXL, surviving, etc., thus resulting in phosphatidyl serine translocation, nuclear condensation, and DNA fragmentation, which are indicative of apoptosis (Hsu et al. 2006; Li et al. 2012; Srinivas, Gopinath, et al. 2004). Plumbagin can induce G2/M arrest via downregulation of the JNK pathway or the EGFR/Akt pathway (Gomathinayagam et al. 2008; Sandur et al. 2006; Hsu et al. 2006; Kuo, Hsu, and Cho 2006; Zhao and Lu 2006). Plumbagin could block DNA synthesis by downregulation of cell proliferation marker PCNA by forming p21/PCNA complex (Hsu et al. 2006; Aziz, Dreckschmidt, and Verma 2008). Plumbagin also could induce apoptosis and inhibit angiogenesis by TNFα pathway mediated by NFKβ downregulation (Subramanyan 2011; Li et al. 2012; Kawiak et al. 2007). NFKβ downregulation can in turn inhibit proliferation, invasion, metastasis, and migration through the downregulation of CXCR4 and CXCL12 (Manu et al. 2011). Several studies have proved that plumbagin could induce growth arrest via downregulating the Akt/mTOR pathway (Kuo, Hsu, and Cho 2006; Pan et al. 2015; Zhou et al. 2015; Li et al. 2014), whereas Sandur et al. (2010) showed that plumbagin could act via JAK/STAT pathway. Plumbagin inhibited angiogenesis and metastasis by downregulating MMP 9, metastatic TF, VEGF, and Glut 1, leading to the inhibition of the NFKB pathway (Aziz, Dreckschmidt, and Verma 2008; Sinha et al. 2013; Zhang et al. 2015). Also, plumbagin inhibited TAP-induced invasion and migration by inhibiting MMPs and uPA (Shieh et al. 2010). Plumbagin is also known to inhibit metastasis by abrogation of RANKL-induced NF-kappaB pathway by blocking RANK association with TRAF6 (Li et al. 2012; Sung, Oyajobi, and Aggarwal 2012).

The above pathways in prostate cancer are targeted using a variety of therapeutic agents, some of which are approved, and some of which are still under trial.

6.9.4 Stem Cells

Certain previous studies have shown the effect of plumbagin on various stem cell signaling pathways. Plumbagin is reported to inhibit a ROS generator, nuclear NAD(P)H oxidase (nNOX4), the regulation of which is significant for the pathophysiologic effect in stem cell proliferation (Guida et al. 2013). Plumbagin has also been reported to inhibit stem cell pathways like Notch1 signaling (Qiao et al. 2015) and Wnt signaling pathways (Raghu and Karunagaran 2014). Studies from our laboratory have proved that plumbagin can reduce cancer stem cell population by downregulating EMT and stem cell markers in prostate cancer as well as breast cancer (unpublished data). Further studies need to be done to evaluate the unexplored roles of plumbagin in combating prostate tumorigenesis by targeting the prostate cancer stem cells.

6.10   RADIOSENSITIZATION AND CHEMOSENSITIZATION POTENTIAL OF PLUMBAGIN

Plumbagin possesses the capability to sensitize cancer cells to various treatments. It has been reported to be a potential radiosensitizer by modulating apoptotic pathways in melanoma cells (Prasad et al. 1996; Rao et al. 2015), Ehrlich ascites carcinoma cells (Devi, Rao, and Solomon 1998), as well as in cervical cancer cells (Nair et al. 2008). It has been proved that the cellular redox status plays a significant role in radioresistance of prostate cancer cells (Checker et al. 2015). Ganasoundari, Zare, and Devi (1997) proved that the radiosensitization potential of plumbagin is not tumor-specific. Radiation needs oxygen to have its effect. Plumbagin is a quinone analogue, which can sequester electrons, thus blocking the electron transport chain. Therefore, oxygen will not be used up in the mitochondria, and this high oxygen content can make the cells sensitive to radiation. Radiation treatments improved overall survival of a subgroup of patients with metastatic castrate-resistant prostate cancer (Harrison et al. 2013). Hence, using radiation therapy in combination with plumbagin might be advantageous in these patients.

Plumbagin has also been proved to be a potent chemosensitizer, as it enhances the response of cancer cells to chemotherapeutic agents like paclitaxel (Sandur et al. 2006), thalidomide, bortezomib (Sandur et al. 2010), mitoxanthrone (Shukla et al. 2007), and finasteride (unpublished data from our lab). Mitoxanthrone and finasteride are drugs currently used in prostate cancer therapy. Qiao et al. (2015) reported that a combination of plumbagin and zoledronic acid synergistically suppressed cancer progression by potentiating cancer cell apoptosis. Studies from our lab have proved that use of PARP inhibitors in combination with plumbagin exhibits synergistic activity (unpublished data). Also, plumbagin has been reported to play a protective role against cell damage induced by dexamethasone by regulating antioxidant and apoptotic markers (Zhang et al. 2015). Cytotoxicity of plumbagin is dose-dependent and specific for cancer cells at specific concentration. A combination of plumbagin with other appropriate therapeutic agents can lead to the designing of potent anticancer drugs against human prostate cancer.

6.11   COMMON TUMOR SUPPRESSOR GENES IN PROSTATE CANCER AS MOLECULAR TARGETS OF PLUMBAGIN

A functional interplay between tumor suppressors BRCA, PTEN, and p53 occurs in prostate cancer. BRCA1 and BRCA2 mutations can increase prostate cancer risk as well as predispose patients to early onset and aggressive BRCA-defective cancers. Defective BRCA dependent DNA repair and constitutive AR signaling act together in CRPC (Sundararajan, Ahmed, and Goodman Jr 2011). BRCA-defective cancers have been reported to be more sensitive to DNA damage caused by topoisomerase II inhibitors (Treszezamsky et al. 2007). Plumbagin has been reported to be more effective in BRCA-defective ovarian cancers (Thasni et al. 2008; Srinivas, Annab, et al. 2004). Similarly, our studies showed an increased sensitivity of BRCA-defective breast and prostate cancer cells to plumbagin (unpublished data from our lab). Various synergistic and antagonistic functions exist between BRCA1 and plumbagin, which can be exploited for effective growth inhibition in BRCA1-defective cancer cells (Somasundaram and Srinivas 2012). Somasundaram and Srinivas (2012) showed that both plumbagin and BRCA1 could inhibit DNA replication, tubulin polymerization and estrogen mediated cell growth, whereas induction of DNA double strand breaks and ROS generation by plumbagin could be counteracted by BRCA1. The increased sensitivity of BRCA 1/2 defective tumor cells to topoisomerase II–mediated double strand damage might be due to double strand brake induction at cell cycle phases where BRCA1/2–mediated homologous recombination is prominent or due to other specific interaction between BRCA1/2 and topoisomerase II (Lou, Minter-Dykhouse, and Chen 2005).

When BRCA is mutant, HR (homologous recombination) and NHEJ (non-homologous end joining) will be defective. This principle is used in PARP inhibition for BRCA1-defective cancers. Here, we propose that plumbagin would be effective in such conditions, as ROS induction by plumbagin causes DNA damage which cannot be repaired in a cell which is HR/NHEJ defective.

The most commonly mutated or inactivated genes in prostate cancer are tumor suppressors PTEN and p53. The role of PTEN dysregulation has provided much insight into the mechanisms underlying prostate cancer initiation and progression. Loss of PTEN expression can also be considered as a starting event in BRCA1 associated cancers. Nuclear PTEN along with BRCA1 plays a significant role in DNA repair cell cycle arrest and genomic stability. Hafeez et al. (2015) proved that a deletion of PTEN in prostate epithelium leads to neoplasia followed by invasive adenocarcinoma, and plumbagin inhibits both early stage and CRPC in PTEN knockout mice.

BRCA can interact with p53, and PTEN can regulate p53 protein level and vice versa; these tumor suppressors can cooperatively function upon conditions of oxidative stress and help in tumor suppression (Ongusaha et al. 2003; Chang et al. 2008; Chen et al. 2005). Various controversial reports exist on plumbagin's effect on p53. Plumbagin has been reported to increase p53 level as well as decrease p53 level and also act in p53-independent pathways (K et al. 2013; Kuo, Hsu, and Cho 2006; Sandur et al. 2006; Gomathinayagam et al. 2008; Hsu et al. 2006; Zhao and Lu 2006). Thus, changes in p53 expression by plumbagin might be cancer-specific (Sinha et al. 2013). Powolny and Singh (2008) reported that plumbagin induces apoptosis in human prostate cancer cells irrespective of their p53 status.

6.12   PLUMBAGIN NANOPARTICLES

Nanoformulation of plumbagin nanoparticles (NP) from *Plumbago zeylanica* in silver NP, gold NP, and bimetallic gold-silver NP have gained potential as a natural drug due to its high surface area-to-volume ratio (Salunke et al. 2014). Srinivas et al. (2011) have reported that fabrication of plumbagin in gold NP can reduce the cytotoxicity of PB. Silver NP conjugated plumbagin has been proved to impart selectivity by targeting towards anionic cancerous cells, as well as sensitivity by inducing apoptosis at a lower concentration (Duraipandy et al. 2014). Nano plumbagin is reported to show biocompatibility with normal prostate cells and induce concentration and pH-dependent cytotoxicity on prostate cancer cells. The antimigration and partial apoptosis induction potential makes plumbagin NP a potential agent against prostate cancer (Harikrishnan et al. 2015).

6.13 SUMMARY

Plumbagin, the napthaquinone derivative extracted from roots of plumbago, has been reported to be of great medicinal value since ancient times. Here we have summarized the mechanisms behind the anticancerous potential of plumbagin; however, many mechanisms remain unexplored.

Many molecules/pathways that are causing the transformation of early-stage prostate cancer to CRPC have been now found to be targets of plumbagin. A number of pathways – both AR-dependent and AR-independent – which are now reported to be novel therapeutic targets in prostate cancer therapies are also proved to be the targets of plumbagin. Many of the therapeutic agents targeting these pathways, either clinically approved or under clinical trial, might possess side effects in either a dose-dependent or time-dependent manner. Plumbagin is selectively cytotoxic to cancer cells, as it is proved to be nontoxic to normal cells at lower concentration. Thus, the cytotoxicity of plumbagin is concentration-dependent and specific to cancer cells at the specific concentration. Recently, nanoformulations of the plumbagin nanoparticle, which helps to increase specificity and reduce cytotoxicity, is under study. The chemosensitization and radiosensitization properties of plumbagin can potentiate the effects of a wide range of therapeutics, both those that are clinically approved and those under development. A combinatorial approach using plumbagin and current treatment modalities can lead to designing of potent anticancer drugs against human prostate cancer, which would pave the way to overcoming the ill effects of existing treatment regimes.

ACKNOWLEDGEMENTS

This work was supported by an intramural grant from Rajiv Gandhi Centre for Biotechnology, Kerala State Council for Science Technology and Environment (No. 016/SRSHS/2011/CSTE), and a grant-in-aid from the Board of Research in Nuclear Sciences (No.37(1)/14/16/2014) and the Indian Council of Medical Research (ICMR) (ICMR Project No. 53/20/2012-BMS to PS. R.R.S acknowledges research fellowship from ICMR. The authors also acknowledge the Council for Scientific and Industrial Research, Government of India, for the senior research fellowship to R.N.

REFERENCES

Abedinpour, P., V. T. Baron, A. Chrastina, J. Welsh, and P. Borgstrom. 2013. The combination of plumbagin with androgen withdrawal causes profound regression of prostate tumors in vivo. *Prostate* 73 (5): 489–99.

Acharya, B. R., B. Bhattacharyya, and G. Chakrabarti. 2008. The natural naphthoquinone plumbagin exhibits antiproliferative activity and disrupts the microtubule network through tubulin binding. *Biochemistry* 47(30): 7838–45.

Ahmad, A., S. Banerjee, Z. Wang, D. Kong, and F. H. Sarkar. 2008. Plumbagin-induced apoptosis of human breast cancer cells is mediated by inactivation of NF-kappaB and Bcl-2. *J Cell Biochem* 105(6): 1461–71.

Anuf, A. R., R. Ramachandran, R. Krishnasamy, P. S. Gandhi, and S. Periyasamy. 2014. Antiproliferative effects of Plumbago rosea and its purified constituent plumbagin on SK-MEL 28 melanoma cell lines. *Pharmacognosy Res* 6(4): 312–9.

Arnold, J. T., and J. T. Isaacs. 2002. Mechanisms involved in the progression of androgen-independent prostate cancers: it is not only the cancer cell's fault. *Endocr Relat Cancer* 9(1): 61–73.

Attar, R. M., M. Jure-Kunkel, A. Balog, M. E. Cvijic, J. Dell-John, C. A. Rizzo, L. Schweizer, T. E. Spires, J. S. Platero, M. Obermeier, W. Shan, M. E. Salvati, W. R. Foster, J. Dinchuk, S. J. Chen, G. Vite, R. Kramer, and M. M. Gottardis. 2009. Discovery of BMS-641988, a novel and potent inhibitor of androgen receptor signaling for the treatment of prostate cancer. *Cancer Res* 69(16): 6522–30.

Aziz, M. H., N. E. Dreckschmidt, and A. K. Verma. 2008. Plumbagin, a medicinal plant-derived naphthoquinone, is a novel inhibitor of the growth and invasion of hormone-refractory prostate cancer. *Cancer Res* 68(21): 9024–32.

Beer, T. M., G. T. Bernstein, J. M. Corman, L. M. Glode, S. J. Hall, W. L. Poll, P. F. Schellhammer, L. A. Jones, Y. Xu, J. W. Kylstra, and M. W. Frohlich. 2011. Randomized trial of autologous cellular immunotherapy with sipuleucel-T in androgen-dependent prostate cancer. *Clin Cancer Res* 17(13): 4558–67.

Bosland, M. C. 2005. The role of estrogens in prostate carcinogenesis: a rationale for chemoprevention. *Rev Urol* 7 Suppl 3:S4-S10.

Bruno, R. D., T. S. Vasaitis, L. K. Gediya, P. Purushottamachar, A. M. Godbole, Z. Ates-Alagoz, A. M. Brodie, and V. C. Njar. 2011. Synthesis and biological evaluations of putative metabolically stable analogs of VN/124-1 (TOK-001): head to head anti-tumor efficacy evaluation of VN/124-1 (TOK-001) and abiraterone in LAPC-4 human prostate cancer xenograft model. *Steroids* 76(12): 1268–79.

Chang, C. J., D. J. Mulholland, B. Valamehr, S. Mosessian, W. R. Sellers, and H. Wu. 2008. PTEN nuclear localization is regulated by oxidative stress and mediates p53-dependent tumor suppression. *Mol Cell Biol* 28(10): 3281–9.

Checker, R., L. Gambhir, D. Sharma, M. Kumar, and S. K. Sandur. 2015. Plumbagin induces apoptosis in lymphoma cells via oxidative stress mediated glutathionylation and inhibition of mitogen-activated protein kinase phosphatases (MKP1/2). *Cancer Lett* 357(1): 265–78.

Chen, C. A., H. H. Chang, C. Y. Kao, T. H. Tsai, and Y. J. Chen. 2009. Plumbagin, isolated from Plumbago zeylanica, induces cell death through apoptosis in human pancreatic cancer cells. *Pancreatology* 9(6): 797–809.

Chen, M. B., Y. Zhang, M. X. Wei, W. Shen, X. Y. Wu, C. Yao, and P. H. Lu. 2013. Activation of AMP-activated protein kinase (AMPK) mediates plumbagin-induced apoptosis and growth inhibition in cultured human colon cancer cells. *Cell Signal* 25(10): 1993–2002.

Chen, Z., L. C. Trotman, D. Shaffer, H. K. Lin, Z. A. Dotan, M. Niki, J. A. Koutcher, H. I. Scher, T. Ludwig, W. Gerald, C. Cordon-Cardo, and P. P. Pandolfi. 2005. Crucial role of p53-dependent cellular senescence in suppression of Pten-deficient tumorigenesis. *Nature* 436(7051): 725–30.

Chesis, P. L., D. E. Levin, M. T. Smith, L. Ernster, and B. N. Ames. 1984. Mutagenicity of quinones: pathways of metabolic activation and detoxification. *Proc Natl Acad Sci U S A* 81(6): 1696–700.

Chung, L. Y., T. C. Cheung, S. K. Kong, K. P. Fung, Y. M. Choy, Z. Y. Chan, and T. T. Kwok. 2001. Induction of apoptosis by green tea catechins in human prostate cancer DU145 cells. *Life Sci* 68(10): 1207–14.

Chuu, C. P., R. A. Hiipakka, J. Fukuchi, J. M. Kokontis, and S. Liao. 2005. Androgen causes growth suppression and reversion of androgen-independent prostate cancer xenografts to an androgen-stimulated phenotype in athymic mice. *Cancer Res* 65(6): 2082–4.

Clegg, N. J., J. Wongvipat, J. D. Joseph, C. Tran, S. Ouk, A. Dilhas, Y. Chen, K. Grillot, E. D. Bischoff, L. Cai, A. Aparicio, S. Dorow, V. Arora, G. Shao, J. Qian, H. Zhao, G. Yang, C. Cao, J. Sensintaffar, T. Wasielewska, M. R. Herbert, C. Bonnefous, B. Darimont, H. I. Scher, P. Smith-Jones, M. Klang, N. D. Smith, E. De Stanchina, N. Wu, O. Ouerfelli, P. J. Rix, R. A. Heyman, M. E. Jung, C. L. Sawyers, and J. H. Hager. 2012. ARN-509: a novel antiandrogen for prostate cancer treatment. *Cancer Res* 72(6): 1494–503.

Cookson, M. S., B. J. Roth, P. Dahm, C. Engstrom, S. J. Freedland, M. Hussain, D. W. Lin, W. T. Lowrance, M. H. Murad, W. K. Oh, D. F. Penson, and A. S. Kibel. 2013. Castration-resistant prostate cancer: AUA Guideline. *J Urol* 190(2): 429–38.

Copeland, R. L., Jr., J. R. Das, O. Bakare, N. M. Enwerem, S. Berhe, K. Hillaire, D. White, D. Beyene, O. O. Kassim, and Y. M. Kanaan. 2007. Cytotoxicity of 2,3-dichloro-5,8-dimethoxy-1,4-naphthoquinone in androgen-dependent and -independent prostate cancer cell lines. *Anticancer Res* 27(3B): 1537–46.

Crawford, E. D., and A. H. Hou. 2009. The role of LHRH antagonists in the treatment of prostate cancer. *Oncology (Williston Park)* 23(7): 626–30.

de Bono, J. S., C. J. Logothetis, A. Molina, K. Fizazi, S. North, L. Chu, K. N. Chi, R. J. Jones, O. B. Goodman, Jr., F. Saad, J. N. Staffurth, P. Mainwaring, S. Harland, T. W. Flaig, T. E. Hutson, T. Cheng, H. Patterson, J. D. Hainsworth, C. J. Ryan, C. N. Sternberg, S. L. Ellard, A. Flechon, M. Saleh, M. Scholz, E. Efstathiou, A. Zivi, D. Bianchini, Y. Loriot, N. Chieffo, T. Kheoh, C. M. Haqq, H. I. Scher, and Cou-Aa-Investigators. 2011. Abiraterone and increased survival in metastatic prostate cancer. *N Engl J Med* 364(21): 1995–2005.

Devi, P. U., B. S. Rao, and F. E. Solomon. 1998. Effect of plumbagin on the radiation induced cytogenetic and cell cycle changes in mouse Ehrlich ascites carcinoma in vivo. *Indian J Exp Biol* 36(9): 891–5.

Duraipandy, N., R. Lakra, S. Kunnavakkam Vinjimur, D. Samanta, P. S. K, and M. S. Kiran. 2014. Caging of plumbagin on silver nanoparticles imparts selectivity and sensitivity to plumbagin for targeted cancer cell apoptosis. *Metallomics* 6(11): 2025–33.

Dutt, S. S., and A. C. Gao. 2009. Molecular mechanisms of castration-resistant prostate cancer progression. *Future Oncol* 5(9): 1403–13.

Eisenberger, M. A., B. A. Blumenstein, E. D. Crawford, G. Miller, D. G. McLeod, P. J. Loehrer, G. Wilding, K. Sears, D. J. Culkin, I. M. Thompson, Jr., A. J. Bueschen, and B. A. Lowe. 1998. Bilateral orchiectomy with or without flutamide for metastatic prostate cancer. *N Engl J Med* 339(15): 1036–42.

Eldhose, B., M. Gunawan, M. Rahman, M. S. Latha, and V. Notario. 2014. Plumbagin reduces human colon cancer cell survival by inducing cell cycle arrest and mitochondria-mediated apoptosis. *Int J Oncol* 45(5): 1913–20.

Eschwege, P., F. Dumas, P. Blanchet, V. Le Maire, G. Benoit, A. Jardin, B. Lacour, and S. Loric. 1995. Haematogenous dissemination of prostatic epithelial cells during radical prostatectomy. *Lancet* 346(8989): 1528–30.

Ferlay, J., I. Soerjomataram, R. Dikshit, S. Eser, C. Mathers, M. Rebelo, D. M. Parkin, D. Forman, and F. Bray. 2015. Cancer incidence and mortality worldwide: sources, methods and major patterns in GLOBOCAN 2012. *Int J Cancer* 136(5): E359–86.

Fujii, N., Y. Yamashita, Y. Arima, M. Nagashima, and H. Nakano. 1992. Induction of topoisomerase II-mediated DNA cleavage by the plant naphthoquinones plumbagin and shikonin. *Antimicrob Agents Chemother* 36(12): 2589–94.

Gaascht, F., M. H. Teiten, C. Cerella, M. Dicato, D. Bagrel, and M. Diederich. 2014. Plumbagin modulates leukemia cell redox status. *Molecules* 19(7): 10011–32.

Ganasoundari, A., S. M. Zare, and P. U. Devi. 1997. Modification of bone marrow radiosensitivity by medicinal plant extracts. *Br J Radiol* 70(834): 599–602.

Gomathinayagam, R., S. Sowmyalakshmi, F. Mardhatillah, R. Kumar, M. A. Akbarsha, and C. Damodaran. 2008. Anticancer mechanism of plumbagin, a natural compound, on non-small cell lung cancer cells. *Anticancer Res* 28(2A): 785–92.

Gravina, G. L., M. Tortoreto, A. Mancini, A. Addis, E. Di Cesare, A. Lenzi, Y. Landesman, D. McCauley, M. Kauffman, S. Shacham, N. Zaffaroni, and C. Festuccia. 2014. XPO1/CRM1-selective inhibitors of nuclear export (SINE) reduce tumor spreading and improve overall survival in preclinical models of prostate cancer (PCa). *J Hematol Oncol* 7: 46.

Guida, M., T. Maraldi, E. Resca, F. Beretti, M. Zavatti, L. Bertoni, G. B. La Sala, and A. De Pol. 2013. Inhibition of nuclear Nox4 activity by plumbagin: effect on proliferative capacity in human amniotic stem cells. *Oxid Med Cell Longev* 2013: 680816.

Gupta-Elera, G., A. R. Garrett, R. A. Robison, and K. L. O'Neill. 2012. The role of oxidative stress in prostate cancer. *Eur J Cancer Prev* 21(2): 155–62.

Habib, N. S., A. A. Bekhit, and J. Y. Park. 2003. Synthesis and biological evaluation of some new substituted naphthoquinones. *Boll Chim Farm* 142(5): 232–8.

Hafeez, B. B., J. W. Fischer, A. Singh, W. Zhong, A. Mustafa, L. Meske, M. O. Sheikhani, and A. K. Verma. 2015. Plumbagin inhibits prostate carcinogenesis in intact and castrated PTEN knockout mice via targeting PKCepsilon, Stat3, and epithelial-to-mesenchymal transition markers. *Cancer Prev Res (Phila)* 8(5): 375–86.

Hafeez, B. B., W. Zhong, J. W. Fischer, A. Mustafa, X. Shi, L. Meske, H. Hong, W. Cai, T. Havighurst, K. Kim, and A. K. Verma. 2013. Plumbagin, a medicinal plant (Plumbago zeylanica)-derived 1,4-naphthoquinone, inhibits growth and metastasis of human prostate cancer PC-3M-luciferase cells in an orthotopic xenograft mouse model. *Mol Oncol* 7(3): 428–39.

Hafeez, B. B., W. Zhong, A. Mustafa, J. W. Fischer, O. Witkowsky, and A. K. Verma. 2012. Plumbagin inhibits prostate cancer development in TRAMP mice via targeting PKCepsilon, Stat3 and neuroendocrine markers. *Carcinogenesis* 33(12): 2586–92.

Hafeez, B. B., W. Zhong, J. Weichert, N. E. Dreckschmidt, M. S. Jamal, and A. K. Verma. 2011. Genetic ablation of PKC epsilon inhibits prostate cancer development and metastasis in transgenic mouse model of prostate adenocarcinoma. *Cancer Res* 71(6): 2318–27.

Hafeez, Bilal B, Laurie A Colson, and Ajit K Verma. 2010. Plumbagin a non-toxic natural agent, induces apoptosis and inhibits the growth of prostate cancer LNCaP and C4-2 cells via blocking of both androgen and non-androgen activation of androgen receptor signaling. *Cancer Res* 70(8 Supplement): 3780.

Harikrishnan, A. N., S. K. Snima, R. C. Kamath, S. V. Nair, and V. K. Lakshmanan. 2015. Plumbagin nanoparticles induce dose and pH dependent toxicity on prostate cancer cells. *Curr Drug Deliv.*

Harrison, M. R., T. Z. Wong, A. J. Armstrong, and D. J. George. 2013. Radium-223 chloride: a potential new treatment for castration-resistant prostate cancer patients with metastatic bone disease. *Cancer Manag Res* 5: 1–14.

Hotte, S. J., and F. Saad. 2010. Current management of castrate-resistant prostate cancer. *Curr Oncol* 17 Suppl 2:S72–9.

Hsu, Y. L., C. Y. Cho, P. L. Kuo, Y. T. Huang, and C. C. Lin. 2006. Plumbagin (5-hydroxy-2-methyl-1,4-naphthoquinone) induces apoptosis and cell cycle arrest in A549 cells through p53 accumulation via c-Jun NH2-terminal kinase-mediated phosphorylation at serine 15 in vitro and in vivo. *J Pharmacol Exp Ther* 318(2): 484–94.

Hurwitz, M. 2015. Chemotherapy in prostate cancer. *Curr Oncol Rep* 17(10): 44.

Hwang, G. H., J. M. Ryu, Y. J. Jeon, J. Choi, H. J. Han, Y. M. Lee, S. Lee, J. S. Bae, J. W. Jung, W. Chang, L. K. Kim, J. G. Jee, and M. Y. Lee. 2015. The role of thioredoxin reductase and glutathione reductase in plumbagin-induced, reactive oxygen species-mediated apoptosis in cancer cell lines. *Eur J Pharmacol* 765: 384–393.

Jeyachandran, R, A Mahesh, L Cindrella, S Sudhakar, and K Pazhanichamy. 2009. Antibacterial activity of Plumbagin and root extracts of Plumbago zeylanica L. *Acta Biologica Cracoviensia Series Botanica* 51(1): 17–22.

Joo, M. K., J. J. Park, S. H. Kim, H. S. Yoo, B. J. Lee, H. J. Chun, S. W. Lee, and Y. T. Bak. 2015. Antitumorigenic effect of plumbagin by induction of SH2-containing protein tyrosine phosphatase 1 in human gastric cancer cells. *Int J Oncol* 46(6): 2380–8.

K, A. T., R. T, R. G, C. S. K, R. S. Nair, S. G, A. Banerji, V. Somasundaram, and P. Srinivas. 2013. Structure activity relationship of plumbagin in BRCA1 related cancer cells. *Mol Carcinog* 52(5): 392–403.

Kaku, T., T. Hitaka, A. Ojida, N. Matsunaga, M. Adachi, T. Tanaka, T. Hara, M. Yamaoka, M. Kusaka, T. Okuda, S. Asahi, S. Furuya, and A. Tasaka. 2011. Discovery of orteronel (TAK-700), a naphthylmethyl-imidazole derivative, as a highly selective 17,20-lyase inhibitor with potential utility in the treatment of prostate cancer. *Bioorg Med Chem* 19(21): 6383–99.

Karantanos, T., P. G. Corn, and T. C. Thompson. 2013. Prostate cancer progression after androgen deprivation therapy: mechanisms of castrate resistance and novel therapeutic approaches. *Oncogene* 32(49): 5501–11.

Kawiak, A., J. Piosik, G. Stasilojc, A. Gwizdek-Wisniewska, L. Marczak, M. Stobiecki, J. Bigda, and E. Lojkowska. 2007. Induction of apoptosis by plumbagin through reactive oxygen species-mediated inhibition of topoisomerase II. *Toxicol Appl Pharmacol* 223(3): 267–76.

Khandrika, L., B. Kumar, S. Koul, P. Maroni, and H. K. Koul. 2009. Oxidative stress in prostate cancer. *Cancer Lett* 282(2): 125–36.

Kumar, B., S. Koul, L. Khandrika, R. B. Meacham, and H. K. Koul. 2008. Oxidative stress is inherent in prostate cancer cells and is required for aggressive phenotype. *Cancer Res* 68(6): 1777–85.

Kuo, P. L., Y. L. Hsu, and C. Y. Cho. 2006. Plumbagin induces G2-M arrest and autophagy by inhibiting the AKT/mammalian target of rapamycin pathway in breast cancer cells. *Mol Cancer Ther* 5(12): 3209–21.

Labrie, F., B. Candas, L. Cusan, J. L. Gomez, P. Diamond, R. Suburu, and M. Lemay. 1996. Diagnosis of advanced or noncurable prostate cancer can be practically eliminated by prostate-specific antigen. *Urology* 47(2): 212–7.

Lee, J. H., J. H. Yeon, H. Kim, W. Roh, J. Chae, H. O. Park, and D. M. Kim. 2012. The natural anticancer agent plumbagin induces potent cytotoxicity in MCF-7 human breast cancer cells by inhibiting a PI-5 kinase for ROS generation. *PLoS One* 7(9): e45023.

Li, J., L. Shen, F. R. Lu, Y. Qin, R. Chen, J. Li, Y. Li, H. Z. Zhan, and Y. Q. He. 2012. Plumbagin inhibits cell growth and potentiates apoptosis in human gastric cancer cells in vitro through the NF-kappaB signaling pathway. *Acta Pharmacol Sin* 33(2): 242–9.

Li, Jiawen, Qin Shen, Rui Peng, Rongyi Chen, Ping Jiang, Yanqiu Li, Li Zhang, and Jingjing Lu. 2010. Plumbagin enhances TRAIL-mediated apoptosis through up-regulation of death receptor in human melanoma A375 cells. *Journal of Huazhong University of Science and Technology [Medical Sciences]* 30: 458–463.

Li, T. K., A. Y. Chen, C. Yu, Y. Mao, H. Wang, and L. F. Liu. 1999. Activation of topoisomerase II-mediated excision of chromosomal DNA loops during oxidative stress. *Genes Dev* 13(12): 1553–60.

Li, Y. C., S. M. He, Z. X. He, M. Li, Y. Yang, J. X. Pang, X. Zhang, K. Chow, Q. Zhou, W. Duan, Z. W. Zhou, T. Yang, G. H. Huang, A. Liu, J. X. Qiu, J. P. Liu, and S. F. Zhou. 2014. Plumbagin induces apoptotic and autophagic cell death through inhibition of the PI3K/Akt/mTOR pathway in human non-small cell lung cancer cells. *Cancer Lett* 344(2): 239–59.

Linja, M. J., K. J. Savinainen, T. L. Tammela, J. J. Isola, and T. Visakorpi. 2003. Expression of ERalpha and ERbeta in prostate cancer. *Prostate* 55(3): 180–6.

Liou, G. Y., and P. Storz. 2010. Reactive oxygen species in cancer. *Free Radic Res* 44(5): 479–96.

Liu, X., M. Niu, X. Xu, W. Cai, L. Zeng, X. Zhou, R. Yu, and K. Xu. 2014. CRM1 is a direct cellular target of the natural anti-cancer agent plumbagin. *J Pharmacol Sci* 124(4): 486–93.

Lou, Z., K. Minter-Dykhouse, and J. Chen. 2005. BRCA1 participates in DNA decatenation. *Nat Struct Mol Biol* 12(7): 589–93.

Madan, R. A., M. Mohebtash, P. M. Arlen, M. Vergati, M. Rauckhorst, S. M. Steinberg, K. Y. Tsang, D. J. Poole, H. L. Parnes, J. J. Wright, W. L. Dahut, J. Schlom, and J. L. Gulley. 2012. Ipilimumab and a poxviral vaccine targeting prostate-specific antigen in metastatic castration-resistant prostate cancer: a phase 1 dose-escalation trial. *Lancet Oncol* 13(5): 501–8.

Manu, K. A., M. K. Shanmugam, P. Rajendran, F. Li, L. Ramachandran, H. S. Hay, R. Kannaiyan, S. N. Swamy, S. Vali, S. Kapoor, B. Ramesh, P. Bist, E. S. Koay, L. H. Lim, K. S. Ahn, A. P. Kumar, and G. Sethi. 2011. Plumbagin inhibits invasion and migration of breast and gastric cancer cells by downregulating the expression of chemokine receptor CXCR4. *Mol Cancer* 10: 107.

Marchetti, M., L. Resnick, E. Gamliel, S. Kesaraju, H. Weissbach, and D. Binninger. 2009. Sulindac enhances the killing of cancer cells exposed to oxidative stress. *PLoS One* 4(6): e5804.

McLean, L., U. Soto, K. Agama, J. Francis, R. Jimenez, Y. Pommier, L. Sowers, and E. Brantley. 2008. Aminoflavone induces oxidative DNA damage and reactive oxidative species-mediated apoptosis in breast cancer cells. *Int J Cancer* 122(7): 1665–74.

Meeran, S. M., S. Katiyar, and S. K. Katiyar. 2008. Berberine-induced apoptosis in human prostate cancer cells is initiated by reactive oxygen species generation. *Toxicol Appl Pharmacol* 229(1): 33–43.

Mitsiades, N., C. C. Sung, N. Schultz, D. C. Danila, B. He, V. K. Eedunuri, M. Fleisher, C. Sander, C. L. Sawyers, and H. I. Scher. 2012. Distinct patterns of dysregulated expression of enzymes involved in androgen synthesis and metabolism in metastatic prostate cancer tumors. *Cancer Res* 72(23): 6142–52.

Mizutani, H., S. Tada-Oikawa, Y. Hiraku, S. Oikawa, M. Kojima, and S. Kawanishi. 2002. Mechanism of apoptosis induced by a new topoisomerase inhibitor through the generation of hydrogen peroxide. *J Biol Chem* 277(34): 30684–9.

Mostaghel, E. A., S. T. Page, D. W. Lin, L. Fazli, I. M. Coleman, L. D. True, B. Knudsen, D. L. Hess, C. C. Nelson, A. M. Matsumoto, W. J. Bremner, M. E. Gleave, and P. S. Nelson. 2007. Intraprostatic androgens and androgen-regulated gene expression persist after testosterone suppression: therapeutic implications for castration-resistant prostate cancer. *Cancer Res* 67(10): 5033–41.

Nair, S., R. R. Nair, P. Srinivas, G. Srinivas, and M. R. Pillai. 2008. Radiosensitizing effects of plumbagin in cervical cancer cells is through modulation of apoptotic pathway. *Mol Carcinog* 47(1): 22–33.

Nazeem, S., A. S. Azmi, S. Hanif, A. Ahmad, R. M. Mohammad, S. M. Hadi, and K. S. Kumar. 2009. Plumbagin induces cell death through a copper-redox cycle mechanism in human cancer cells. *Mutagenesis* 24(5): 413–8.

Oh, W. K. 2002. The evolving role of estrogen therapy in prostate cancer. *Clin Prostate Cancer* 1(2): 81–9.

Ongusaha, P. P., T. Ouchi, K. T. Kim, E. Nytko, J. C. Kwak, R. B. Duda, C. X. Deng, and S. W. Lee. 2003. BRCA1 shifts p53-mediated cellular outcomes towards irreversible growth arrest. *Oncogene* 22(24): 3749–58.

Ono, T., A. Ota, K. Ito, T. Nakaoka, S. Karnan, H. Konishi, A. Furuhashi, T. Hayashi, Y. Yamada, Y. Hosokawa, and Y. Kazaoka. 2015. Plumbagin suppresses tumor cell growth in oral squamous cell carcinoma cell lines. *Oral Dis* 21(4): 501–11.

Padhye, S., P. Dandawate, M. Yusufi, A. Ahmad, and F. H. Sarkar. 2012. Perspectives on medicinal properties of plumbagin and its analogs. *Med Res Rev* 32(6): 1131–58.

Pan, S. T., Y. Qin, Z. W. Zhou, Z. X. He, X. Zhang, T. Yang, Y. X. Yang, D. Wang, J. X. Qiu, and S. F. Zhou. 2015. Plumbagin induces G2/M arrest, apoptosis, and autophagy via p38 MAPK- and PI3K/Akt/mTOR-mediated pathways in human tongue squamous cell carcinoma cells. *Drug Des Devel Ther* 9: 1601–26.

Parker, C., S. Nilsson, D. Heinrich, S. I. Helle, J. M. O'Sullivan, S. D. Fossa, A. Chodacki, P. Wiechno, J. Logue, M. Seke, A. Widmark, D. C. Johannessen, P. Hoskin, D. Bottomley, N. D. James, A. Solberg, I. Syndikus, J. Kliment, S. Wedel, S. Boehmer, M. Dall'Oglio, L. Franzen, R. Coleman, N. J. Vogelzang, C. G. O'Bryan-Tear, K. Staudacher, J. Garcia-Vargas, M. Shan, O. S. Bruland, O. Sartor, and Alsympca Investigators. 2013. Alpha emitter radium-223 and survival in metastatic prostate cancer. *N Engl J Med* 369(3): 213–23.

Paschos, A., R. Pandya, W. C. Duivenvoorden, and J. H. Pinthus. 2013. Oxidative stress in prostate cancer: changing research concepts towards a novel paradigm for prevention and therapeutics. *Prostate Cancer Prostatic Dis* 16(3): 217–25.

Powolny, A. A., and S. V. Singh. 2008. Plumbagin-induced apoptosis in human prostate cancer cells is associated with modulation of cellular redox status and generation of reactive oxygen species. *Pharm Res* 25(9): 2171–80.

Prasad, V. S., P. U. Devi, B. S. Rao, and R. Kamath. 1996. Radiosensitizing effect of plumbagin on mouse melanoma cells grown in vitro. *Indian J Exp Biol* 34(9): 857–8.

Qiao, H., T. Y. Wang, W. Yan, A. Qin, Q. M. Fan, X. G. Han, Y. G. Wang, and T. T. Tang. 2015. Synergistic suppression of human breast cancer cells by combination of plumbagin and zoledronic acid in vitro. *Acta Pharmacol Sin* 36(9): 1085–98.

Qiu, J. X., Y. Q. He, Y. Wang, R. L. Xu, Y. Qin, X. Shen, S. F. Zhou, and Z. F. Mao. 2013. Plumbagin induces the apoptosis of human tongue carcinoma cells through the mitochondria-mediated pathway. *Med Sci Monit Basic Res* 19: 228–36.

Qiu, J. X., Z. W. Zhou, Z. X. He, R. J. Zhao, X. Zhang, L. Yang, S. F. Zhou, and Z. F. Mao. 2015. Plumbagin elicits differential proteomic responses mainly involving cell cycle, apoptosis, autophagy, and epithelial-to-mesenchymal transition pathways in human prostate cancer PC-3 and DU145 cells. *Drug Des Devel Ther* 9: 349–417.

Raghu, D., and D. Karunagaran. 2014. Plumbagin downregulates Wnt signaling independent of p53 in human colorectal cancer cells. *J Nat Prod* 77(5): 1130–4.

Rao, Bola Sadashiva Satish, Mandala Rayabandla Sunil Kumar, Shubhankar Das, Kiran Aithal, and Nayanabhirama Udupa. 2015. Radiosensitizing potential of Plumbagin in B16F1 melanoma tumor cells through mitochondrial mediated programmed cell death. *Journal of Applied Biomedicine*.

Ross, D., H. Thor, S. Orrenius, and P. Moldeus. 1985. Interaction of menadione (2-methyl-1,4-naphthoquinone) with glutathione. *Chem Biol Interact* 55(1–2): 177–84.

Saad, F., and S. J. Hotte. 2010. Guidelines for the management of castrate-resistant prostate cancer. *Can Urol Assoc J* 4(6): 380–4.

Salunke, G. R., S. Ghosh, R. J. Santosh Kumar, S. Khade, P. Vashisth, T. Kale, S. Chopade, V. Pruthi, G. Kundu, J. R. Bellare, and B. A. Chopade. 2014. Rapid efficient synthesis and characterization of silver, gold, and bimetallic nanoparticles from the medicinal plant Plumbago zeylanica and their application in biofilm control. *Int J Nanomedicine* 9: 2635–53.

Sandur, S. K., H. Ichikawa, G. Sethi, K. S. Ahn, and B. B. Aggarwal. 2006. Plumbagin (5-hydroxy-2-methyl-1 ,4-naphthoquinone) suppresses NF-kappaB activation and NF-kappaB-regulated gene products through modulation of p65 and IkappaBalpha kinase activation, leading to potentiation of apoptosis induced by cytokine and chemotherapeutic agents. *J Biol Chem* 281(25): 17023–33.

Sandur, S. K., M. K. Pandey, B. Sung, and B. B. Aggarwal. 2010. 5-hydroxy-2-methyl-1,4-naphthoquinone, a vitamin K3 analogue, suppresses STAT3 activation pathway through induction of protein tyrosine phosphatase, SHP-1: potential role in chemosensitization. *Mol Cancer Res* 8(1): 107–18.

Sauer, H., M. Wartenberg, and J. Hescheler. 2001. Reactive oxygen species as intracellular messengers during cell growth and differentiation. *Cell Physiol Biochem* 11(4): 173–86.

Scher, H. I., T. M. Beer, C. S. Higano, A. Anand, M. E. Taplin, E. Efstathiou, D. Rathkopf, J. Shelkey, E. Y. Yu, J. Alumkal, D. Hung, M. Hirmand, L. Seely, M. J. Morris, D. C. Danila, J. Humm, S. Larson, M. Fleisher, C. L. Sawyers, and Consortium Prostate Cancer Foundation/Department of Defense Prostate Cancer Clinical Trials. 2010. Antitumour activity of MDV3100 in castration-resistant prostate cancer: a phase 1–2 study. *Lancet* 375(9724): 1437–46.

Scher, H. I., and C. L. Sawyers. 2005. Biology of progressive, castration-resistant prostate cancer: directed therapies targeting the androgen-receptor signaling axis. *J Clin Oncol* 23(32): 8253–61.

Schmid, H. P., J. E. McNeal, and T. A. Stamey. 1993. Observations on the doubling time of prostate cancer. The use of serial prostate-specific antigen in patients with untreated disease as a measure of increasing cancer volume. *Cancer* 71(6): 2031–40.

Schmitt, B., T. J. Wilt, P. F. Schellhammer, V. DeMasi, O. Sartor, E. D. Crawford, and C. L. Bennett. 2001. Combined androgen blockade with nonsteroidal antiandrogens for advanced prostate cancer: a systematic review. *Urology* 57(4): 727–32.

Schumacker, P. T. 2006. Reactive oxygen species in cancer cells: live by the sword, die by the sword. *Cancer Cell* 10(3): 175–6.

Seifried, H. E., D. E. Anderson, E. I. Fisher, and J. A. Milner. 2007. A review of the interaction among dietary antioxidants and reactive oxygen species. *J Nutr Biochem* 18(9): 567–79.

Shankar, S., G. Suthakar, and R. K. Srivastava. 2007. Epigallocatechin-3-gallate inhibits cell cycle and induces apoptosis in pancreatic cancer. *Front Biosci* 12: 5039–51.

Shieh, J. M., T. A. Chiang, W. T. Chang, C. H. Chao, Y. C. Lee, G. Y. Huang, Y. X. Shih, and Y. W. Shih. 2010. Plumbagin inhibits TPA-induced MMP-2 and u-PA expressions by reducing binding activities of NF-kappaB and AP-1 via ERK signaling pathway in A549 human lung cancer cells. *Mol Cell Biochem* 335(1–2): 181–93.

Shih, Y. W., Y. C. Lee, P. F. Wu, Y. B. Lee, and T. A. Chiang. 2009. Plumbagin inhibits invasion and migration of liver cancer HepG2 cells by decreasing productions of matrix metalloproteinase-2 and urokinase-plasminogen activator. *Hepatol Res* 39(10): 998–1009.

Shukla, S., C. P. Wu, K. Nandigama, and S. V. Ambudkar. 2007. The naphthoquinones, vitamin K3 and its structural analogue plumbagin, are substrates of the multidrug resistance linked ATP binding cassette drug transporter ABCG2. *Mol Cancer Ther* 6(12 Pt 1): 3279–86.

Silvestris, N., B. Leone, G. Numico, V. Lorusso, and M. De Lena. 2005. Present status and perspectives in the treatment of hormone-refractory prostate cancer. *Oncology* 69(4): 273–82.

Singh, S. V., S. K. Srivastava, S. Choi, K. L. Lew, J. Antosiewicz, D. Xiao, Y. Zeng, S. C. Watkins, C. S. Johnson, D. L. Trump, Y. J. Lee, H. Xiao, and A. Herman-Antosiewicz. 2005. Sulforaphane-induced cell death in human prostate cancer cells is initiated by reactive oxygen species. *J Biol Chem* 280(20): 19911–24.

Sinha, S., K. Pal, A. Elkhanany, S. Dutta, Y. Cao, G. Mondal, S. Iyer, V. Somasundaram, F. J. Couch, V. Shridhar, R. Bhattacharya, D. Mukhopadhyay, and P. Srinivas. 2013. Plumbagin inhibits tumorigenesis and angiogenesis of ovarian cancer cells in vivo. *Int J Cancer* 132(5): 1201–12.

Small, E. J., S. Halabi, N. A. Dawson, W. M. Stadler, B. I. Rini, J. Picus, P. Gable, F. M. Torti, E. Kaplan, and N. J. Vogelzang. 2004. Antiandrogen withdrawal alone or in combination with ketoconazole in androgen-independent prostate cancer patients: a phase III trial (CALGB 9583). *J Clin Oncol* 22(6): 1025–33.

Somasundaram, V., and P. Srinivas. 2012. Insights into the targeted elimination of BRCA1-defective cancer stem cells. *Med Res Rev* 32(5): 948–67.

Son, T. G., S. Camandola, T. V. Arumugam, R. G. Cutler, R. S. Telljohann, M. R. Mughal, T. A. Moore, W. Luo, Q. S. Yu, D. A. Johnson, J. A. Johnson, N. H. Greig, and M. P. Mattson. 2010. Plumbagin, a novel Nrf2/ARE activator, protects against cerebral ischemia. *J Neurochem* 112(5): 1316–26.

Srinivas, G., L. A. Annab, G. Gopinath, A. Banerji, and P. Srinivas. 2004. Antisense blocking of BRCA1 enhances sensitivity to plumbagin but not tamoxifen in BG-1 ovarian cancer cells. *Mol Carcinog* 39(1): 15–25.

Srinivas, P., G. Gopinath, A. Banerji, A. Dinakar, and G. Srinivas. 2004. Plumbagin induces reactive oxygen species, which mediate apoptosis in human cervical cancer cells. *Mol Carcinog* 40(4): 201–11.

Srinivas, P., C. R. Patra, S. Bhattacharya, and D. Mukhopadhyay. 2011. Cytotoxicity of naphthoquinones and their capacity to generate reactive oxygen species is quenched when conjugated with gold nanoparticles. *Int J Nanomedicine* 6: 2113–22.

Srivastava, S. K., and S. V. Singh. 2004. Cell cycle arrest, apoptosis induction and inhibition of nuclear factor kappa B activation in anti-proliferative activity of benzyl isothiocyanate against human pancreatic cancer cells. *Carcinogenesis* 25(9): 1701–9.

Sternberg, C. N., P. Whelan, J. Hetherington, B. Paluchowska, P. H. Slee, K. Vekemans, P. Van Erps, C. Theodore, O. Koriakine, T. Oliver, D. Lebwohl, M. Debois, A. Zurlo, L. Collette, and Eortc Genitourinary Tract Group of the. 2005. Phase III trial of satraplatin, an oral platinum plus prednisone vs. prednisone alone in patients with hormone-refractory prostate cancer. *Oncology* 68(1): 2–9.

Subramanyan, R. 2011. Operability in transposition of great arteries with ventricular septal defect: A difficult question – is the answer really so simple? *Ann Pediatr Cardiol* 4(1): 45–6.

Sun, J., and R. J. McKallip. 2011. Plumbagin treatment leads to apoptosis in human K562 leukemia cells through increased ROS and elevated TRAIL receptor expression. *Leuk Res* 35(10): 1402–8.

Sundararajan, Srinath, Aisha Ahmed, and Oscar B Goodman Jr. 2011. The relevance of BRCA genetics to prostate cancer pathogenesis and treatment. *Clin Adv Hematol Oncol* 9(10): 748–55.

Sung, B., B. Oyajobi, and B. B. Aggarwal. 2012. Plumbagin inhibits osteoclastogenesis and reduces human breast cancer-induced osteolytic bone metastasis in mice through suppression of RANKL signaling. *Mol Cancer Ther* 11(2): 350–9.

Tannock, I. F., R. de Wit, W. R. Berry, J. Horti, A. Pluzanska, K. N. Chi, S. Oudard, C. Theodore, N. D. James, I. Turesson, M. A. Rosenthal, M. A. Eisenberger, and T. A. X. Investigators. 2004. Docetaxel plus prednisone or mitoxantrone plus prednisone for advanced prostate cancer. *N Engl J Med* 351(15): 1502–12.

Thasni, K. A., S. Rakesh, G. Rojini, T. Ratheeshkumar, G. Srinivas, and S. Priya. 2008. Estrogen-dependent cell signaling and apoptosis in BRCA1-blocked BG1 ovarian cancer cells in response to plumbagin and other chemotherapeutic agents. *Ann Oncol* 19(4): 696–705.

Thasni, K. A., T. Ratheeshkumar, G. Rojini, K. C. Sivakumar, R. S. Nair, G. Srinivas, Asoke Banerji, V. Somasundaram, and P. Srinivas. 2013. Structure activity relationship of plumbagin in BRCA1 related cancer cells. *Mol Carcinog* 52(5): 392–403.

Tian, L., D. Yin, Y. Ren, C. Gong, A. Chen, and F. J. Guo. 2012. Plumbagin induces apoptosis via the p53 pathway and generation of reactive oxygen species in human osteosarcoma cells. *Mol Med Rep* 5(1): 126–32.

Treszezamsky, A. D., L. A. Kachnic, Z. Feng, J. Zhang, C. Tokadjian, and S. N. Powell. 2007. BRCA1- and BRCA2-deficient cells are sensitive to etoposide-induced DNA double-strand breaks via topoisomerase II. *Cancer Res* 67(15): 7078–81.

Vaverkova, V., O. Vrana, V. Adam, T. Pekarek, J. Jampilek, and P. Babula. 2014. The study of naphthoquinones and their complexes with DNA by using Raman spectroscopy and surface enhanced Raman spectroscopy: new insight into interactions of DNA with plant secondary metabolites. *Biomed Res Int* 2014: 461393.

Wang, C. C., Y. M. Chiang, S. C. Sung, Y. L. Hsu, J. K. Chang, and P. L. Kuo. 2008. Plumbagin induces cell cycle arrest and apoptosis through reactive oxygen species/c-Jun N-terminal kinase pathways in human melanoma A375.S2 cells. *Cancer Lett* 259(1): 82–98.

Wang, F., Q. Wang, Z. W. Zhou, S. N. Yu, S. T. Pan, Z. X. He, X. Zhang, D. Wang, Y. X. Yang, T. Yang, T. Sun, M. Li, J. X. Qiu, and S. F. Zhou. 2015. Plumbagin induces cell cycle arrest and autophagy and suppresses epithelial to mesenchymal transition involving PI3K/Akt/mTOR-mediated pathway in human pancreatic cancer cells. *Drug Des Devel Ther* 9: 537–60.

Wang, H., Y. Mao, A. Y. Chen, N. Zhou, E. J. LaVoie, L. F. Liu. 2001. Stimulation of topoisomerase II-mediated DNA damage via a mechanism involving protein thiolation. *Biochemistry* 40(11): 3316–3323.

Waris, G., and H. Ahsan. 2006. Reactive oxygen species: role in the development of cancer and various chronic conditions. *J Carcinog* 5: 14.

Weckermann, D., and R. Harzmann. 2004. Hormone therapy in prostate cancer: LHRH antagonists versus LHRH analogues. *Eur Urol* 46(3): 279–83; discussion 283–4.

Xu, K. H., and D. P. Lu. 2010. Plumbagin induces ROS-mediated apoptosis in human promyelocytic leukemia cells in vivo. *Leuk Res* 34(5): 658–65.

Xu, T. P., H. Shen, L. X. Liu, and Y. Q. Shu. 2013. Plumbagin from Plumbago zeylanica L induces apoptosis in human non-small cell lung cancer cell lines through NF-kappaB inactivation. *Asian Pac J Cancer Prev* 14(4): 2325–31.

Yan, W., B. Tu, Y. Y. Liu, T. Y. Wang, H. Qiao, Z. J. Zhai, H. W. Li, and T. T. Tang. 2013. Suppressive effects of plumbagin on invasion and migration of breast cancer cells via the inhibition of STAT3 signaling and down-regulation of inflammatory cytokine expressions. *Bone Res* 1(4): 362–70.

Zhang, S., D. Li, J. Y. Yang, and T. B. Yan. 2015. Plumbagin protects against glucocorticoid-induced osteoporosis through Nrf-2 pathway. *Cell Stress Chaperones* 20(4): 621–9.

Zhao, Y. L., and D. P. Lu. 2006. [Effects of plumbagin on the human acute promyelocytic leukemia cells in vitro]. *Zhongguo Shi Yan Xue Ye Xue Za Zhi* 14(2): 208–11.

Zhou, Z. W., X. X. Li, Z. X. He, S. T. Pan, Y. Yang, X. Zhang, K. Chow, T. Yang, J. X. Qiu, Q. Zhou, J. Tan, D. Wang, and S. F. Zhou. 2015. Induction of apoptosis and autophagy via sirtuin1- and PI3K/Akt/mTOR-mediated pathways by plumbagin in human prostate cancer cells. *Drug Des Devel Ther* 9: 1511–54.

CHAPTER 7

Neem and Prostate Cancer Therapy

Krishna Vanaja Donkena and Charles Y.F. Young

CONTENTS

7.1 PROSTATE CANCER

Cancer is the second leading cause of death in the United States after heart disease. The American Cancer Society (ACS) estimates that a total of 1,658,370 new cancer cases and 589,430 cancer deaths are projected to occur in the United States in 2015 (Siegel et al., 2015). Prostate cancer is the most commonly diagnosed cancer and the second leading cause of death after lung and bronchus cancer among men. The estimated new prostate cancer cases and deaths are 220,800 and 27,540, respectively, in 2015, according to ACS (Siegel et al., 2015).

The U.S. Prevention Services Task Force comprises a panel of experts that provides cancer screening recommendations and continually reviews the scientific evidence for the potential benefits and harms of screening (Thomas et al., 2015). Comprehensive lifestyle modifications in diet, activity, stress management, weight control, and social support offer opportunities to reduce the risk of developing prostate cancer (Cuzick et al., 2014). Because of the advances in early diagnosis and treatment, the mortality rate of prostate cancer has declined since the 1970s. Today, the 10-year relative survival rate is about 98%, and the 15-year survival rate is about 90% (Brawley, 2012a; Heidenreich et al., 2014). This means that patients with organ-localized prostate cancer could potentially be cured. Surgery or radiation may be the main optional treatment for prostate-localized cancer. However, studies have shown that about 30% of men who were diagnosed with "apparently" localized disease and treated with radical prostatectomy eventually had relapse. Prostate cancer relapse is commonly detected as a rise of serum prostate-specific antigen (*PSA*) levels (Lu-Yao et al., 1996; Wright et al., 2009). The recurrent cancer may progress to (or already be in) a metastatic state, by which time the cancer has usually become incurable. Unfortunately, less than one-third of men diagnosed with metastatic disease survive 5 years (Brawley, 2012a; 2012b; Howlander et al., 2010).

As indicated above, advanced prostate cancer is deadly; recurrent metastatic prostate cancer is almost incurable. Because androgen signaling is vital for the development, maintenance, and progression of the prostate, androgen deprivation therapy (ADT) was initially proposed by Huggins and Hodges (1941) in the 1940s as an option for treating prostate cancer. Even today, ADT (including the use of antiandrogens or surgical castration) is a critical component as a first-line standard therapy for treating advanced or metastatic prostate cancer. Although ADT is usually effective, it only works for a short duration of treatment. Prostate cancer can evolve to regain the ability to grow despite low levels of circulating androgens (Sun et al., 2010; Chen et al., 2008). Clinical and laboratory evidence strongly indicates that the nuclear androgen receptor (*AR*), the central player of androgen signaling, still plays a critical role in recurrent prostate cancer, which becomes unresponsive to the initial ADT (Attar et al., 2009; Ross et al., 2008; Quintela et al., 2015; Wyatt and Gleave, 2015). Recently, because the majority of these recurrent cancerous tissues persistently express functional *AR* (Vis and Schroder, 2009; Schroder et al., 2010), the term "castration-resistant prostate cancer" (CRPC) has been suggested to replace "hormone refractory prostate cancer" or "androgen-independent prostate cancer" for these unresponsive cancers (Heemers and Mohler, 2014). Intriguingly, these CRPC patients also became resistant to many anti-prostate cancer drugs, including docetaxel, abiraterone, and enzalutamide, which have shown modest but significant improvement of ADT patient survival time (Petrylak et al., 2004; Vaishampayan et al., 2009; Loriot et al., 2013).

Recently, innovative systemic treatments of CRPC have been rapidly developed. CRPC patients may still respond to new second-line therapy of androgen-related treatment with the use of androgen synthesis– or *AR* function–inhibiting drugs (e.g., abiraterone and enzalutamide), then followed, if required, by a sequential or combination treatment with neoadjuvant chemotherapy agents (e.g., docetaxel and cabazitaxel), immunotherapy agents (e.g., sipuleucel-T), or radionuclides (e.g., radium-223) (Quintela et al., 2015; van Dodewaard-de Jong et al., 2015; Nouri et al., 2014; Mukherji et al., 2014; Hoskin et al., 2014). Clearly, CRPC patients have more new options for treatment with significant benefits. Nevertheless, there are still problems that concern patients such as side effects or toxicities (Crawford and Moul, 2015; Nguyen et al., 2015), and the more problematic issue of therapy resistance or disease recurrence after these treatments (Quintela et al., 2015; Wyatt and Gleave, 2015; Loriot et al., 2013; Schrader et al., 2014). Thus, it is urgent that novel and more effective treatments for CRPC be developed.

7.2 NEEM AND ANTICANCER ACTIVITIES

Neem (*Azadirachta indica*) is an evergreen plant native to India and the surrounding countries of Nepal, Pakistan, Bangladesh, and Sri Lanka. Today, neem trees can also be found in parts of Africa and America, as well as other parts of Asia. Neem has important uses in the fields of agriculture, industry, medicine, and the environment (Brahmachari, 2004; Ogbuewu et al., 2011). The tender shoots and flowers of neem plants have also been used as vegetables in some Southeast Asian countries and India (Hao et al., 2014). Neem is one of the main medicinal plants in India, and has been used in Ayurvedic, Unani, and homoeopathy traditional medicine systems for centuries. Its presumably pharmacological properties make it an ideal choice as an antiseptic, antiviral, antipyretic, anti-inflammatory, antiulcer, or antifungal agent (Subapriya and Nagini, 2005; Bodduluru et al., 2014; Veitch et al., 2008).

In traditional medicine, crude extracts have been prepared from different parts of the tree and used for treating various human diseases. Because of its relative safety and its compatibility with other bioactive ingredients that are used in treating human diseases (Paul et al., 2011; Meeran et al., 2013), the extracts, especially from leaves, have been studied to understand their pharmacological actions and molecular mechanisms (Hao et al., 2014; Subapriya and Nagini, 2005; Paul et al., 2011;

Meeran et al., 2013; Subapriya et al., 2005a; Kumar et al., 2006). Neem contains a vast number of bioactive compounds with diverse chemical structures. There are more than 140 chemicals found in various parts of the tree, including leaves, flowers, seeds, fruits, roots, and bark. For convenience, these compounds may be divided into two major groups: isoprenoids and non-isoprenoids (Subapriya and Nagini, 2005; Takagi et al., 2014).

The isoprenoids are mainly diterpenoids and triterpenoids, including protomeliacins, limonoids, azadirone and its derivatives, genudin and its derivatives, vilarin compounds, and csecomeliacins such as nimbin, salannin, and azadirachtin. The non-isoprenoids include polyphenolics such as flavonoids and their glycosides, dihydrochalcone, coumarin, and tannins, aliphatic compounds, phenolic acids, and macro-molecules such as proteins (amino acids) and carbohydrates (polysaccharides), among others (Bandopadhyay et al., 2002; Govindachari et al., 1996; Luo et al., 1999; Siddiqui et al., 2004; Singh et al., 2005).

Neem extracts, as used in traditional medicine, have long been recognized for their ability to reduce cancerous phenotypes. Neem is currently being studied for its anticancer activities in cancer prevention and therapeutic aspects. Neem extracts can be prepared with various solvents including water, or organic solvents such as ethanol, methanol, ether, petrol ether, ethyl acetate, dimethyl sulfoxide, and acetone in which ethanol, methanol, and water are the popular means of preparing the extract for anticancer studies (Hao et al., 2014; Beuth et al., 2006; Schumacher et al., 2011; Udeinya et al., 2008; Sharma et al., 2014b). Accordingly, composition of bioactive components in extracts varies depending on the process of extraction, which will affect the interpretation of the results and present difficulties for comparisons across multiple studies. Also, the involvement and function of individual compounds and their combining action have not been well studied.

Neem leaf extracts prepared mainly by ethanol extraction have shown anti-oxidative, tumor-suppressive, anti-proliferative, apoptosis-inducing, and antiangiogenic activities through modulation of multiple biochemical signaling pathways. These activities and their potential molecular targets have been evaluated by using several *in vitro* cancer cell systems or *in vivo* models. *In vitro* cultured cancer cell systems include prostate (Kumar et al., 2006; Mahapatra et al., 2011; Gunadharini et al., 2011), leukemia (Schumacher et al., 2011; Chitta et al., 2014; Pangjit et al., 2014), pancreas (Veeraraghavan et al., 2011a), breast, and cervix (Sharma et al., 2014b). Neem leaf extract exhibits its capacity to modulate multiple cellular and biochemical pathways. The neem leaf extracts used in these cells or animal models showed anti-proliferative activity by inducing cell cycle arrest via p53-dependent p21 accumulation and downregulation of the cell cycle regulatory proteins cyclin B, cyclin D1, p53, and proliferating cell nuclear antigen (*PCNA*) (Chitta et al., 2014; Subapriya et al; 2006; Elumalai et al., 2012, Sharma et al., 2014a), or other proliferation-related proteins such as phosphoinositide 3-kinase (*PI3K*), p-*Akt* (Gunadharini et al., 2011), and *NF-κB* activity (Schumacher et al., 2011). Eventually cell death may be induced via apoptosis pathway by upregulating pro-apoptotic events or proteins like poly ADP-ribose polymerase 1 (*PARP-1*) and caspase 3 cleavage, *Bax*, and downregulating cell survival signaling-related genes such as *Bcl-2* (Kumar et al., 2006; Sharma et al., 2014b; Mahapatra et al., 2011). One study (Chitta et al., 2014) also suggests that neem extract-induced cell death may be caused, in addition to apoptosis, by autophagy as shown by an increase in LC3-I cleavage. Anticancer or cancer prevention activity of neem extracts by ethanol or methanol extraction may also be associated with its strong free radical scavenging power (Pangjit et al., 2014), and capability of induction of a number of antioxidant enzymes such as glutathione S-transferase (*GST*) cytochrome P450 monooxygenases (*CYP1A1* and *CYP1A2*), and aldo-keto reductase AKR1 family members (*AKR1C1, AKR1C2, AKR1C3,* and *AKR1B10*) (Sharma et al., 2014b; Mahapatra et al., 2011; Vinothini et al., 2009; Manikandan et al., 2008; Wu et al., 2014; Mahapatra et al., 2012) in cultured cell or animal models. In chemically induced carcinogenesis models of mice (Dasgupta et al., 2004), rats (Subapriya et al., 2003; Arumugam et al., 2014; Arakaki et al., 2006), hamsters (Subapriya et al., 2005b; 2006; Balasenthil et al., 1999; Manikandan et al., 2012), or animal tumor models (Mahapatra et al., 2011; Veeraragavan et al., 2011a; Wu et al., 2014; Othman et al., 2011), neem leaf extract demonstrated its high potency in cancer prevention or therapeutic effects by targeting various cellular and biochemical pathways that seem consistent with the findings in cultured cancer cell systems described above. Moreover, neem leaf extract may confer its combining effects by potentiating therapeutic effects of radiotherapy on cultured pancreatic cancer cells or human neuroblastoma xenograft or cisplatin-based chemotherapy on cultured breast and cervical cancer cells via promoting pro-apoptotic signaling and antioxidant enzymes and suppressing survival signaling including *NF-κB* activity (Sharma et al., 2014b; Veeraraghavan et al., 2011a, 2011b). Thus, potentially, neem leaf extract alone or in combination with radiation or chemical therapy can be used to treat radiation- or drug-resistant cancer.

There are many different limonoids/terpenoids identified from the neem leaf or other parts of the tree plant (Takagi et al., 2014; Mahapatra et al., 2011; 2012; Wu et al., 2014; Subapriya and Nagini, 2005; Akihisa et al., 2011). Only a few limonoids, such as azadirachtin, nimbolide, and gedunin, have been studied for their anticancer activities. Both azadirachtin and nimbolide exhibited preventive effects on the development of chemical-induced carcinogenesis by modulating multiple mechanisms, including prevention of procarcinogen activation and oxidative DNA damage, upregulation of antioxidant and carcinogen detoxification enzymes, and inhibition of tumor growth and angiogenesis in an animal model (Priyadarsini et al., 2009; Harish Kumar et al., 2009; 2010). In cell-based studies, these two limonoids showed cancer cell cytotoxicity or induction of cell cycle arrest and apoptosis (Priyadarsini et al., 2009; Akudugu et al., 2001; Cohen et al., 1996; Gupta et al., 2010; 2013). For the above systems tested, nimbolide demonstrated a greater potency than azadirachtin (Priyadarsini et al., 2009; 2010). Nimbolide has been extensively evaluated for its anticancer activities by using several types of tumor cells *in vitro* or *in vivo*, such as neuroblastoma, osteosarcoma, choriocarcinoma, leukemia, and melanoma cells (Harish Kumar et al., 2010; Cohen et al., 1996; Gupta et al., 2010; Roy et al., 2007), glioblastoma (Karkare et al., 2014), and colon cancer cells (Gupta et al., 2013; Roy et al., 2007; Gupta et al., 2011), to demonstrate its tumor inhibition effects through modulating multiple cellular and biochemical pathways. However, gedunin seems to possess a different anticancer action from nimbolide or azadirachtin by acting as an hsp90 inhibitor (Brandt et al., 2008) via direct binding and inactivating the co-chaperone p23 protein (Patwardhan et al., 2013) to cause inhibition of cancer cell proliferation (Uddin et al., 2007; Kamath et al., 2009; Hieronymus et al., 2006).

In addition to organic solvent-based extracts as described above, water-based neem extracts have been prepared to examine anticancer activities. The obvious difference of aqueous neem leaf extract from organic neem leaf extract is its contents, which are mainly water-soluble nonisoprenoids, including proteins, polysaccharides, and other small molecules like amino acids, polyphenols, etc. (Baral et al., 2004; Sarkar et al., 2007). It has been known that various extract preparations of the neem plant may have immunomodulation activities (Roy et al., 2013; Chakraborty et al., 2012; 2011). Aqueous neem leaf extract has been shown to activate humoral and cell-mediated immune responses (Ray et al., 1996) through various immunocompetent cells in order to retard tumor growth (Paul et al., 2011). Aqueous neem leaf extract has shown its potent anticancer activity by enhancing immunogenicity of poorly immunogenic murine Ehrlich's carcinoma, B16 melanoma (Baral et al., 2004), breast tumor-associated antigen (Mandal-Ghosh et al., 2007), sarcoma L-1 cells, and lymphosarcoma RAW cells (Beuth et al., 2006). This immune activation includes stimulation of NK/NK-T cells, macrophage, and the secretion of *TNF-α* (Haque and Baral, 2006) and *IFN-γ* (Bose et al., 2007). Moreover, aqueous neem leaf extract mediates immune activation and protects mice from leukopenia caused by cancer chemotherapy (Ghosh et al., 2006). It has also been shown that glycoproteins, whose molecular weights range from 22 to 65 kDa (Sarkar et al., 2007), isolated from aqueous neem leaf extract, may be the key component contributing to immune-modulating activities of aqueous neem leaf extract against cancer (Sarkar et al., 2008; Chakraborty et al., 2008; Mallick et al., 2013; Goswami et al., 2014; Banerjee et al., 2014).

7.3 NEEM LEAF EXTRACT AND PROSTATE CANCER THERAPY

The anti-androgenic property of neem leaves is evident from the initial studies of Kasturi et al., who showed regression of seminal vesicles and ventral prostate in rats after oral administration of neem leaf powder (Kasturi et al., 2002; 1995). Most of the studies on prostate cancer cells focus on the anticancer activity of nimbolide, a limonoid (Gupta et al., 2011; Babykutty et al., 2012). Nimbolide represents a small fraction (<2%) of the entire neem leaf extract (Gangar and Koul, 2007; Silva et al., 2007). Approximately 77% of compounds present in neem leaves with anticancer activity are unknown. Anti-proliferative activity of both the crude ethanol extract of neem leaves and the isolated compound nimbolide in androgen-independent PC3 prostate cancer cells were mediated through inhibition of *PI3K* and *AKT* pathways that play a vital role in development and progression of prostate cancer (Raja Singh et al., 2014). Bax is an inducer and *Bcl2* is an inhibitor of apoptosis. Ethanol extract of neem leaves induced apoptosis in PC3 cells by inducing *Bax* and inhibiting *Bcl2* expression (Kumar et al., 2006).

In our initial studies, we used ethanol extracts of neem leaves (EENL) obtained by Soxhlet extraction to study anti-cancer effects. Analysis of the components in EENL by mass spectrometry suggested the presence of 2′, 3′-dehydrosalannol, 6-desacetyl nimbinene, and nimolinone. EENL inhibited proliferation of the castration-resistant prostate cancer cells C4-2B and PC3. Genome-wide gene expression changes of these human prostate cancer cells treated with EENL revealed that most of the upregulated genes were associated with functions of cell death and drug metabolism, and the downregulated genes were associated with cell cycle, DNA replication, recombination, and repair functions. We demonstrated the upregulation of the *HMOX1*, *AKR1C1*, *AKR1C2*, *AKR1C3*, and *AKR1B10* in castration-resistant prostate cancer cells C4-2B and PC3 (Mahapatra et al., 2011).

Numerous studies have focused on androgen ablation, by decreased androgen synthesis and blockade of *AR*, as the major treatment for hormone-sensitive prostate cancer (Buchan and Goldenberg, 2010; Quon and Loblaw, 2010). Finasteride and dutasteride are 5α-reductase inhibitors. Despite androgen deprivation therapy in prostate cancer patients, prostatic dihydrotestosterone (DHT) levels were found to be 25% of the pretreatment levels (Nishiyama et al., 2004). Steady-state levels of intracellular DHT are maintained through a balance between local synthetic and catabolic rates. However, little emphasis has been placed on the importance of DHT catabolism in prostate cancer. *AKRs* are phase I drug-metabolizing enzymes for a variety of carbonyl-containing drugs (Jin and Penning, 2007). Compared to paired benign tissues, prostate cancer tissues showed a reduced metabolism of DHT, which corresponded with a loss of *AKR1C2* expression (Ji et al., 2003). Transient expression of *AKR1C2* reduced DHT-stimulated proliferation of LAPC-4 prostate cancer cells (Ji et al., 2007). *AKR1C2* is responsible for the majority of DHT catabolism and predominately reduces DHT to the weak androgen 3α-androstanediol. *AKR1C1* also catalyzes the stereospecific reduction of DHT to the weak androgen 3β-androstanediol. 3β-diol is a ligand for estrogen receptor-β, which promotes anti-proliferative response in the prostate (Ji et al., 2007; Guerini et al., 2005). Cellular proliferation experiments showed that increased *AKR1C2* expression can reduce DHT-stimulated cell growth, and increased metabolism of DHT can block the activation of *AR* (Chakraborty et al., 2008). Thus, androgen catabolism can indirectly regulate the activity of *AR* and thereby provides new therapeutic targets for the treatment of prostate cancer. In early stages of well and moderately differentiated primary malignant tumors *AKR1B10* is overexpressed whereas in advanced tumor stages with low grade of differentiation it is downregulated, implying that *AKR1B10* may be a helpful marker for differentiation (Heringlake et al., 2010). Castration-resistant prostate cancer cells C4-2B and PC3 treated with EENL showed highly significant upregulation in the RNA and protein expression levels of *AKR1C2*, *AKR1C3*, and *AKR1B10* (Mahapatra et al., 2011). We further evaluated the antitumor effects of the EENL using the xenograft prostate cancer models. Mice treated with intraperitoneal injection of EENL (100 and 200 mg/kg body weight) exhibited a drastic reduction in C4-2B and

PC3 xenograft tumor growth (Mahapatra et al., 2011). The increase in *AKRs* could contribute to the suppression of DHT levels observed in the C4-2B tumor tissues of EENL-treated mice. No DHT was detected in the PC3 luciferase-expressing (PC-3M-luc2) tumors, which supports the previous finding that PC-3 cells do not express 5-reductase type II for conversion of testosterone to DHT (Negri-Cesi et al., 1999). We speculate that upregulation of *AKR* expression with EENL treatment, via inactivation of *AR* signaling or activation of non-*AR* pathways, could inhibit cellular proliferation by inducing apoptosis and reduce tumor growth. The proposed model of the AR signaling and the regulation of EENL is depicted (Figure 7.1). EENL promotes degradation of DHT and deactivation of AR by upregulating DHT catabolizing enzymes AKR1C1 and AKR1C2.

Angiogenesis is the growth of blood vessels from the existing vasculature, which is a necessary process for tumor progression. Recognition that inhibiting angiogenesis could lead to cancer therapies has stimulated intensive research in the field and emerged as a valid therapeutic target for solid malignancies (Boehm et al., 2010). Effective targeting of tumor vasculature by the angiogenesis inhibitors could provide crucial suppression of not only tumor growth but also tumor metastasis. Antiangiogenic therapy has been established as a modality in cancer treatment, and the most prominent target of the antiangiogenic compounds is vascular endothelial growth factor (*VEGF*) and its receptors. The safety of the approved antiangiogenic agents (e.g., bavacizumab, sunitnib, and sorafenib) is of special concern when taking these agents for longer-term adjuvant or maintenance treatments (Boehm et al., 2010). A process of angiogenesis comprises several major steps, including proliferation, sprouting, elongation, and migration of endothelial cells. Hence, to control tumor angiogenesis with targeted therapy, a major concern is the side effects from these drugs, which depend largely on what each drug targets. Plant extracts and natural compounds possess various bioactive phytochemicals usually targeting multiple signaling pathways, exhibit less toxicity, and thus are ideal as alternative and complementary forms of cancer treatments that involve the dysregulation of multiple genes (Ng et al., 2010). This has prompted the recent testing for anticancer and antiangiogenic potential of numerous plant extracts such as those from green tea, grape seed, pomegranate juice, soy, garlic, and neem (Varinska et al., 2010). Pomegranate extract is an example having potential clinical effects on treating advanced prostate cancer by prolonging PSA doubling time (Pantuck et al., 2006). These studies indicate that plant extracts could be well-tolerated and inexpensive natural antiangiogenic agents and could potentially be used in cancer prevention and treatment.

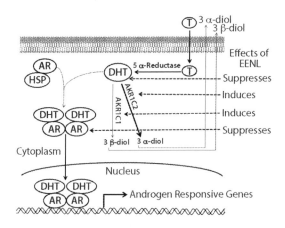

Figure 7.1 Proposed model of the *AR* signaling and the regulation of EENL is depicted. EENL promotes degradation of DHT and deactivation of *AR* by upregulating DHT-catabolizing enzymes *AKR1C1* and *AKR1C2*.

We used EENL to study the effects on angiogenesis because a combination of neem compounds could have a multitargeted approach for regulation of multiple signaling pathways in cancer progression. EENL effects were evaluated on angiogenesis by assessing the tube formation of endothelial cells using a matrigel culture system (Mahapatra et al., 2012). EENL inhibited *VEGF* induced *in vitro* tube formation of human umbilical vein endothelial cells (HUVECs) and blocked the development of vasculature essential for new vessel development *in vivo* necessary for tumor cell proliferation and invasion. The antiangiogenesis activity of EENL is associated with inhibition of *VEGF* activity. Treatment of HUVECs with EENL inhibited proliferation, migration, and invasion. We demonstrated the upregulation of the Heme-oxygenase-1 (*HMOX1*), activating transcription factor 3 (*ATF3*), and early growth response protein 1 (*EGR1*) mRNA and protein expression in HUVECs with EENL treatment. *HMOX1* is an enzyme that catalyzes degradation of heme to carbon monoxide, iron, and biliverdin. It plays a crucial role in vascular disease and cellular defense against stressful conditions (Loboda et al., 2008). A large number of plant extracts and pharmacological compounds (e.g., green tea, curcumin, and statins) have been demonstrated to induce *HMOX1* in various cells (Abdel Aziz et al., 2010; Lee et al., 2004; Wu et al., 2011). Inhibition of *HMOX1* induces leukocyte infiltration and enhances VEGF-induced angiogenesis (Bussolati et al., 2004). Overexpression of *HMOX1* downregulates the *MMP9* expression and decreases the invasive potential in prostate cancer cells (Gueron et al., 2009). Increase in the RNA and protein expression levels of *HMOX1* is associated with inhibition of invasion and migration of HUVECs. The induction of *HMOX1* by EENL treatment could be a possible mechanism to attenuate the excess formation of blood vessels in inflammatory angiogenesis of the cancer. *ATF3* is a stress-inducible transcription factor which regulates genes in processes such as calcium signaling, Wnt, and p53 pathways. It provides the cell with a means of responding to a wide range of environmental insult, thus maintaining DNA integrity and protecting the cell against transformation (Yan et al., 2005). *ATF3* has been demonstrated to play a role in diverse cellular processes such as metabolic pathways, anabolic and catabolic processes, energy generation, cell cycle, apoptosis, adhesion, and cytoskeleton pathways critical for cancer progression (Wang et al. 2010). We demonstrated that EENL treatment increased the expression of *ATF3* in HUVECs. Enforced expression of *ATF3* can restore p53 activity and induce apoptosis of cells; targeting *ATF3* expression through EENL could be a promising strategy for cancer therapy. *EGR-1* is an early response transcription factor with DNA binding activity that activates the transcription of several hundred genes (Khachigian et al., 1996). *EGR-1* controls the expression of genes, many of which play a pivotal role in the regulation of cell growth, differentiation, and apoptosis (Abdel-Malak et al., 2009). Regulation of *HMOX1, ATF3,* and *EGR1* by EENL indicates the importance for further validation of these pathways and antiangiogenic potential in preclinical models and in clinical trials, for successful translation of nontoxic neem treatment into clinical practice to prevent tumor progression.

To obtain higher extraction efficiencies of bioactive compounds present in neem leaves, we adopted a supercritical extraction method (Girotra et al., 2013). The extraction was carried out using supercritical CO_2 (Wu et al., 2014). The supercritical process is a gentle way to extract these delicate plant compounds in order to optimally preserve their potency and stability. During the extraction process we collected volatile oils from the neem leaves. Volatile oils are rich in hydrocarbons consisting of monoterpenes and sesquiterpenes. For example, volatile oils from Nagami kumquats inhibit prostate cancer cell proliferation (Jayaprakasha et al., 2012). Volatile oils can reduce acute and chronic inflammation and, more importantly, help in absorption of other compounds in humans (Jurenka, 2009). The relatively low temperature of the process and the stability of CO_2 allows most compounds to be extracted with little damage or denaturing. This extraction results in a concentrated and potent extract. The half maximal inhibitory concentration (IC_{50}) of EENL to inhibit PC3 cells is 25 µg/mL, whereas the supercritical extraction of neem leaf (SENL) is 15 µg/mL. Compared to EENL, extraction efficacy of compounds were improved with SENL (Wu et al., 2014). Chromatographic separation of

Table 7.1   Major Compounds Identified by Mass-Spectrometric Analysis in HPLC Fractions of SENL

Fraction No.	Major Compounds
2	Nimbandiol and nimbolide
3	2′,3′-Dihydronimbolide
4	Nimbolide, 2′,3′-Dihydronimbolide, and desacetylnimbin
5	Desacetylnimbin and 28-deoxonimbolide
6	28-deoxonimbolide and desacetylSalannin
7	DesacetylSalannin and salannin

compounds in SENL was performed using HPLC column (Figure 7.2 in color insert). Major compounds identified in the SENL are nimbandiol, nimbolide, 2′,3′-dihydronimbolide, desacetylnimbin, 28-deoxonimbolide, desacetyl salannin, and salannin (Table 7.1).

The androgen-dependent LNCaP-luc2 cells were slightly more sensitive to SENL treatment compared to androgen-independent PC3 cells (Wu et al., 2014). This could be due to the differential expression of genes in the cell lines (Chakrabarti et al., 2002). DHT is the most effective androgen to activate *AR* functions (Chang et al., 2011). SENL treatment significantly decreased the expression of DHT-induced *PSA* and intracellular DHT levels in LNCaP cells. To address the role of SENL in suppression of PSA and DHT levels, we analyzed the modulation of DHT-induced *AR* expression levels. SENL significantly inhibited DHT-induced *AR* Serine 81 phosphorylation and total *AR* levels in LNCaP-luc2 cells (Wu et al., 2014).

We showed previously that ethanol extracts from neem leaves induces *AKR1C2* in prostate cancer cells and suppresses DHT levels in xenograft prostate tumor tissues of mice (Mahapatra et al., 2011). *AKR1C2* plays a prominent role in DHT catabolism (Ji et al., 2007). We speculate that an increase in the *AKR1C2* levels with SENL treatment induces degradation of DHT. Reduction in the DHT levels affects ligand-induced stability of the *AR* levels. The effects of SENL on the inhibition of androgen-dependent LNCaP-luc2 cell growth could be partially mediated by downregulation of the androgen-regulated pathways; however, the inhibition of *AR*-negative PC3 cell growth indicates that *AR*-independent mechanisms may be affected by SENL treatment.

Many studies have reported focal adhesion kinase (*FAK*) as a positive regulator of tumor progression (Lechertier and Hodivala-Dilke, 2012; Chang et al., 2007). *FAK* is the primary enzyme involved in the engagement of integrins and assembly of focal adhesion (Infusino and Jacobson, 2012). Phosphorylation of *FAK* at Y-397 has been shown to be elevated in tumor metastasis (Miyazaki et al., 2003). We demonstrated that activation of *FAK* at Y-397 and integrin β1 levels were reduced in SENL-treated cells. Further evidence of inactivation of *FAK* by SENL is demonstrated by our immunofluorescence staining, which reveals inhibition in the formation of focal adhesions in LNCaP-luc2 and PC3 cells (Wu et al., 2014). Our data indicate that SENL may contribute to anti-migration, anti-invasion, and growth-inhibitory effects by suppressing integrin and *FAK* signaling. While the exact mechanism of SENL on inhibition of prostate cancer cells is not completely understood, it appears to entail *FAK* inactivation, *AR* downregulation, and DHT degradation pathways. We postulate that one of the main SENL effects is mediated through regulation of *FAK* required for tumor cell migration and metastasis.

We also demonstrated that oral administration of SENL suppressed prostate cancer xenograft tumor growth (Figure 7.3 in color insert). There were no significant changes in body weight in the SENL-treated groups compared with the control group, which confirms that SENL at both 100 and 200 mg/kg body weight has no adverse physiological effects (Wu et al., 2014). The most significant histologic change observed after SENL treatment in mice was the formation of hyalinized tumor tissue in more than 80% of the mice (200 mg/kg body weight) (Figure 7.4 in color insert).

In our previous study, we observed a similar histological change in the C4-2B and PC3 xenograft tumor tissues of mice treated intraperitoneally with EENL (Mahapatra et al., 2012). Fibrous tissue formation is an indicator of decreased tumor invasiveness and improved tumor regression (Okano et al., 2000; Yamamoto et al., 1999). This histologic feature of hyalinization confirms the tumor regression with SENL treatment. We have shown that SENL treatment of prostate cancer cells *in vitro* reduces *PSA* and increases *AKR1C2* levels (Mahapatra et al., 2011). Immunohistochemistry analysis of SENL-treated mouse tumor tissues revealed reduction in the *PSA* and increase in *AKR1C2* levels, which further supports our *in vitro* findings (Mahapatra et al., 2011). Mass spectrometric analysis of tumor tissues and plasma suggests 28-deoxonimbolide and nimbolide as the bioavailable compound after SENL treatment. We anticipate that SENL can mediate antitumor activity *in vivo* by modulating multiple pathways in tumor development and progression. We speculate that neem, with its low risk of toxicity, can be used safely for prostate cancer prevention and treatment trials.

Terpenoids constitute the largest class of natural compounds for drug discovery (Huang et al., 2012; Yared and Tkaczuk, 2012; Cunningham et al., 2013). More than 70 terpenoids have been identified in the neem plant (Paul et al., 2011; Akhila and Rani, 1999). To our knowledge, nimbolide is the only neem terpenoid reported to have anticancer activity (Gupta et al., 2010; 2013). In addition to nimbolide, we have shown the anticancer activity of other terpenoids from neem leaves, which includes nimbandiol, 2′,3′-dihydronimbolide, and 28-deoxynimbolide in prostate cancer cells (Wu et al., 2014). Therefore these compounds can be further exploited to study their anticancer efficacy. We have shown that terpenoids in SENL are active compounds for inhibition of cancer growth. Anticancer activities of SENL are mediated through regulation of *AR* and *FAK* levels. We have demonstrated the *in vivo* therapeutic potential of SENL in a preclinical prostate cancer model. Further studies are required to elucidate the mechanism of action of isolated neem compounds on inhibition of tumor progression individually and in combinations.

Finally, we would like to emphasize the antioxidant properties of neem for the treatment of cancer and other chronic degenerative diseases such as atherosclerosis, diabetes, heart disease, Alzheimer disease, and Parkinson disease. The protective effects of fruits, vegetables, and other foods on prostate cancer may be due to their antioxidant properties. Antioxidants are chemicals that interact with and neutralize free radicals, thus preventing them from causing damage. The oxygen radical absorbance capacity is a method to measure antioxidant capacity of the samples.

Prostatic inflammation can cause the generation of free radicals (Minciullo et al., 2015). Cellular targets at risk from free radical damage depend on the nature of the radicals and its site of generation. Mitochondria, peroxisomes, and inflammatory cell activation, exogenous sources including

Table 7.2   Antioxidant Levels in Neem and Other Foods

Nutrient	ORAC* per gram
Neem bark	476.00
Neem oil	430.06
Neem leaf	357.00
Cranberry	94.56
Plum	63.39
Blueberry	62.20
Spinach	26.40
Broccoli	15.90
Grapefruit	15.48
Tomato	4.6

*Oxygen radical absorbance capacity

environmental agents, pharmaceuticals, and industrial chemicals can produce reactive oxygen species. Oxidative stress is an imbalance between the production and detoxification of reactive oxygen species that can cause tissue damage. It has been associated with prostate cancer development and progression due to an increase of reactive oxygen species (Freitas et al., 2012). Oxygen radicals are associated with different steps of carcinogenesis, including structural DNA damage, epigenetic changes, protein, and lipid damage, which lead to changes in chromosome instability, genetic mutation, and modulation of cell growth that may result in cancer. During the development of cancer, the body's resources for quenching these free radicals or repairing the damage they cause are inadequate. In laboratory and animal studies, the presence of increased levels of exogenous antioxidants has been shown to prevent the development of cancer (Donkena et al., 2010). As shown in Table 7.2, neem bark, oil, and leaves have high antioxidant effects. Neem leaf compounds, or fractions, have been shown to modulate cellular processes of cancer cells through their antioxidant properties (Manikandan et al., 2008). We conclude that, along with its immune-boosting properties, the presence of high antioxidant levels may help to explain the chemotherapeutic effects of neem on cancer.

7.5 SUMMARY

The reports described above using either EENL or SENL have only identified the major known compounds. Further studies are required to profile and characterize all the compounds present in these extracts. Substantial numbers of current treatment strategies are focused to study single-agent therapy of cancer, but tumorigenesis and progression is a multi-step process, and cancer cells adapt to alternative pathways to survive when a single target is blocked. The most significant of these disadvantages is tumor drug resistance, as this was found to be the most common reason for treatment failure. The improved therapeutic effects of combination chemotherapy or the use of extracts containing multiple compounds may result from both the additive and synergistic effects of the combination of compounds. For successful therapy of heterogeneous prostate cancer with marked variability in patient outcomes, we need to consider further studies to demonstrate how the combination of compounds present in the neem extracts would be beneficial to reduce the risk of resistance and improve therapeutic efficacy with least toxicity.

REFERENCES

Abdel Aziz, M.T. El-Asmar, M.F. El Nadi, E.G. et al. 2010. The effect of curcumin on insulin release in rat-isolated pancreatic islets. *Angiology* 61: 557–566.

Abdel-Malak, N.A. Mofarrahi, M. Mayaki, D. et al. 2009. Early growth response-1 regulates angiopoietin-1-induced endothelial cell proliferation, migration, and differentiation. *Arterioscler Thromb Vasc Biol* 29: 209–216.

Akhila, A. Rani, K. 1999. Chemistry of the neem tree (Azadirachta indica A. Juss.). *Fortschr Chem Org Naturst* 78: 47–149.

Akihisa, T. Takahashi, A. Kikuchi, T. et al. 2011. The melanogenesis-inhibitory, anti-inflammatory, and chemopreventive effects of limonoids in n-hexane extract of Azadirachta indica A. Juss. (neem) seeds. *J Oleo Sci* 60: 53–59.

Akudugu, J. Gade, G. Bohm, L. 2001. Cytotoxicity of azadirachtin A in human glioblastoma cell lines. *Life Sci* 68: 1153–1160.

Arakaki, J. Suzui, M. Morioka, T. et al. 2006. Antioxidative and modifying effects of a tropical plant Azadirachta indica (Neem) on azoxymethane-induced preneoplastic lesions in the rat colon. *Asian Pac J Cancer Prev* 7: 467–471.

Arumugam, A. Agullo, P. Boopalan, T. et al. 2014. Neem leaf extract inhibits mammary carcinogenesis by altering cell proliferation, apoptosis, and angiogenesis. *Cancer Biol Ther* 15: 26–34.

Attar, R.M. Takimoto, C.H. Gottardis, M.M. 2009. Castration-resistant prostate cancer: locking up the molecular escape routes. *Clin Cancer Res* 15: 3251–3255.

Babykutty, S. S, P.P. J, N.R. et al. 2012. Nimbolide retards tumor cell migration, invasion, and angiogenesis by downregulating MMP-2/9 expression via inhibiting ERK1/2 and reducing DNA-binding activity of NF-kappaB in colon cancer cells. *Mol Carcinog* 51: 475–490.

Balasenthil, S. Arivazhagan, S. Ramachandran, C.R. et al. 1999. Chemopreventive potential of neem (Azadirachta indica) on 7,12-dimethylbenz[a]anthracene (DMBA) induced hamster buccal pouch carcinogenesis. *J Ethnopharmacol* 67: 189–195.

Bandyopadhyay, U. Biswas, K. Chatterjee, R. et al. 2002. Gastroprotective effect of Neem (Azadirachta indica) bark extract: possible involvement of H(+)-K(+)-ATPase inhibition and scavenging of hydroxyl radical. *Life Sci* 71: 2845–2865.

Banerjee, S. Ghosh, T. Barik, S. et al. 2014. Neem leaf glycoprotein prophylaxis transduces immune dependent stop signal for tumor angiogenic switch within tumor microenvironment. *PLoS One* 9: e110040.

Baral, R. Chattopadhyay, U. 2004. Neem (Azadirachta indica) leaf mediated immune activation causes prophylactic growth inhibition of murine Ehrlich carcinoma and B16 melanoma. *Int Immunopharmacol* 4: 355–366.

Beuth, J. Schneider, H. Ko, H.L. 2006. Enhancement of immune responses to neem leaf extract (Azadirachta indica) correlates with antineoplastic activity in BALB/c-mice. *In Vivo* 20: 247–251.

Bodduluru, L.N. Kasala, E.R. Thota, N. et al. 2014. Chemopreventive and therapeutic effects of nimbolide in cancer: the underlying mechanisms. *Toxicol In Vitro* 28: 1026–1035.

Boehm, S. Rothermundt, C. Hess, D. et al. 2010. Antiangiogenic drugs in oncology: a focus on drug safety and the elderly – a mini-review. *Gerontology* 56: 303–309.

Bose, A. Haque, E. Baral, R. 2007. Neem leaf preparation induces apoptosis of tumor cells by releasing cytotoxic cytokines from human peripheral blood mononuclear cells. *Phytother Res* 21: 914–920.

Brahmachari, G. 2004. Neem – an omnipotent plant: a retrospection. *Chem BioChem* 5: 408–421.

Brandt, G.E. Schmidt, M.D. Prisinzano, T.E. et al. 2008. Gedunin, a novel hsp90 inhibitor: semisynthesis of derivatives and preliminary structure-activity relationships. *J Med Chem* 51: 6495–6502.

Brawley, O.W. 2012a. Trends in prostate cancer in the United States. *J Natl Cancer Inst Monogr* 2012: 152–6.

Brawley, O.W. 2012b. Prostate cancer epidemiology in the United States. *World J Urol* 30: 195–200.

Buchan, N.C. Goldenberg, S.L. 2010. Intermittent androgen suppression for prostate cancer. *Nat Rev Urol* 7: 552–560.

Bussolati, B. Ahmed, A. Pemberton, H. et al. 2004. Bifunctional role for VEGF-induced heme oxygenase-1 in vivo: induction of angiogenesis and inhibition of leukocytic infiltration. *Blood* 103: 761–766.

Chakrabarti, R. Robles, L.D. Gibson, J. Muroski, M. 2002. Profiling of differential expression of messenger RNA in normal, benign, and metastatic prostate cell lines. *Cancer Genet Cytogenet* 139: 115–125.

Chakraborty, K. Bose, A. Pal, S. et al. 2008. Neem leaf glycoprotein restores the impaired chemotactic activity of peripheral blood mononuclear cells from head and neck squamous cell carcinoma patients by maintaining CXCR3/CXCL10 balance. *Int Immunopharmacol* 8: 330–340.

Chakraborty, T. Bose, A. Barik, S. et al. 2011. Neem leaf glycoprotein inhibits CD4+CD25+Foxp3+ Tregs to restrict murine tumor growth. *Immunotherapy* 3: 949–969.

Chakraborty, T. Bose, A. Goswami, K.K. et al. 2012. Neem leaf glycoprotein suppresses regulatory T cell mediated suppression of monocyte/macrophage functions. *Int Immunopharmacol* 12: 326–333.

Chang, K.H. Li, R. Papari-Zareei, M. et al. 2011. Dihydrotestosterone synthesis bypasses testosterone to drive castration-resistant prostate cancer. *Proc Natl Acad Sci U S A* 108: 13728–13733.

Chang, Y.M. Kung, H.J. Evans, C.P. 2007. Nonreceptor tyrosine kinases in prostate cancer. *Neoplasia* 9: 90–100.

Chen, Y. Sawyers, C.L. Scher, H.I. 2008. Targeting the androgen receptor pathway in prostate cancer. *Curr Opin Pharmacol* 8: 440–448.

Chitta, K.S. Khan, A.N. Ersing, N. et al. 2014. Neem leaf extract induces cell death by apoptosis and autophagy in B-chronic lymphocytic leukemia cells. *Leuk Lymphoma* 55: 652–661.

Cohen, E. Quistad, G.B. Casida, J.E. 1996. Cytotoxicity of nimbolide, epoxyazadiradione and other limonoids from neem insecticide. *Life Sci* 58: 1075–1081.

Crawford, E.D. Moul, J.W. 2015. ADT risks and side effects in advanced prostate cancer: cardiovascular and acute renal injury. *Oncology* 29: 55–58, 65–66.

Cunningham, D. Hawkes, E.A. Jack, A. et al. 2013. Rituximab plus cyclophosphamide, doxorubicin, vincristine, and prednisolone in patients with newly diagnosed diffuse large B-cell non-Hodgkin lymphoma: a phase 3 comparison of dose intensification with 14-day versus 21-day cycles. *Lancet* 381: 1817–1826.

Cuzick, J. Thorat, M.A. Andriole, G. et al. 2014. Prevention and early detection of prostate cancer. *The Lancet Oncol* 15: e484–492.

Dasgupta, T. Banerjee, S. Yadava, P.K. et al. 2004. Chemopreventive potential of Azadirachta indica (Neem) leaf extract in murine carcinogenesis model systems. *J Ethnopharmacol* 92: 23–36.

Donkena, K.V. Young, C.Y. Tindall, D.J. 2010. Oxidative stress and DNA methylation in prostate cancer. *Obstet Gynecol Int* 2010: 302051.

Elumalai, P. Gunadharini, D.N. Senthilkumar, K. et al. 2012. Induction of apoptosis in human breast cancer cells by nimbolide through extrinsic and intrinsic pathway. *Toxicol Lett* 215: 131–142.

Freitas, M. Baldeiras, I. Proenca, T.et al. 2012. Oxidative stress adaptation in aggressive prostate cancer may be counteracted by the reduction of glutathione reductase. *FEBS Open Bio* 2: 119–128.

Gangar, S.C. Koul, A. 2007. Azadirachta indica leaf extract modulates initiation phase of murine forestomach tumorigenesis. *Indian J Biochem Biophys* 44: 209–215.

Ghosh, D. Bose, A. Haque, E. et al. 2006. Pretreatment with neem (Azadirachta indica) leaf preparation in Swiss mice diminishes leukopenia and enhances the antitumor activity of cyclophosphamide. *Phytother Res* 20: 814–818.

Girotra, P. Singh, S.K. Nagpal, K. 2013. Supercritical fluid technology: a promising approach in pharmaceutical research. *Pharm Dev Technol* 18: 22–38.

Goswami, K.K. Barik, S. Sarkar, M. et al. 2014. Targeting STAT3 phosphorylation by neem leaf glycoprotein prevents immune evasion exerted by supraglottic laryngeal tumor induced M2 macrophages. *Mol Immunol* 59: 119–127.

Govindachari, T.R. Narasimhan, N.S. Suresh, G. et al. 1996. Insect antifeedant and growth-regulating activities of Salannin and other c-seco limonoids from neem oil in relation to Azadirachtin. *J Chem Ecol* 22: 1453–1461.

Guerini, V. Sau, D. Scaccianoce, E. et al. 2005. The androgen derivative 5alpha-androstane-3beta,17beta-diol inhibits prostate cancer cell migration through activation of the estrogen receptor beta subtype. *Cancer Res* 65: 5445–5453.

Gueron, G. De Siervi, A. Ferrando, M. et al. 2009. Critical role of endogenous heme oxygenase 1 as a tuner of the invasive potential of prostate cancer cells. *Mol Cancer Res* 7: 1745–1755.

Gunadharini, D.N. Elumalai, P. Arunkumar, R. et al. 2011. Induction of apoptosis and inhibition of PI3K/Akt pathway in PC-3 and LNCaP prostate cancer cells by ethanolic neem leaf extract. *J Ethnopharmacol* 134: 644–650.

Gupta, S.C. Prasad, S. Reuter, S. et al. 2010. Modification of cysteine 179 of IkappaBalpha kinase by nimbolide leads to down-regulation of NF-kappaB-regulated cell survival and proliferative proteins and sensitization of tumor cells to chemotherapeutic agents. *J Biol Chem* 285: 35406–35417.

Gupta, S.C. Prasad, S. Sethumadhavan, D.R. et al. 2013. Nimbolide, a limonoid triterpene, inhibits growth of human colorectal cancer xenografts by suppressing the proinflammatory microenvironment. *Clin Cancer Res* 19: 4465–4476.

Gupta, S.C. Reuter, S. Phromnoi, K. et al. 2011. Nimbolide sensitizes human colon cancer cells to TRAIL through reactive oxygen species- and ERK-dependent up-regulation of death receptors, p53, and Bax. J Biol Chem. 286: 1134–1146.

Hao, F. Kumar, S. Yadav, N. et al. 2014. Neem components as potential agents for cancer prevention and treatment. *BBA* 1846: 247–257.

Haque, E. Baral, R. 2006. Neem (Azadirachta indica) leaf preparation induces prophylactic growth inhibition of murine Ehrlich carcinoma in Swiss and C57BL/6 mice by activation of NK cells and NK-T cells. *Immunobiology* 211: 721–731.

Harish Kumar, G. Chandra Mohan, K.V. Jagannadha Rao, A. et al. 2009. Nimbolide a limonoid from Azadirachta indica inhibits proliferation and induces apoptosis of human choriocarcinoma (BeWo) cells. *Invest New Drugs* 27: 246–252.

Harish Kumar, G. Vidya Priyadarsini, R. Vinothini, G. et al. 2010. The neem limonoids azadirachtin and nimbolide inhibit cell proliferation and induce apoptosis in an animal model of oral oncogenesis. *Invest New Drugs* 28: 392–401.

Heemers, H.V. Mohler, J.L. 2014. Revisiting nomenclature for the description of prostate cancer androgen-responsiveness. *Am J Clin Exp Urol* 2: 121–126.

Heidenreich, A. Bastian, P.J. Bellmunt, J. et al. 2014. EAU guidelines on prostate cancer. Part II: treatment of advanced, relapsing, and castration-resistant prostate cancer. *Eur Urol* 65: 467–479.

Heringlake, S. Hofdmann, M. Fiebeler, A. et al. 2010. Identification and expression analysis of the aldo-ketoreductase1-B10 gene in primary malignant liver tumours. *J Hepatol* 52: 220–227.

Hieronymus, H. Lamb, J. Ross, K.N. et al. 2006. Gene expression signature-based chemical genomic prediction identifies a novel class of HSP90 pathway modulators. *Cancer Cell* 10: 321–330.

Hoskin, P. Sartor, O. O'Sullivan, J.M. et al. 2014. Efficacy and safety of radium-223 dichloride in patients with castration-resistant prostate cancer and symptomatic bone metastases, with or without previous docetaxel use: a prespecified subgroup analysis from the randomised, double-blind, phase 3 ALSYMPCA trial. *The Lancet Oncol* 15: 1397–1406.

Howlader, N. Ries, L.A. Mariotto, A.B. et al. 2010. Improved estimates of cancer-specific survival rates from population-based data. *J Natl Cancer Inst* 102: 1584–1598.

Huang, M. Lu, J.J. Huang, M.Q. et al. 2012. Terpenoids: natural products for cancer therapy. *Expert Opin Investig Drug* 21: 1801–1818.

Huggins, C. Hodges, C.V. 1941. Studies on prostatic cancer: I. The effect of castration, of estrogen and of androgen injection on serum phosphatases in metastatic carcinoma of the prostate. *J Urol* 168: 9–12.

Infusino, G.A. Jacobson, J.R. 2012. Endothelial FAK as a therapeutic target in disease. *Microvasc Res*. 83: 89–96.

Jayaprakasha, G.K. Murthy, K.N. Demarais, R. et al. 2012. Inhibition of prostate cancer (LNCaP) cell proliferation by volatile components from Nagami kumquats. *Planta Med* 78: 974–980.

Ji, Q. Chang, L. Stanczyk, F.Z. et al. 2007. Impaired dihydrotestosterone catabolism in human prostate cancer: critical role of AKR1C2 as a pre-receptor regulator of androgen receptor signaling. *Cancer Res* 67: 1361–1369.

Ji, Q. Chang, L. VanDenBerg, D. et al. 2003. Selective reduction of AKR1C2 in prostate cancer and its role in DHT metabolism. *Prostate* 54: 275–289.

Jin, Y. Penning, T.M. 2007. Aldo-keto reductases and bioactivation/detoxication. *Annu Rev Pharmacol Toxicol* 47: 263–292.

Jurenka, J.S. 2009. Anti-inflammatory properties of curcumin, a major constituent of Curcuma longa: a review of preclinical and clinical research. *Altern Med Rev* 14: 141–153.

Kamath, S.G. Chen, N. Xiong, Y. et al. 2009. Gedunin, a novel natural substance, inhibits ovarian cancer cell proliferation. *Int J Gynecol Cancer* 19: 1564–1569.

Karkare, S. Chhipa, R.R. Anderson, J. et al. 2014. Direct inhibition of retinoblastoma phosphorylation by nimbolide causes cell-cycle arrest and suppresses glioblastoma growth. *Clin Cancer Res* 20: 199–212.

Kasturi, M. Ahamed, R.N. Pathan, K.M. et al. 2002. Ultrastructural changes induced by leaves of Azadirachta indica (Neem) in the testis of albino rats. *J Basic Clin Physiol Pharmacol* 13: 311–328.

Kasturi, M. Manivannan, B. Ahamed, R.N. et al. 1995. Changes in epididymal structure and function of albino rat treated with Azadirachta indica leaves. *Indian J Exp Biol* 33: 725–729.

Khachigian, L.M. Lindner, V. Williams, A.J. et al. 1996. Egr-1-induced endothelial gene expression: a common theme in vascular injury. *Science* 271: 1427–1431.

Kumar, S. Suresh, P.K. Vijayababu, M.R. et al. 2006. Anticancer effects of ethanolic neem leaf extract on prostate cancer cell line (PC-3). *J Ethnopharmacol* 105: 246–250.

Lechertier, T. Hodivala-Dilke, K. 2012. Focal adhesion kinase and tumour *angiogenesis*. *J Pathol* 226: 404–412.

Lee, T.S. Chang, C.C. Zhu, Y. et al. 2004. Simvastatin induces heme oxygenase-1: a novel mechanism of vessel protection. *Circulation* 110: 1296–1302.

Loboda, A. Jazwa, A. Grochot-Przeczek, A. et al. 2008. Heme oxygenase-1 and the vascular bed: from molecular mechanisms to therapeutic opportunities. *Antioxid Redox Signal* 10: 1767–1812.

Loriot, Y. Bianchini, D. Ileana, E. et al. 2013. Antitumour activity of abiraterone acetate against metastatic castration-resistant prostate cancer progressing after docetaxel and enzalutamide (MDV3100). *Ann Oncol* 24: 1807–1812.

Luo, X. Ma, Y. Wu, S. et al. 1999. Two novel azadirachtin derivatives from azadirachta indica. *J Nat Prod* 62: 102210–102214.

Lu-Yao, G.L. Potosky, A.L. Albertsen, P.C. et al. 1996. Follow-up prostate cancer treatments after radical prostatectomy: a population-based study. *J Natl Cancer Inst* 88: 166–173.

Mahapatra, S. Karnes, R.J. Holmes, M.W. et al. 2011. Novel molecular targets of Azadirachta indica associated with inhibition of tumor growth in prostate cancer. *AAPS J* 13: 365–377.

Mahapatra, S. Young, C.Y. Kohli, M. et al. 2012. Antiangiogenic effects and therapeutic targets of Azadirachta indica leaf extract in endothelial cells. *Evid Based Complementary Altern Med* 2012: 303019.

Mallick, A. Barik, S. Goswami, K.K. et al. 2013. Neem leaf glycoprotein activates CD8(+) T cells to promote therapeutic anti-tumor immunity inhibiting the growth of mouse sarcoma. *PLoS One* 8: e47434.

Mandal-Ghosh, I. Chattopadhyay, U. Baral, R. 2007. Neem leaf preparation enhances Th1 type immune response and anti-tumor immunity against breast tumor associated antigen. *Cancer Immun* 7: 8.

Manikandan, P. Ramalingam, S.M. Vinothini, G. et al. 2012. Investigation of the chemopreventive potential of neem leaf subfractions in the hamster buccal pouch model and phytochemical characterization. *Eur J Med Chem* 56: 271–281.

Manikandan, P. Letchoumy, P.V. Gopalakrishnan, M. et al. 2008. Evaluation of Azadirachta indica leaf fractions for in vitro antioxidant potential and in vivo modulation of biomarkers of chemoprevention in the hamster buccal pouch carcinogenesis model. *Food Chem Toxicol* 46: 2332–2343.

Meeran, M. Murali, A. Balakrishnan, R. Narasimhan, D. 2013. "Herbal remedy is natural and safe" – truth or myth? *J Assoc Physicians India* 61: 848–650.

Minciullo, P.L. Inferrera, A. Navarra, M. et al. 2015. Oxidative stress in benign prostatic hyperplasia: a systematic review. *Urol Int* 94: 249–254.

Miyazaki, T. Kato, H. Nakajima, M. et al. 2003. FAK overexpression is correlated with tumour invasiveness and lymph node metastasis in oesophageal squamous cell carcinoma. *Br J Cancer* 89: 140–5.

Mukherji, D. Omlin, A. Pezaro, C. et al. 2014. Metastatic castration-resistant prostate cancer (CRPC): preclinical and clinical evidence for the sequential use of novel therapeutics. *Cancer Metastasis Rev* 33: 555–566.

Negri-Cesi, P. Colciago, A. Poletti, A. et al. 1999. 5alpha-reductase isozymes and aromatase are differentially expressed and active in the androgen-independent human prostate cancer cell lines DU145 and PC3. *Prostate* 41: 224–232.

Ng, K.W. Salhimi, S.M. Majid, A.M. et al. 2010. Anti-angiogenic and cytotoxicity studies of some medicinal plants. *Planta Med* 76: 935–940.

Nguyen, P.L. Alibhai, S.M. Basaria, S. et al. 2015. Adverse effects of androgen deprivation therapy and strategies to mitigate them. *Eur Urol* 7: 825–836.

Nishiyama, T. Hashimoto, Y. Takahashi, K. 2004. The influence of androgen deprivation therapy on dihydrotestosterone levels in the prostatic tissue of patients with prostate cancer. *Clin Cancer Res* 10: 7121–7126.

Nouri, M. Ratther, E. Stylianou, N. et al. 2014. Androgen-targeted therapy-induced epithelial mesenchymal plasticity and neuroendocrine transdifferentiation in prostate cancer: an opportunity for intervention. *Front Oncol* 4: 370.

Ogbuewu, I.P. Unamba-Oparah, I.C. Odoemenam, V.U. et al. 2011. The potentiality of medicinal plants as the source of new contraceptive principles in males. *N Am J Med Sci* 3: 255–263.

Okano, K. Yamamoto, J. Kosuge, T. et al. 2000. Fibrous pseudocapsule of metastatic liver tumors from colorectal carcinoma. Clinicopathologic study of 152 first resection cases. *Cancer* 89: 267–75.

Othman, F. Motalleb, G. Lam Tsuey Peng, S. et al. 2011. Extract of Azadirachta indica (neem) leaf induces apoptosis in 4T1 breast cancer BALB/c mice. *Cell J* 13: 107–116.

Pangjit, K. Tantiphaipunwong, P. Sajjapong, W. et al. 2014. Iron-chelating, free radical scavenging and antiproliferative activities of Azadirachta indica. *J Med Assoc Thai* 97 Suppl 4: S36–S43.

Pantuck, A.J. Leppert, J.T. Zomorodian, N. et al. 2006. Phase II study of pomegranate juice for men with rising prostate-specific antigen following surgery or radiation for prostate cancer. *Clin Cancer Res* 12: 4018–4026.

Patwardhan, C.A. Fauq, A. Peterson, L.B. et al. 2013. Gedunin inactivates the co-chaperone p23 protein causing cancer cell death by apoptosis. *J Biol Chem* 288: 7313–7325.

Paul, R. Prasad, M. Sah, N.K. 2011. Anticancer biology of Azadirachta indica L (neem): a mini review. *Cancer Biol Ther* 12: 467–476.

Petrylak, D.P. Tangen, C.M. Hussain, M.H. et al. 2004. Docetaxel and estramustine compared with mitoxantrone and prednisone for advanced refractory prostate cancer. *N Engl J Med* 351: 1513–1520.

Priyadarsini, R.V. Manikandan, P. Kumar, G.H. et al. 2009. The neem limonoids azadirachtin and nimbolide inhibit hamster cheek pouch carcinogenesis by modulating xenobiotic-metabolizing enzymes, DNA damage, antioxidants, invasion and angiogenesis. *Free Radic Res* 43: 492–504.

Priyadarsini, R.V. Murugan, R.S. Sripriya, P. et al. 2010. The neem limonoids azadirachtin and nimbolide induce cell cycle arrest and mitochondria-mediated apoptosis in human cervical cancer (HeLa) cells. *Free Radic Res* 44: 624–634.

Quintela, M.L. Mateos, L.L. Estevez, S.V. et al. 2015. Enzalutamide: a new prostate cancer targeted therapy against the androgen receptor. *Cancer Treat Rev* 41: 247–253.

Quon, H. Loblaw, D.A. 2010. Androgen deprivation therapy for prostate cancer-review of indications in 2010. *Curr Oncol* 17 Suppl 2:S38–44.

Raja Singh, P. Arunkumar, R. Sivakamasundari, V. et al. 2014. Anti-proliferative and apoptosis inducing effect of nimbolide by altering molecules involved in apoptosis and IGF signalling via PI3K/Akt in prostate cancer (PC-3) cell line. *Cell Biochem Funct* 32: 217–228.

Ray, A. Banerjee, B.D. Sen, P. 1996. Modulation of humoral and cell-mediated immune responses by Azadirachta indica (Neem) in mice. *Indian J Exp Biol* 34: 698–701.

Ross, R.W. Oh, W.K. Xie, W. et al. 2008. Inherited variation in the androgen pathway is associated with the efficacy of androgen-deprivation therapy in men with prostate cancer. *J Clin Oncol* 26: 842–847.

Roy, M.K. Kobori, M. Takenaka, M. et al. 2007. Antiproliferative effect on human cancer cell lines after treatment with nimbolide extracted from an edible part of the neem tree (Azadirachta indica). *Phytother Res* 21: 245–250.

Roy, S. Barik, S. Banerjee, S. et al. 2013. Neem leaf glycoprotein overcomes indoleamine 2,3 dioxygenase mediated tolerance in dendritic cells by attenuating hyperactive regulatory T cells in cervical cancer stage IIIB patients. *Hum Immunol* 74: 1015–1023.

Sarkar, K. Bose, A. Chakraborty, K. et al. 2008. Neem leaf glycoprotein helps to generate carcinoembryonic antigen specific anti-tumor immune responses utilizing macrophage-mediated antigen presentation. *Vaccine* 26: 4352–62.

Sarkar, K. Bose, A. Laskar, S. et al. 2007. Antibody response against neem leaf preparation recognizes carcinoembryonic antigen. *Int Immunopharmacol* 7: 306–312.

Schrader, A.J. Boegemann, M. Ohlmann, C.H. et al. 2014. Enzalutamide in castration-resistant prostate cancer patients progressing after docetaxel and abiraterone. *Eur Urol* 65: 30–36.

Schroder, F.H. van den Bergh, R.C. Wolters, T. et al. 2010. Eleven-year outcome of patients with prostate cancers diagnosed during screening after initial negative sextant biopsies. *Eur Urol* 57: 256–266.

Schumacher, M. Cerella, C. Reuter, S. et al. 2011. Anti-inflammatory, pro-apoptotic, and anti-proliferative effects of a methanolic neem (Azadirachta indica) leaf extract are mediated via modulation of the nuclear factor-kappaB pathway. *Genes Nutr* 6: 149–160.

Sharma, C. Mansoori, M.N. Dixit, M. et al. 2014a. Ethanolic extract of Coelogyne cristata Lindley (Orchidaceae) and its compound coelogin promote osteoprotective activity in ovariectomized estrogen deficient mice. *Phytomedicine* 21: 1702–1707.

Sharma, C. Vas, A.J. Goala, P. et al. 2014b. Ethanolic neem (Azadirachta indica) leaf extract prevents growth of MCF-7 and HeLa cells and potentiates the therapeutic index of cisplatin. *J Oncol* 2014: 321754.

Siddiqui, B.S. Afshan, F. Gulzar, T. et al. 2004. Tetracyclic triterpenoids from the leaves of Azadirachta indica. *Phytochemistry* 65: 2363–2367.

Siegel, R.L. Miller, K.D. Jemal, A. 2015. Cancer statistics, 2015. *CA: Cancer J Clin* 65: 5–29.

Silva, J.C. Jham, G.N. Oliveira, R.D. et al. 2007. Purification of the seven tetranortriterpenoids in neem (Azadirachta indica) seed by counter-current chromatography sequentially followed by isocratic preparative reversed-phase high-performance liquid chromatography. *J Chromatogr* 1151: 203–210.

Singh, U.P. Maurya, S. Singh, D.P. 2005. Phenolic acids in neem (Azadirachta indica): a major pre-existing secondary metabolite. *J Herb Pharmacother* 5: 35–43.

Subapriya, R. Bhuvaneswari, V. Nagini, S. 2005a. Ethanolic neem (Azadirachta indica) leaf extract induces apoptosis in the hamster buccal pouch carcinogenesis model by modulation of Bcl-2, Bim, caspase 8 and caspase 3. *Asian Pac J Cancer Prev* 6: 515–520.

Subapriya, R. Bhuvaneswari, V. Ramesh, V. et al. 2005b. Ethanolic leaf extract of neem (Azadirachta indica) inhibits buccal pouch carcinogenesis in hamsters. *Cell Biochem Funct* 23: 229–238.

Subapriya, R. Kumaraguruparan, R. Chandramohan, K.V. et al. 2003. Chemoprotective effects of ethanolic extract of neem leaf against MNNG-induced oxidative stress. *Pharmazie* 58: 512–517.

Subapriya, R. Kumaraguruparan, R. Nagini, S. 2006. Expression of PCNA, cytokeratin, Bcl-2 and p53 during chemoprevention of hamster buccal pouch carcinogenesis by ethanolic neem (Azadirachta indica) leaf extract. *Clin Biochem* 39: 1080–1087.

Subapriya, R. Nagini, S. 2005. Medicinal properties of neem leaves: a review. *Curr Med Chem Anticancer Agents* 5: 149–146.

Sun, S. Sprenger, C.C. Vessella, R.L. et al. 2010. Castration resistance in human prostate cancer is conferred by a frequently occurring androgen receptor splice variant. *J Clin Invest* 120: 2715–2730.

Takagi, M. Tachi, Y. Zhang, J. et al. 2014. Cytotoxic and melanogenesis-inhibitory activities of limonoids from the leaves of Azadirachta indica (Neem). *Chem Biodiv* 11: 451–468.

Thomas, C.C. Richards, T.B. Plescia, M. et al. 2015. CDC Grand Rounds: the future of cancer screening. *Morb Mortal Wkly Rep* 64: 324–327.

Uddin, S.J. Nahar, L. Shilpi, J.A. et al. 2007. Gedunin, a limonoid from Xylocarpus granatum, inhibits the growth of CaCo-2 colon cancer cell line in vitro. *Phytother Res* 21: 757–761.

Udeinya, J.I. Shu, E.N. Quakyi, I. et al. 2008. An antimalarial neem leaf extract has both schizonticidal and gametocytocidal activities. *Am J Ther* 15: 108–110.

Vaishampayan, U.N. Marur, S. Heilbrun, L.K. et al. 2009. Phase II trial of capecitabine and weekly docetaxel for metastatic castrate resistant prostate cancer. *J Urol* 182: 317–323.

van Dodewaard-de Jong, J.M. Verheul, H.M. Bloemendal, H.J. et al. 2015. New treatment options for patients with metastatic prostate cancer: what is the optimal sequence? *Clin Genitourin Cancer* 13: 271–279.

Varinska, L. Mirossay, L. Mojzisova, G. et al. 2010. Antiangogenic effect of selected phytochemicals. *Pharmazie* 65: 57–63.

Veeraraghavan, J. Aravindan, S. Natarajan, M. et al. 2011a. Neem leaf extract induces radiosensitization in human neuroblastoma xenograft through modulation of apoptotic pathway. *Anticancer Res* 31: 161–170.

Veeraraghavan, J. Natarajan, M. Lagisetty, P. et al. 2011b. Impact of curcumin, raspberry extract, and neem leaf extract on rel protein-regulated cell death/radiosensitization in pancreatic cancer cells. *Pancreas* 40: 1107–1119.

Veitch, G.E. Pinto, A. Boyer, A. et al. 2008. Synthesis of natural products from the Indian neem tree Azadirachta indica. *Org Lett* 10: 569–572.

Vinothini, G. Manikandan, P. Anandan, R. et al. 2009. Chemoprevention of rat mammary carcinogenesis by Azadirachta indica leaf fractions: modulation of hormone status, xenobiotic-metabolizing enzymes, oxidative stress, cell proliferation and apoptosis. *Food Chem Toxicol* 47: 1852–1863.

Vis, A.N. Schroder, F.H. 2009. Key targets of hormonal treatment of prostate cancer. Part 2: the androgen receptor and 5alpha-reductase. *BJU Int* 104: 1191–1197.

Wang, H. Mo, P. Ren, S. Yan, C. 2010. Activating transcription factor 3 activates p53 by preventing E6-associated protein from binding to E6. *J Biol Chem* 285: 13201–13210.

Wright, J.L. Salinas, C.A. Lin, D.W. et al. 2009. Prostate cancer specific mortality and Gleason 7 disease differences in prostate cancer outcomes between cases with Gleason 4 + 3 and Gleason 3 + 4 tumors in a population based cohort. *J Urol* 182: 2702–2777.

Wu, Q. Kohli, M. Bergen, H.R. 3rd. et al. 2014. Preclinical evaluation of the supercritical extract of azadirachta indica (neem) leaves in vitro and in vivo on inhibition of prostate cancer tumor growth. *Mol Cancer Ther* 13: 1067–1077.

Wu, T.Y. Khor, T.O. Saw, C.L. et al. 2011. Anti-inflammatory/anti-oxidative stress activities and differential regulation of Nrf2-mediated genes by non-polar fractions of tea Chrysanthemum zawadskii and licorice Glycyrrhiza uralensis. *AAPS J* 13: 1–13.

Wyatt, A.W. Gleave, M.E. 2015. Targeting the adaptive molecular landscape of castration-resistant prostate cancer. *EMBO Mol Med* 7: 878–894.

Yamamoto, J. Shimada, K. Kosuge, T. et al. 1999. Factors influencing survival of patients undergoing hepatectomy for colorectal metastases. *Br J Surg* 86: 332–337.

Yan, C. Lu, D. Hai, T. et al. 2005. Activating transcription factor 3, a stress sensor, activates p53 by blocking its ubiquitination. *EMBO J* 24: 2425–2435.

Yared, J.A. Tkaczuk, K.H. 2012. Update on taxane development: new analogs and new formulations. *Drug Des Devel Ther* 6: 371–384.

CHAPTER 8

Kava in Prostate Cancer Prevention and Treatment

Arman Walia, Nikta Rezakahn Khajeh, Michael Wu, Cyrus Khoyilar, and Xiaolin Zi

CONTENTS

ABBREVIATIONS

AR:	androgen receptor
ADT:	androgen deprivation therapy
CRPC:	castration-resistant prostate cancer
CYP17A1:	cytochrome P450, family 17, subfamily A, polypeptide 1
DBD:	DNA-binding domain
DHT:	dihydrotestosterone
GnRH:	gonadotropin-releasing hormone
HR:	hinge region

LBD: carboxyl ligand-binding domain
LH: luteinizing hormone
NAE: NEDDylation activation enzyme
NEDD8: precursor cell-expressed developmentally downregulated 8
NTD: amino terminal activation domain
PCa: prostate cancer
PIN: prostatic intraepithelial neoplasia
PSA: prostate-specific antigen
Pten: phosphatase and tensin homolog
Rb: retinoblastoma protein
Skp2: S-phase kinase-associated protein 2
TMPRSS2: transmembrane protease, serine 2
TRAIL: TNF-related apoptosis-inducing ligand
TRAMP: The autochthonous transgenic adenocarcinoma of the mouse prostate

8.1 KAVA ROOT EXTRACTS AND ITS ACTIVE COMPONENTS

Kava-kava, scientifically recognized as *Piper methysticum*, is a plant that originates from the Pacific Islands. For thousands of years it has been embedded in the culture of the region, extracted and served frequently, from informal social gatherings to traditional ceremonies (Kuchta et al. 2015). Kava's appeal stems from its neuropharmacologic properties: an intoxicating agent that produces sedative, anxiolytic, and analgesic effects. As a result, the plant has been studied and utilized for its therapeutic value across the globe. In certain areas of the Pacific (Micronesia, Melanesia, and Polynesia) (Figure 8.1 in color insert), kava is reportedly used to calm nerves, prevent fatigue, and treat insomnia. The Western world has also adopted the substance as a commercialized health supplement. The understanding of kava's therapeutic reach is still growing, which indicates a need for continued study.

Kava root extracts are composed of a complex mixture of phytochemicals. Kavalactones are the most abundant components in kava root extracts (Dharmaratne et al. 2002). They are a group of naturally-occurring stereoisomers, mainly including Kawain, Yangonin, Dihydrokawain, Methysticin, Demethoxyyangonin, and Dihydromethysticin (Figure 8.2). For over 2,000 years, the traditional method of extraction involved removing the root, cleaning, cutting, and macerating it (Singh 1992). Then the root is infused with water and coconut milk; it is strained and then ready to drink. More standardized methods of extraction involve 60% of either ethanol, which yields approximately 30% kavalactones or acetone, which yields 70% kavalactones (Côté et al. 2004). Such methods are used industrially to extract kavalactones, specifically for dietary supplement use in countries like Germany, Australia, and the United States.

Chalcones, the other main components of kava extracts, are a mixture of three diastereomers: flavokawains A, B, and C (Dharmaratne et al. 2002). These structures substitute as 5, 6-dihydro-alpha-pyrones with similar backbones but different side chains (Figure 8.2). Flavokawain A is the most abundant chalcone found in kava root extracts, at an average concentration of 0.46%, while flavokawain B and C constitute up to 0.015 and 0.012%, respectively (Dharmaratne et al. 2002). Flavokawains are derived from flavonoids and can be synthesized out of plant roots by the Claisen-Schmidt condensation method (Jandial et al. 2014).

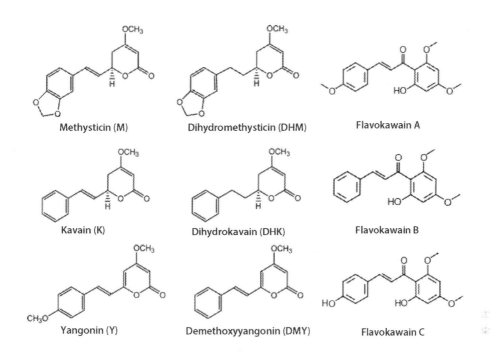

Figure 8.2 Chemical structures of main kava components.

8.2 KAVA CONSUMPTION AND PROSTATE CANCER

Interest in kava's potential role in cancer prevention and treatment sparked from epidemiologic analysis of kava consumption in populations of the Pacific Islands. Tobacco is a known leading cause of cancer, and despite widespread use of tobacco in the region cancer incidence in the South Pacific island nations has remained low (Henderson et al. 1985; Rasanathan and Tukuitonga 2007). Fiji, for example, has significantly higher smoking rates but just 5–10% of the incidence of lung cancer as compared to the United States. Uniquely, in three kava drinking countries (Vanuatu, Fiji, and Western Samoa) more men drink kava and smoke than do women, yet there is a lower incidence of cancer for men than for women (Steiner 2000). The Cancer Council in New South Wales released a particularly interesting report on migrants during 1991–2001, stating that the occurrence of prostate cancer (PCa) in Fijian men who migrated to New South Wales, Australia increased by 5 times (Supramaniam et al. 2006). This emphasized the importance of investigating the influences of the environment and dietary habits on cancer prevention in the region. An epidemiological study observed an inverse relationship between kava consumption and cancer incidence in the South Pacific Islands (Steiner 2000). It reported that the age-standardized cancer incidence in countries with the highest kava consumption (Vanuatu, Fiji, and Western Samoa) was one-third to one-fourth the rate of that in non-kava–drinking countries in the region such as New Zealand and Maoris (Steiner 2000; Rasanathan and Tukuitonga 2007). Kava has therefore been increasingly studied for its potential as a cancer preventive and therapeutic agent.

8.3 PROSTATE CANCER

PCa is responsible for 3% of men's total deaths and 10% of men's deaths by cancer in the United States (US). One-sixth of US men will be diagnosed with PCa and more than two million are living with it (Tabayoyong and Abouassaly 2015). Thus, PCa is a major public health burden. Asian/Pacific men who consume a low fat and plant-based diet have the lowest rates of clinical PCa in the world (Jemal et al. 2010). However, when Asian men migrate to the US, rates of clinical PCa increase (Haenszel and Kurihara 1968). These observations implicate both environmental factors and dietary habits (such as consumption of low-fat and plant-based diet) in PCa development. Therefore, one of the strategies for prevention and treatment of PCa has focused on the use of natural and synthetic bioactive food components.

A PCa diagnosis holds different meaning for different patients. It can be detected early or late, which determines the severity of the disease as well as the treatment course. Early-stage PCa is typically treated by some combination of active surveillance, radiation therapy, and radical prosta-tectomy (Akram et al. 2015). Late-stage PCa generally requires a more aggressive approach with hormone therapy.

Healthy prostatic tissue utilizes androgenic stimulation for growth and maintenance, a char-acteristic retained by most PCa cells. Hormone therapy, or androgen deprivation therapy (ADT), manipulates the androgen receptor (AR)–signaling axis to inhibit tumor growth. There are two main types of ADT. The first aims to reduce circulating androgen levels, specifically testosterone and dihydrotestosterone (DHT), which act as ligands to activate the AR. Androgen production in the testes is regulated by luteinizing hormone (LH) released from the pituitary. Gonadotropin-releasing hormone (GnRH) agonists/antagonists (i.e. Leuprolide, Degarelix) are delivered to suppress LH and ultimately reduce gonadal androgen production. However, the gonads are not the body's only androgen factory; the adrenal glands contribute as well. The other form of ADT, termed antiandro-gen therapy, uses antiandrogens (i.e. flutamide, bicalutamide, nilutamide) to prevent the binding of androgens to the AR, and can therefore serve as a complementary treatment to LH suppression.

Despite the short-term efficacy of ADT, many PCa patients inevitably develop resistance to the attempted androgen signaling blockade, resulting in castration-resistant prostate cancer (CRPC). Prostate-specific antigen (PSA) is used as a serum marker for PCa, and is expressed as an andro-gen dependent gene (Penning 2014). Increased levels of PSA in CRPC patients therefore indicates continued, adaptive AR signaling in the presence of lowered androgen levels (Kasper and Cookson 2006). Studies have shown aberrant AR activation in CRPC can be accomplished through mul-tiple mechanisms including AR amplification, AR mutation, AR splice variation, and intratumoral androgen biosynthesis (Visakorpi et al. 1995). The importance of AR function in CRPC indicates a need for further investigation of the AR as a target for treatment.

There have been recent developments in this regard, particularly drugs capable of either AR dysfunction or inhibition of extragonadal androgen biosynthesis. The AR is a ligand-activated transcription factor that consists of four domains: an amino terminal activation domain (NTD), DNA-binding domain (DBD), hinge region (HR), and carboxyl ligand-binding domain (LBD) (Eisermann et al. 2013). Androgens bind the LBD to promote dissociation of the AR from heat shock proteins and translocation into the nucleus (Dar et al. 2014). Subsequent dimerization and DNA binding allow the NTD to promote transcriptional activation of target genes (Jenster et al. 1991). Enzalutamide (XTANDIÒ), a currently prescribed treatment for metastatic CRPC patients, competitively binds to the LBD of the AR. It not only prevents binding of androgen to the AR, but also is able to disrupt nuclear localization and transcriptional activation of AR target genes (Tran et al. 2009). Abiraterone (ZYTIGAÒ), another recently introduced drug, reduces androgen production to a greater extent than standard ADT by inhibiting the enzyme cytochrome P450, family 17, sub-family A, polypeptide 1 (CYP17A1). CYP17A1 catalyzes androgen synthesis in testicular, adrenal, and prostatic tumor tissues; thus, abiraterone reduces intratumoral and adrenal androgen synthesis in addition to suppression of gonadal testosterone synthesis (O'Donnell et al. 2004).

Similar to primary ADT, second-generation hormone therapies like enzalutamide and abiraterone are also temporally limited. The leading method of treatment evasion by CRPC cells is androgen insensitivity, in the form of overactive AR splice variants and, in a minority of patients, AR-negative PCa cells (Mosca et al. 2005).

8.4 SUPPRESSION OF ANDROGEN RECEPTOR EXPRESSION BY KAVA ROOT EXTRACTS AND ITS ACTIVE COMPONENTS

AR plays a key role in PCa development and progression. AR signaling has been a valid and critical target for development of both preventive and therapeutic agents against PCa at different stages (Siddique et al. 2012). The kava root extract and its active components have therefore been studied individually and in combination, and exhibit differential mechanisms of AR downregulation (Li et al. 2012).

In PCa cell lines, the kava root extract and individual kavalactones, including kawain, 5′, 6′-dehydrokawain, yangonin, and methysticin, markedly decrease mRNA expression of the AR target genes PSA and TMPRSS2, whereas AR mRNA levels remain largely unaffected. Western blotting analysis revealed both the kava root extract and individual kavalactones decrease AR and PSA protein expression through reduction of the AR protein stability.

In contrast to the kava extract and kavalactone, flavokawain B, a kava chalcone, inhibits AR mRNA expression by downregulating protein expression of an AR transcriptional factor Sp1 and its binding to the AR promoter. In addition, flavokawain B downregulates the expression of AR in prostate stromal cells.

The AR splice variant V7, lacking the ligand-binding domain and a constitutively active transcription factor, has been shown to predict the resistance to the second generation of anti-androgen drugs enzalutamide and abiraterone (Antonarakis et al. 2014). We have shown that both flavokawain B and 5′, 6′-dehydrokawain are more effective in decreasing the expression of the AR-splicing variant V7 than that of the AR full length (Li et al. 2012). Moreover, kavalactones and flavokawain B act synergistically or additively to downregulate protein expression of both AR and the AR splice variant V7, leading to lower PSA levels (Li et al. 2012). These results suggested that in the kava root extract, kavalactones in combination with flavokawain B may play a dominant role for inhibiting expression of ARs and their target genes.

Approaches that target androgen synthesis or androgen-AR interactions frequently result in development of drug resistance. In responding to lower levels of androgens, PCa and stromal cells overexpress AR, interact with coactivators, and generate AR mutations or splice variant to adapt for the low androgen environment (Watson et al. 2015). The demonstrated effect of the kava root extract and its active components on downregulation of AR and its splice variant expression in both epithelial cells and stromal cells around tumor microenvironment may have the potential to overcome or prevent resistance to current anti-androgen therapies.

8.5 *IN VITRO* GROWTH INHIBITION OF PROSTATE CANCER CELL LINES BY KAVA ROOT EXTRACTS AND ITS ACTIVE COMPONENTS

The kava root extract similarly inhibited androgen sensitive (LNCaP and LAPC-4) and insensitive PCa cell lines (C4-2B, 22Rv1, PC3 and DU145) with IC_{50s} ranging from 5.3 to 46 µg/mL (Li et al. 2012). The kava root extract was more potent than kavalactones but less potent than flavokawain B in inhibiting the growth. Among the kavalactones, 5´, 6´-dehydrokawain is the most potent agent in inhibiting the growth of PCa cell lines. Flavokawain B is about 6–2.5 and 11–1.5 times more effective than the kava root extract and 5´, 6´-dehydrokawain, respectively, in inhibition of PCa cell growth except for LNCaP cells (Li et al. 2012). The kava root extract is equally effective in inhibiting the growth of androgen-sensitive LNCaP and its CRPC derivative C4-2B, while flavokawain B is about 4.5 times more effective in reducing the growth of C4-2B cells than the growth of LNCaP cells (Li et al. 2012).

Interestingly, flavokawain B exhibits greater inhibition in AR-negative CRPC cells than AR-positive PCa cells, with minimal effect on normal prostate epithelial and stromal cells (Tang et al. 2010). Furthermore, both flavokawains A and B selectively inhibit the growth of Rb-deficient cells and PCa cell lines with overexpression of Skp2 (Li et al. 2015). Skp2 expression can be induced by ADT and plays a role in castration resistance (Chuu et al. 2011). These results suggested that Skp2 may be a main target for flavokawains A and B's inhibitory effect on PCa cell growth.

8.6 A KAVA CHALCONE FLAVOKAWAIN B INDUCES APOPTOSIS IN PROSTATE CANCER CELLS

The growth-inhibitory effect of flavokawain B is due to induction of apoptosis. Flavokawain B activates an extrinsic apoptotic pathway through increasing the mRNA and protein expression of death receptor 5 (DR5) (Tang et al. 2010). Flavokawain B also acts synergistically with TNF-related apoptosis-inducing ligand (TRAIL), a ligand for death receptor, to induce apoptosis (Tang et al. 2010). In addition, flavokawain B induces mitochondrial-mediated apoptosis via increasing the expression of proapoptotic proteins Bax, Puma, and Bim and downregulating the expression of anti-apoptotic proteins XIAP and surviving (Tang et al. 2010). Flavokawain A, another kava chalcone, induces apoptosis in cancer cells by similar mechanisms of action (Zi and Simoneau 2005). These results indicate that flavokawains A and B are robust apoptosis inducers.

8.7 FLAVOKAWAIN A IS A NOVEL NEDDYLATION INHIBITOR AND DEGRADES SKP2 PROTEIN

Skp2 is a critical oncogene and overexpressed in human PCa (Robbins et al. 2011; Yang et al. 2002; Nguyen et al. 2011). Skp2 was shown to be required for spontaneous tumor development that occurs in the pRb, the p19Arf, and Pten deficient mouse models (Wang et al. 2010; Lin et al. 2010). Since either mutated or silenced Pten and Rb are common in PCa (Suzuki et al. 1998; Kubota et al. 1995; Bettendorf et al. 2008), Skp2 represents an appealing drug target for PCa prevention and therapy. We have shown that flavokawain A, a kava chalcone, downregulated the protein expression of Skp2 in all tested cancer cell lines that were derived from prostate, breast, renal, liver, lung, colon, and cervical cancers, melanoma, and osteosarcoma regardless of their genetic background (Li et al. 2015). Flavokawain A induces a proteasome-dependent and ubiquitination-mediated Skp2 degradation (Li et al. 2015). Skp2 ubiquitination and degradation can be mediated either (1) by the Cdh1/APC E3 complex (Bashir et al. 2004) or (2) through an autocatalytic mechanism involving a Skp2-bound Cullin1-based core ubiquitin ligase (Wirbelauer et al. 2000). Similar to ubiquitination, NEDDylation of Cullin1 is involved in sequential attachment of NEDD8 to a thiolester within a specific cysteine site of NEDD8-E1 (NEDDylation activation enzyme, NAE) and NEDD8-E2 (Ubc12) (Soucy et al. 2009). Degradation of Skp2 by flavokawain A was found to be involved in a functional Cullin1, but independent of Cdh1 expression. Further studies have demonstrated that FKA docked into the ATP-binding pocket of the NAE complex, inhibited NEDD8 conjugations to both Cullin1 and Ubc12 in PC3 cells and Ubc12 NEDDylation in an *in vitro* assay. These results indicate that flavokawain A is a novel cell active inhibitor for targeting Skp2 degradation in PCa prevention and treatment.

8.8 *IN VIVO* INHIBITION OF TUMOR GROWTH BY KAVA ROOT EXTRACTS AND ITS ACTIVE COMPONENTS

8.8.1   DU145 Xenograft Model (Tang et al. 2010)

Oral administration of 50 mg/kg flavokawain B daily for 24 days on mice bearing established DU145 tumors resulted in a significant decrease in the growth rate of tumors compared with control group. Flavokawain B treatment reduced tumor growth by 67%. Oral administration of flavokawain B did not affect the body weight gain and diet and water consumption. The mice also did not show any gross abnormalities on necropsy at the end of the treatment. Immunohistochemical and Western blotting analysis shows that flavokawain B treatment induces the expression of pro-apoptotic protein Bim in tumor tissues.

8.8.2   Prostate Cancer Patient-Derived Xenograft Model (Li et al. 2012)

The use of PCa patient-derived xenograft models is thought to be more clinically relevant than the current use of cell lines and transgenic mouse model of PCa, as these models faithfully preserve the histopathological and genotypical characteristics of the original clinical samples (Lin et al. 2014). Two PCa patient-derived xengrafts lines, GM0308 and RC0309, were established by using a subrenal xenograft technique. The GM0308 line was derived from a high-grade (Gleason score sum = 5+5) PCa prostatectomy specimen obtained from a patient who was previously treated with ADT, docetaxel plus carboplatin, and etoposide plus cisplatin. The RC0309 line was derived from a high-grade (Gleason score sum = 5+4) PCa prostatectomy specimen obtained from a patient who had no previous treatments. Both lines secrete PSA into the host mouse serum. The GM0308 line expresses a truncated AR around 80 KDa, without missense mutations in exons 3, 4, or 5. In contrast, RC0309 holds the full length AR.

200 mg/kg flavokawain B daily by intraperitoneal injection into mice bearing GM0308 tumors for 28 days markedly reduced tumor growth by 77.3% and decreased the serum PSA levels by 68% at the end of the treatment. The body weight gain and diet and water consumption of the flavokawain B–treated mice were similar to the control group of mice. In addition, the mice did not show any gross abnormalities on necropsy.

Similarly, dietary feeding of 6 g/kg kava root extract to mice bearing RC0309 tumors for 18 days also resulted in a significant decrease in the growth rate of tumors by approximately 60.1% and the serum PSA levels by 42%. However, dietary feeding of the commercial kava extract also resulted in a decrease in food uptake, wet spleen and kidney weight, and body weight, as well as an increase in wet liver weight. These results suggest that unidentified components of the kava extract, but not flavokawain B, may be toxic to immunodeficient mice.

Immunohistochemical analysis shows that tumor sections from the flavokawain B or the kava root extract treated PCa xenografts exhibited a significant decrease in both density and the number of positive AR staining cells compared to those of vehicle control treatments. In addition, both flavokawain B and kava root extract treatments downregulated mRNA expression of AR target genes PSA and TMPRSS2.

8.8.3 The TRAMP Transgenic Mouse Model (Li et al. 2015)

The autochthonous transgenic adenocarcinoma of the mouse prostate (TRAMP) model develops histological prostatic intraepithelial neoplasia (PIN) that progress to adenocarcinoma with distant site metastases, which recapitulates many salient aspects of human PCa (Gingrich et al. 1996). The model is useful to understand stage-specific effects of agents for prevention and treatment of PCa. To examine whether flavokawain A will inhibit different stages of PCa development, a cohort of TRAMP mice were treated under two different protocols: (1) a prevention protocol in which mice were fed with food supplemented with vehicle control or 0.3% flavokawian A (3 g/kg food) starting from 6 weeks of age and ending at 12 weeks of age; and (2) an intervention protocol in which mice were fed with food that was supplemented with vehicle control or 0.6% flavokawain A (3 g/kg food) starting from 12 weeks of age (when overt cancers are established) and ending at 24 weeks of age (Li et al. 2015). Dietary feeding of 0.3% flavokawain A inhibited high grade (HG)-PIN by 69%. In addition, 12-week FKA feeding of TRAMP mice from the age of 12 weeks significantly decreased the tumor burden. The number of palpable tumors was decreased by about 73% in TRAMP mice fed with 0.6% FKA food compared to those fed with vehicle control, and no metastasis was seen in 0.6% FKA–fed mice.

The *in vivo* mechanisms of the action of flavokawain A are associated with anti-proliferation and induction of apoptosis. Immunohistochemistry and Western blotting studies revealed that Skp2 is strongly expressed in the hyperplastic/dysplastic regions whereas dietary feeding with flavokawain A significantly decreases Skp2 and NEDD8 expression and increases the expression of p27/Kip1 in the prostate of TRAMP mice. Flavokawain A treatment did not result in a decrease in expression of the transgene SV40T and body weight or the weight of liver and kidney. No other signs of toxicity were identified with flavokawain A treatments.

Similarly, in the prevention protocol, TRAMP mice were fed with 3 or 6 g (0.3% or 0.6%) kava root extract/kg food starting at 6 weeks of age and ending at 12 weeks of age, resulting in decreased numbers of HG-PIN and moderately differentiated adenocarcinomas compared to the mice fed with control food (Li et al. 2014). In the intervention protocol, in which TRAMP mice were fed with 0.3% or 0.6% kava root extract food starting at 6 weeks of age and ending at 24 weeks of age, the average genitourinary (GU) weight of 0.6% kava root extract–fed mice was significantly reduced when compared to control food–fed mice (Li et al. 2014). The percentages of large tumors (GU weight >0.9 gram) were also decreased from 86.4% in the control group to 52.2% and 43.5% in 0.3 and 0.6% kava food groups, respectively (Li et al. 2014).

8.9 KAVA TOXICITY AND SAFETIES OF ITS ACTIVE COMPONENTS

Traditional kava preparation has been safely consumed on a daily basis for thousands of years (Currie and Clough 2003). However, there were rare reported cases of hepatotoxicity (0.25/1,000,000) linked to the use of commercial kava extracts in Western countries, which is lower than the rate of hepatic adverse effects (0.90–2.12 cases/1,000,000) for many daily-use drugs (e.g., anxiolytic benzodiazepines) (Clouatre 2004). Currently very little research has been done to prove or disprove the toxicity of kava root extracts. Given a long history of human kava use in the South Pacific Islands, it is unlikely that all active kava components are toxic to humans. Recent studies in preclinical settings have been focused on the safety of active components, mainly kavalactones and flavokawains, in kava root extracts.

In a study to identify nontoxic chemopreventive candidates for lung cancer from kava, methysticin demonstrated the highest NF-κB inhibitory activity ($IC_{50} = 0.19 \pm 0.01$ µg/ml) among the tested kavalactones with no toxicity towards a liver cell line, Hepa 1c1c7 ($IC_{50} \sim 400$ µg/ml) (Shaik et al.

2009). Also in a cytotoxicity test against normal rat hepatocytes, methysticin had an IC_{50} of 63 μg/mL. However, achievable kavalactone concentration in human blood was reported to be only about 3 μg/ml (Mathews et al. 2005). Toxicological studies in animals and human hepatocytes have found no evidence of hepatotoxicity for aqueous kava extracts or kavalactones (Singh et al. 2003). These studies suggest that kavalactones, in particular methysticin alone, are less likely to be the hepatoxic agents due to a long tradition of kava consumption without report of hepatotoxicity.

Flavokawain A is a chalcone that constitutes up to 0.46% of the kava extract (Dharmaratne et al. 2002). Chalcones are α, β-unsaturated ketones and are unique in the flavonoid family (Calliste et al. 2001). Citrus fruits and apples are rich dietary sources of chalcones (Barreca et al. 2014; Khan et al. 2011). Li et al. (2008) have reported that 100 μM flavokawain A has no toxic effect on human normal liver cells L-02 and hepatoma cells HepG2. We have recently carried out extensive *in vitro* and *in vivo* studies of flavokawain A's safety profile, demonstrating that dietary feeding of flavokawain A for up to 13 months did not affect food consumption and body weight, as well as exhibited no adverse effects on major organ function (including liver function) and homoeostasis in mice (Liu et al. 2013; Li et al. 2014). These results indicated that flavokawain A has an excellent profile.

Currently, there is not sufficient evidence that active kava components (kavalactones and flavokawains) rather than the alkaloid pipermethystine from wrong plant parts such as leaves or stems, or mold hepatotoxins from contaminated raw kava materials, may be the culprits of the adverse hepatic reactions (Dragull et al. 2003; Teschke et al. 2012).

8.10 CONCLUSIONS AND PERSPECTIVES

Since PSA testing was introduced in the late 1980s, more men are being diagnosed with early-stage PCa. A group of PCa patients with slow-growing, localized cancers who are not experiencing symptoms related to their cancer are currently undergoing active surveillance but without therapies such as chemotherapy, radiation therapy, or surgery unless their cancer appears to be growing or getting worse. Since about 20 to 30% of patients with PCa in active surveillance groups progress to more aggressive disease, there is a need for development of novel strategies for prolonging the surveillance period and preventing rapid progression. Naturally-occurring compounds with excellent safety profiles would be a reasonable choice.

The kava root extract and its active components have, individually and in combination, demonstrated differential mechanisms of AR downregulation. Therapeutic strategies that target the synthesis of androgen and/or binding to androgen to AR are often associated with development of resistance due to acquired overexpression or overactivity of AR. Approaches for downregulation of AR expression may have the advantage over current anti-androgen drugs (i.e., finasteride, flutamide, leuprolide, abiraterone, and enzalutamide) for overcoming drug resistance. Flavokawains have been shown to be more potent than the kava root extracts or kavalactones in downregulation of AR expression and inhibition of tumor growth in patient-derived xenograft models and transgenic models.

In addition, flavokawain A selectively inhibits the growth of Rb-deficient cells and PCa cells with overexpression of Skp2. Summarization of the mechanisms of action of flavokawain A is shown in Figure 8.3 in the color insert. Flavokawain A is a robust apoptosis inducer via activation of the Bim/Bax–mediated mitochondria pathway and downregulation of expression of the anti-apoptotic proteins survivin and XIAP. Flavokawain A transcriptionally downregulates AR expression via inhibiting the protein expression of transcriptional factor Sp1. Both Sp1 and survivin are substrates of SCF E3 ligase β-TrCP that can also be degraded by Skp2. These multiple downstream targets (i.e., p27, Sp1, AR, surviving, and Bim) of flavokawain A are either directly regulated by Skp2 or indirectly regulated by Skp2 substrates, which suggested that Skp2 is the main target of flavokawain

A for its anticancer effect. Flavokawain A functions as a novel NEDDylation inhibitor for Skp2 degradation. The potential use of flavokawain A with an excellent safety profile is a major plus in the planning of translational development of flavokawain A–based prevention and therapy.

ACKNOWLEDGEMENTS

Work cited from our laboratory was supported by the US PHS grant CA101753 and CA193967, awarded by the National Cancer Institute. Contributions of the present (Christopher Blair, Noriko Yokoyama, Andria Denmon, and Saiyang Zhang) and past (Zhongbo Liu, Xuesen Li, Xia Xu, Shuman Liu, Jun Xie, Xuejiao Tian, Ke Yu, Chunli Wu, Lixia Chen, Yaxiong Tang) members of the Zi laboratory for *in vitro* and *in vivo* studies on flavokawains cited in this article are greatly appreciated.

REFERENCES

Akram, O.N. Mushtaq, G. Kamal, M.A. 2015. An overview of current screening and management approaches for prostate cancer. *Curr Drug Metab* 16: 713–718.

Antonarakis, E.S. Lu, C. Wang, H. et al. 2014. AR-V7 and resistance to enzalutamide and abiraterone in prostate cancer. *N Engl J Med* 371: 1028–1038.

Barreca, D. Bellocco, E. Laganà, G. et al. 2014. Biochemical and antimicrobial activity of phloretin and its glycosilated derivatives present in apple and kumquat. *Food Chem* 160: 292–297.

Bashir, T. Dorrello, N.V. Amador, V. et al. 2004. Control of the SCF(Skp2-Cks1) ubiquitin ligase by the APC/C(Cdh1) ubiquitin ligase. *Nature* 428: 190–193.

Bettendorf, O. Schmidt, H. Staebler, A. et al. 2008. Chromosomal imbalances, loss of heterozygosity, and immunohistochemical expression of TP53, RB1, and PTEN in intraductal cancer, intraepithelial neoplasia, and invasive adenocarcinoma of the prostate. *Genes Chromosomes Cancer* 47: 565–572.

Calliste, C.A. Le Bail, J.C. Trouillas, P. et al. 2001. Chalcones: structural requirements for antioxidant, estrogenic and antiproliferative activities. *Anticancer Res* 21: 3949–3956.

Chuu, C.P. Kokontis, J.M. Hiipakka, R.A. et al. 2011. Androgen suppresses proliferation of castration-resistant LNCaP 104-R2 prostate cancer cells through androgen receptor, Skp2, and c-Myc. *Cancer Sci* 102: 2022–2028.

Clouatre D.L. 2004. Kava kava: examining new reports of toxicity. *Toxicol Lett* 150: 85–96.

Côté, C.S. Kor, C. Cohen, J. et al. 2004. Composition and biological activity of traditional and commercial kava extracts. *Biochem Biophys Res Commun* 322: 147–152.

Currie, B.J. Clough, A.R. 2003. Kava hepatotoxicity with western herbal products: does it occur with traditional kava use? *Med J Aust* 178: 421–422.

Dar, J.A. Masoodi, K.Z. Eisermann, K. et al. 2014. The N-terminal domain of the androgen receptor drives its nuclear localization in castration-resistant prostate cancer cells. *J Steroid Biochem* 143: 473–480.

Dharmaratne, H.R. Nanayakkara, N.P. Khan, I.A. 2002. Kavalactones from Piper methysticum, and their 13C NMR spectroscopic analyses. *Phytochemistry* 59: 429–433.

Dragull, K. Yoshida, W.Y. Tang, C.S. 2003. Piperidine alkaloids from Piper methysticum. *Phytochemistry* 63: 193–198.

Eisermann, K. Wang, D. Jing, Y. et al. 2013. Androgen receptor gene mutation, rearrangement, polymorphism. *Transl Androl Urol* 2: 137–147.

Gingrich, J.R. Barrios, R.J. Morton, R.A. et al. 1996. Metastatic prostate cancer in a transgenic mouse. *Cancer Res* 56: 4096–4102.

Haenszel, W. Kurihara, M. 1968. Studies of Japanese migrants. I. Mortality from cancer and other diseases among Japanese in the United States. *J Natl Cancer Inst* 40: 43–68.

Henderson, B.E. Kolonel, L.N. Dworsky, R. et al. 1985. Cancer incidence in the islands of the Pacific. *Natl Cancer Inst Monogr* 69: 73–81.

Jandial, D.D. Blair, C.A. Zhang, S. et al. 2014. Molecular targeted approaches to cancer therapy and prevention using chalcones. *Curr Cancer Drug Targets* 14: 181–200.

Jemal, A. Center, M.M. DeSantis, C. et al. 2010. Global patterns of cancer incidence and mortality rates and trends. *Cancer Epidemiol Biomarkers Prev* 19: 1893–1907.

Jenster, G. van der Korput, H.A. can Croonhove, C. et al. 1991. Domains of the human androgen receptor involved in steroid binding, transcriptional activation, and subcellular localization. *Mol Endocrinol* 5: 1396.

Kasper, S. Cookson, M.S. 2006. Mechanisms leading to the development of hormone-resistant prostate cancer. *Urol Clin North Am* 33: 201–210.

Khan, M.K. Rakotomanomana, N. Dufour, C. et al. 2011. Binding of citrus flavanones and their glucuronides and chalcones to human serum albumin. *Food Funct* 2: 617–626.

Kubota, Y. Fujinami, K. Uemura, H. et al. 1995. Retinoblastoma gene mutations in primary human prostate cancer. *Prostate* 27: 314–320.

Kuchta, K. Schmidt, M. Nahrstedt, A. 2015. German kava ban lifted by court: the alleged hepatotoxicity of kava (Piper methysticum) as a case of ill-defined herbal drug identity, lacking quality control, and misguided regulatory politics. *Planta Med* 81: 1647–1653.

Li, N. Liu, J.H. Zhang, J. et al. 2008. Comparative evaluation of cytotoxicity and antioxidative activity of 20 flavonoids. *J Agric Food Chem* 56: 3876–3883.

Li, X. Xu, X. Ji, T. et al. 2014. Dietary feeding of Flavokawain A, a Kava chalcone, exhibits a satisfactory safety profile and its association with enhancement of phase II enzymes in mice. *Toxicol Rep* 1: 2–11.

Li, X. Liu, Z. Xu, X. et al. 2012. Kava components down-regulate expression of AR and AR splice variants and reduce growth in patient-derived prostate cancer xenografts in mice. *PLoS One* 7: e31213.

Li, X. Yokoyama, N.N. Zhang, S. et al. 2015. Flavokawain A induces deNEDDylation and Skp2 degradation leading to inhibition of tumorigenesis and cancer progression in the TRAMP transgenic mouse model. *Oncotarget* 6: 41809–41824.

Lin, D. Wyatt, A. W. Xue, H. et al. 2014. High fidelity patient-derived xenografts for accelerating prostate cancer discovery and drug development. *Cancer Res* 74: 1272–1283.

Lin, H.K. Chen, Z. Wang, G. 2010. Skp2 targeting suppresses tumorigenesis by Arf-p53-independent cellular senescence. *Nature* 464: 374–379.

Liu, Z. Xu, X. Li, X. et al. 2013. Kava chalcone, flavokawain A, inhibits urothelial tumorigenesis in the UPII-SV40T transgenic mouse model. *Cancer Prev Res (Phila)* 6: 1365–1375.

Mathews, J.M. Etheridge, A.S. Valentine, J.L. et al. 2005. Pharmacokinetics and disposition of the kavalactone kawain: interaction with kava extract and kavalactones in vivo and in vitro. *Drug Metab Dispos* 33: 1555–1563.

Mosca A. Berruti A. Russo L. et al. 2005. The neuroendocrine phenotype in prostate cancer: basic and clinical aspects. *J Endocrinol Invest* 28: 141–145.

Nguyen, P. L. Lin, D. I. Lei, J. et al. 2011. The impact of Skp2 overexpression on recurrence-free survival following radical prostatectomy. *Urol Oncol* 29: 302–308.

O'Donnell, A. Judson, I. Dowsett, M. et al. 2004. Hormonal impact of the 17alpha-hydroxylas/C17, 20-lyase inhibitor abiraterone acetate (CB7630) in patients with prostate cancer. *Br J Cancer* 90: 2317–2325.

Penning, T.M. 2014. Androgen biosynthesis in castration-resistant prostate cancer. *Endocr Relat Cancer* 21: 67–78.

Rasanathan, K. Tukuitonga, C.F. 2007. Tobacco smoking prevalence in Pacific Island countries and territories: a review. *N Z Med J* 120: U2742.

Robbins, C.M. Tembe, W.A. Baker, A. et al. 2011. Copy number and targeted mutational analysis reveals novel somatic events in metastatic prostate tumors. *Genome Res* 21: 47–55.

Shaik, A.A. Hermanson, D.L. Xing, C. 2009. Identification of methysticin as a potent and non-toxic NF-kappaB inhibitor from kava, potentially responsible for kava's chemopreventive activity. *Bioorg Med Chem Lett* 19: 5732–5736.

Siddique, H.R. Nanda, S. Parray, A. et al. 2012. Androgen receptor in human health: a potential therapeutic target. *Curr Drug Targets* 13: 1907–1916.

Singh, Y.N. 1992. Kava: an overview. *J Ethnopharmacol* 37: 13–45.

Singh, Y.N. Devkota, A.K. 2003. Aqueous kava extracts do not affect liver function tests in rats. *Planta Med* 69: 496–499.

Soucy, T.A. Smith, P.G. Milhollen, M.A. et al. 2009. An inhibitor of NEDD8-activating enzyme as a new approach to treat cancer. *Nature* 458: 732–736.

Steiner GG. 2000. The correlation between cancer incidence and kava consumption. *Hawaii Med J* 59: 420–422.

Supramaniam Rajah; NSW Cancer Council; et al. eds. *Cancer in New South Wales Migrants 1991 to 2001.* Vol 1 Page 33. 2006.

Suzuki, H. Freije, D. Nusskern, D.R. et al. 1998. Interfocal heterogeneity of PTEN/MMAC1 gene alterations in multiple metastatic prostate cancer tissues. *Cancer Res* 58: 204–209.

Tabayoyong, W. Abouassaly, R. 2015. Prostate cancer screening and the associated controversy. *Surg Clin North Am* 95: 1023–1039.

Tang, Y. Li, X. Liu, Z. et al. 2010. Flavokawain B, a kava chalcone, exhibits robust apoptotic mechanisms on androgen receptor-negative, hormone refractory prostate cancer cell lines and reduces tumor growth in a preclinical model. *Int J Cancer* 127: 1758–1768.

Teschke, R. Sarris, J. Schweitzer, I. 2012. Kava hepatotoxicity in traditional and modern use: the presumed Pacific kava paradox hypothesis revisited. *Br J Clin Pharmacol* 73: 170–174.

Tran, C. Ouk, S. Clegg, N.J. et al. 2009. Development of a second-generation antiandrogen for treatment of advanced prostate cancer. *Science* 324: 787–790.

Visakorpi, T. Hyytinen, E. Koivisto, P. et al. 1995. In vivo amplification of the androgen receptor gene and progression of human prostate cancer. *Nat Genet* 9: 401–406.

Wang, H. Bauzon, F. Ji, P. et al. 2010. Skp2 is required for survival of aberrantly proliferating Rb1-deficient cells and for tumorigenesis in Rb1+/- mice. *Nat Genet* 42: 83–88.

Watson, P.A. Arora, V.K. Sawyers, C.L. 2015. Emerging mechanisms of resistance to androgen receptor inhibitors in prostate cancer. *Nat Rev Cancer* 15: 701–711.

Wirbelauer, C. Sutterlüty, H. Blondel, M. et al. 2000. The F-box protein Skp2 is a ubiquitylation target of a Cul1-based core ubiquitin ligase complex: evidence for a role of Cul1 in the suppression of Skp2 expression in quiescent fibroblasts. *EMBO J* 19: 5362–5375.

Yang, G. Ayala, G. De Marzo, A. et al. 2002. Elevated Skp2 protein expression in human prostate cancer: association with loss of the cyclin-dependent kinase inhibitor p27 and PTEN and with reduced recurrence-free survival. *Clin Cancer Res* 8: 3419–3426.

Zi, X. Simoneau, A.R. 2005. Flavokawain A, a novel chalcone from kava extract, induces apoptosis in bladder cancer cells by involvement of Bax protein-dependent and mitochondria-dependent apoptotic pathway and suppresses tumor growth in mice. *Cancer Res* 65: 3479–3486.

CHAPTER 9

Bitter Melon Extract and Prostate Cancer Therapy

Ratna B. Ray and Sourav Bhattacharya

CONTENTS

9.1 PROSTATE CANCER: THE MALE DISEASE

Prostate cancer is the most common male malignancy and the second leading cause of cancer death among men in the United States. Although prostate cancer is frequently curable in its early stage by surgical or radiation ablation, many patients present locally advanced or metastatic disease for which there are no curative treatment options (Nelson et al., 2003; Albertsen, 2008). The American Cancer Society estimates about 220,800 new cases of prostate cancer and about 27,540 deaths from prostate cancer in the United States in 2015. Prostate cancer occurs more commonly in African-American men and in Caribbean men of African ancestry than in men of other races. African-American men are also more than twice as likely to die of prostate cancer as compared to Caucasian men. The reason for this difference is not clear. More intensive screening in some developed countries probably accounts for at least part of this difference, but other factors such as lifestyle (i.e., diet) are likely to be important as well. Genetic factors, smoking, obesity, inflammation of the prostate, sexually transmitted infections, and vasectomy may also contribute to the disease progression.

Prostate cancer becomes lethal when cancer cells develop into castration-resistant prostate cancer (CRPC). Androgen receptor (AR) gene mutation, altered AR regulation, or overexpression of

AR are often found in CRPC, and are believed to become some of the key factors of the lethal phenotype. Recent studies have suggested that advancing prostate cancer is not uniformly refractory to further hormonal manipulation (Ryan and Tindall, 2011). Although the importance of treatment-mediated selection pressure has been appreciated for some time, it is unclear whether the emergence of the lethal phenotype is a function of androgen deprivation therapy itself or a function of factors initiated at the time of carcinogenesis. Therefore, more effective therapies that can cure localized tumors and prevent their metastasis are urgently needed.

9.2 COMPLEMENTARY AND ALTERNATIVE MEDICINE

Complementary and alternative medicines have been historically practiced for over thousands of years to treat various diseases. Before the introduction of high-throughput screening and genomic tools, the discovery of more than 80% of drugs was either made directly from natural products or influenced by them (Harvey et al., 2015). The use of natural products is still common, and is cost effective for many diseases. Statistical data has shown that among all the new drugs discovered from 1981 to 2007, 50% of them are based on natural products. Thirteen natural product–based drugs were discovered between 2005 and 2007 (Butler, 2008). The term *nutraceutical* has been coined to describe this class of drugs.

Discovery of new drugs from edible substances is gaining more importance due to less toxicity. Many edible fruits and vegetables are examined for their therapeutic and disease-preventive functions. With more and more lab-based research and characterization of active compounds, these functional foods are now used as therapeutic nutraceuticals with higher potency to treat various diseases, including cancer. Several epidemiological studies as well as laboratory research reveal that high intake of fruits and vegetables are linked with a reduced susceptibility to cancer (Key, 2011; Hardin et al., 2012).

9.3 *MOMORDICA CHARANTIA* (BITTER MELON)

Momordica charantia, commonly known as bitter melon, balsam pear, or karela (Figure 9.1), is widely cultivated in Asia, Africa, and South America. This fruit has traditionally been used by alternative medicine practitioners as a remedy for diabetes in India, China, and Central America (Basch et al., 2003). Laboratory research data with animal studies also confirmed that either fresh bitter melon extract (BME) or crude organic fractions isolated from it have beneficial effects on glucose metabolism and on plasma and hepatic lipids (Nerurkar and Ray, 2010). All parts of the plant have been studied for hypoglycemic activity (Sarkar et al., 1996; Jaysooriya et al., 2000),

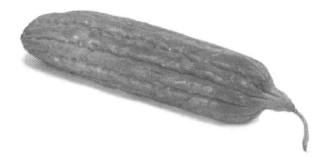

Figure 9.1   Bitter melon fruit.

antihyperglycemic activity in alloxan (Rathi et al., 2002; Kar et al., 2003), or streptozotacine-induced models of diabetes (Grover et al., 2002; Rathi et al., 2002). Similar types of studies were also performed on genetic models of diabetes (Miura et al., 2001). This plant also has some folk-loric uses against psoriasis, infertility, gastrointestinal cramps, and infections (Khan et al., 1998). Different parts of the bitter melon vine including bitter melon flesh, seeds, and leaves, are used for therapy. Based on experimental data, bitter melon has also been proposed as an antiviral and anti-neoplastic agent (Foa-Tomasi et al., 1982: Lee Huang et al., 1990; Nerurkar and Ray, 2010).

9.4 BITTER MELON TREATMENT MODULATES CELL CYCLE PROGRESSION

Cancer is a multistep process in which cells present with uncontrolled proliferative potential. In general, the growth rate of cancer cells exceeds that of normal cells due to deregulation of their homeostasis machineries. Tumor cells represent the culmination of multiple genetic abnormalities. Thus, targeting multiple signaling pathways may be more effective for preventive or therapeutic approaches.

Prostate cancer cells treated with bitter melon extract (made from flesh of bitter melon) died (>90%) within 96 h, whereas primary prostate epithelial cells do not exhibit significant toxicity. To understand the mechanism of BME-mediated proliferation inhibition on prostate cancer cells, cell cycle analysis was performed by flow cytometry. Cell populations in the G0-G1 and S phases were 51% and 35%, respectively, in control PC3 cells (Ru et al., 2011). However, after 24 h incubation with BME, the S-phase population was noticeably enhanced to 45%, whereas the G0-G1 population was decreased to 35%. No significant change was observed in the G2/M phase of cell cycle. The effect observed in prostate cancer cells was not cell type–specific, because both PC3 (androgen receptor-negative and mutant p53) and LNCaP (androgen receptor-positive and wild-type p53) cells displayed similar results. Kuguacin J (KuJ), a purified component of bitter melon (*Momordica charantia*) leaf extract, also displayed an antiproliferative effect on prostate cancer PC3 cells (Pitchakarn et al., 2012).

9.5 MECHANISM OF ACTION OF BME AGAINST PROSTATE CANCER

BME treatment in prostate cancer cells strongly modulates cyclins and inhibits their normal reg-ulation of cell-cycle progression. Cell-cycle progression in eukaryotic cells is controlled by a series of protein complexes composed of cyclins and cyclin-dependent kinases (CDKs). Cyclins are central regulators of the cell cycle. D-type cyclins interact with CDK4 and CDK6 to drive the progression through early/mid-G1 in response to mitogen stimulation. Cyclin E-cdk2 is active in mid G1 close to the restriction point, cyclin A-cdk2 from the beginning of S to M, whereas cyclin B-cdc2 is active at the G2/M transition. The treatment of BME led to a significant downregulation of cyclin D1 and cyclin E in prostate cancer cell lines (Ru et al., 2011). Further, a significant increase of p21 protein in both the prostate cancer cell lines suggested an S phase arrest. To further understand the molecular pathways, the activation of p38MAPK and ERK1/2, which are important upstream regulators of p21, was examined. Activation of p38MAPK and ERK1/2 is also correlated with the promotion of cell-cycle arrest in prostate cancer (Mukhopadhyay et al., 2006; Robertson et al., 2010). Furthermore, phospho-p38, the activated form of p38MAPK, was significantly (2-4.6 fold) induced following BME treatment in both PC3 and LNCaP cell lines (Ru et al., 2011). Prostate cancer cells treated with BME also displayed upregulation of phospho-ERK1/2 expression. Together these results indicated that BME treatment in prostate cancer cells activates MEK-ERK or p38MAPK signaling pathway.

9.6   BITTER MELON TREATMENT AND APOPTOSIS

Cell death plays an important role in development, tissue homeostasis, and degenerative diseases. The two major forms of cell death are apoptosis and necrosis. Apoptosis, a morphologically and biochemically distinct form of cell death, is an important physiologic process in both normal development and pathological consequences. Necrosis is the unregulated digestion of cell components. A diverse set of stimuli can trigger the apoptotic process in virtually all nucleated cells. One of the key regulatory steps for apoptosis is the activation of caspases. Active caspases then cleave many important intracellular substrates, leading to the characteristic morphological changes associated with apoptotic cells. Cell-cycle arrest has been correlated with apoptosis (Xia et al., 2000). BME induces pro-apoptotic mitochondrial changes by altering the expression of Bcl-2, which in turn induces apoptosis (such as PARP cleavage and activation of Caspase 9/3) in prostate cancer cell lines.

9.7   ACTIVE COMPOUND ISOLATED FROM BITTER MELON RESPONSIBLE FOR ANTIPROLIFERATIVE ACTIVITY

Several chemical constituents from bitter melon (seeds, leaves, or fruits) have been reported for their anticancer potential. Significant among the constituents are cucurbitane triterpenes and their glycosides, flavonoids, particularly fisetin, and fatty acids, such as α-eleostearic acid (Horax et al., 2010; Wu and Ng, 2008). MAP30, a 30-kDa single-stranded ribosome-inactivating protein isolated from bitter melon seed, displayed antiproliferative activity against human breast and colon cancer cells (Lee-Huang et al., 2000; Xiong et al., 2009; Li et al., 2009), although further studies are needed to evaluate its *in vivo* effect. Alpha-eleostearic acid (α-ESA), a conjugated linolenic acid, which makes up approximately 60% of bitter melon seed oil, inhibits the proliferation of breast cancer cells *in vitro* (Horax et al., 2010; Grossmann et al., 2009). Although a-ESA strongly induced apoptosis in HL60 cells, the acetone extract of bitter melon seed, which is probably rich in α-ESA acid, did not induce apoptosis in the cells. Lipophilic components of pericarp and placenta in the acetone extract may blunt the apoptosis of HL60 cells. In fact, the acetone extract also did not suppress colon cancer growth in the xenograft model (Tsuzuki et al., 2004). Akihisa et al. (2007) have isolated 13 cucurbitane-type triterpene glycosides, including eight new compounds named charantosides I, II, III, IV, V, VI, VII, and VIII, and five known compounds, 8, 9, 14, 15, and 18, from a methanol extract of the fruits of the Japanese *Momordica charantia*. Compounds 1 and 2 exhibited marked inhibitory effects in both 7,12-dimethylbenz[a]anthracene- and peroxynitrite-induced mouse skin cancer. KuJ has been isolated from the leaf of bitter melon and also can be found in the stem (Pitchakarn et al., 2011). This compound has an effect against prostate cancer, and works via p53-dependent cell-cycle arrest in the G1 phase and induction of apoptosis. KuJ treatment has been shown to reduce the levels of cyclins (D1 and E), cyclin-dependent kinases (Cdk2 and Cdk4), and proliferating cell nuclear antigen. It has been shown to reduce the androgen receptors in prostate cells, which reduces prostate-specific antigens. However, very little follow-up information is available about these compounds, and *in vivo* efficacy remains unknown. We have isolated one new sterol and a peroxide compound (C2) from the flesh part of the fruit of *M. charantia*. This compound displays antiproliferative activity against several cancer cells, including prostate cancer cells (unpublished results; Figure 9.2). The EC_{50} of this compound is 35 uM In Pc3 cells. However, more work will be necessary to understand the *in vivo* activity of bitter melon active components.

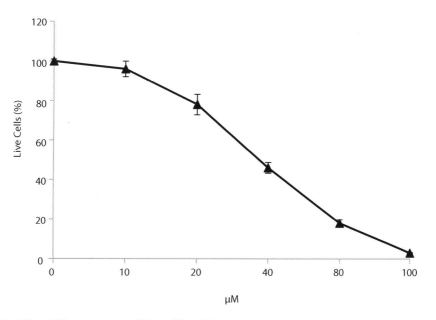

Figure 9.2 EC_{50} of C2 compound on PC3 cell line. Cells were treated with indicated concentration of purified C2 compound and cell viability was measured 24 h post-treatment.

9.8 CHEMOPREVENTIVE EFFECT OF BITTER MELON EXTRACT

Prevention is always better than therapy. Genetically manipulated animal models have emerged as useful resources for developing strategies against many pathological conditions, including cancer. For prostate cancer, one such model is TRAMP (Greenberg et al., 1995; Gingrich et al., 1997). The transgene construct in these mice is a PB-Tag gene consisting of the minimal −426/+28 bp regulatory sequence of the rat probasin promoter directing prostate-specific epithelial expression of the SV-40 early genes introduced into the C57BL/6 mouse. TRAMP males develop spontaneous multistage prostate carcinogenesis that exhibits both histological and molecular features recapitulating many salient aspects of human prostate cancer. TRAMP males characteristically express the PB-Tag transgene by 8 weeks of age and display high-grade prostatic neoplasia or well-differentiated prostate cancer by 10–12 weeks of age. Distant site metastasis can be detected by 20 weeks of male TRAMP mice, and by 30 weeks of age some animals harbor prostate cancer that metastasizes to the lymph node and lungs. We have used the TRAMP mouse model for a chemoprevention study (Ru et al., 2011). The body weights of the control and BME-fed mice did not differ significantly throughout the experimental time frame. All animals were examined for gross pathology at the time of sacrifice and demonstrated no evidence of global edema, abnormal organ size, or appearance in non-target organs. Further, a significant weight difference of the prostate (70%) was observed between control and experimental groups.

The incidence of normal gland on the prostate section from the BME-fed group was significantly higher than observed in control group, although the incidence of low-grade PIN was similar in both groups. Importantly, the incidence of high-grade PIN from the BME-fed group was significantly lower than the control group (Figure 9.3, panels A and B; see color insert). Also, approximately a 21% area of the prostate gland was histologically normal in BME-fed group, as compared with approximately 12% normal glands in the control group (Ru et al., 2011). In addition, BME treatment in TRAMP mice strongly reduces PCNA expression that may prevent prostate tumor progression in TRAMP mice (Figure 9.3, panel C). A subsequent study revealed that there is no difference in SV40 T-antigen expression in control and BME-fed mice prostate tissues (Figure 9.3, panel D).

9.9 BITTER MELON AS A THERAPEUTIC AGENT

Limited information is available about the therapeutic efficacy of bitter melon in prostate cancer in the preclinical model. Intravenous inoculation of the rat prostate cancer cell line (PLS10) into nude mice resulted in a 100% survival rate in the mice given a bitter melon leaf extract (BMLE) diet as compared with 80% in the controls (Pitchakarn et al., 2010). However, in this study, the incidence of lung metastasis did not show any difference (Pitchakarn et al., 2010). Subsequently, this group showed that 1% and 5% BMLE in the diet resulted in 63% and 57% inhibition of PC3 xenograft growth without adverse effect on host body weight (Pitchakarn et al., 2012). Although these studies provided important information, it was difficult to judge when the BMLE was started in the diet of these mice. We also examined whether BME feeding could regress prostate cancer xenograft tumor growth. For this, human prostate cancer PC3 cells were implanted into Balb/c athymic nude mice. When tumor volume was ~100 mm^3, mice were divided into two groups. The experimental group was gavaged with BME for 5 days a week, and the control group similarly received water. A reduction in tumor growth and volume was observed in BME-fed mice as compared to control mice (unpublished results; Figure 9.4 in color insert). Thus, these results indicated that bitter melon can be used as a therapeutic agent along with standard treatment in prostate cancer, although combination therapy data from preclinical study is not available currently.

9.10 CONCLUSION

The use of dietary products for managing the carcinogenic process provides an opportunity for additional therapy along with conventional medicine for treatment of the disease. Studies from our laboratory and others strongly suggest a promising antitumor effect of bitter melon (Ray et al., 2010; Fang et al., 2012; Rajamoorthi et al., 2013; Singh et al., 2014). Further, we need to evaluate the anticancer efficacy of bitter melon in different prostate cancer mouse models. This result will further emphasize the effect of bitter melon in prostate cancer therapy. This natural product serves as a potent agent for enhancing the therapeutic effects of chemotherapy, radiotherapy, or other standard therapeutics for the treatment of human cancers. We have put forth our best effort to cite the most relevant references on bitter melon and prostate cancer therapy; however, we could not include all the citations. The active constituents of bitter melon for cancer prevention and therapy are in their infancy stage. Several candidate components are identified as anticancer agents; however, preclinical validation is needed. Thus, in spite of great progress, much more work is required to optimize the *in vivo* activity of bitter melon. The consumption of bitter melon in diets has a translational potential in the fight against several cancers, including prostate, and has a beneficial effect on the general population.

REFERENCES

Akihisa, T. Higo, N. Tokuda, H. et al. 2007. Cucurbitane-type triterpenoids from the fruits of Momordica charantia and their cancer chemopreventive effects. *J Nat Prod* 70: 1233–1239.
Albertsen, P.C. 2008. The face of high risk prostate cancer. *World J Urol* 26(3): 205–210.

Basch, E. Gabard, S. Ulbricht, C. 2003. Bitter melon (*Momordica charantia*): a review of efficacy and safety. *Am J Health Syst Pharm* 60: 356–359.

Butler, M.S. 2008. Natural products to drugs: natural product-derived compounds in clinical trials. *Nat Prod Rep* 25: 475–516.

Fang, E.F. Zhang, C.Z. Zhang, L. et al. 2012. In vitro and in vivo anticarcinogenic effects of RNase MC2, a ribonuclease isolated from dietary bitter gourd, toward human liver cancer cells. *Int J Biochem Cell Biol* 44: 1351–1360.

Foa-Tomasi, L. Campadelli-Fiume, G. Barbieri, L. et al. 1982. Effect of ribosome-inactivating proteins on virus-infected cells. Inhibition of virus multiplication and of protein synthesis. *Arch Virol* 71: 323–332.

Gingrich, J.R. Barrios, R.J. Kattan, M.W. et al. 1997. Androgen-independent prostate cancer progression in the TRAMP model. *Cancer Res* 57(21): 4687–4691.

Greenberg, N.M. DeMayo, F. Finegold, M.J et al. 1995. Prostate cancer in a transgenic mouse. *Proc Natl Acad Sci* 92: 3439–3443.

Grossmann, M.E. Mizuno, N.K. Dammen, M.L. et al. 2009. Eleostearic acid inhibits breast cancer proliferation by means of an oxidation-dependent mechanism. *Cancer Prev Res (Phila)* 2(10): 879–886.

Grover, J.K. Rathi, S.S. Vats, V. 2002. Amelioration of experimental diabetic neuropathy and gastropathy in rats following oral administration of plant (Eugenia jambolana, Mucuna pruriens and Tinospora cordifolia) extracts. *Indian J Exp Biol* 40: 273–276.

Hardin, J. Cheng, I. Witte J.S. 2012. Impact of consumption of vegetable, fruit, grain, and high glycemic index foods on aggressive prostate cancer risk. *Nutr Cancer* 63(6): 860–872.

Harvey, A.L. Edrada-Ebel, R. Quinn, R.J. 2015. The re-emergence of natural products for drug discovery in the genomics era. *Nat Rev Drug Discov* 14: 111–129.

Horax, R. Hettiarachchy, N. Chen, P. 2010. Extraction, quantification, and antioxidant activities of phenolics from pericarp and seeds of bitter melons (*Momordica charantia*) harvested at three maturity stages (immature, mature, and ripe). *J Agric Food Chem* 58(7): 4428–4433.

Jayasooriya, A.P. Sakono, M. Yukizaki, C. et al. 2000. Effects of Momordica charantia powder on serum glucose levels and various lipid parameters in rats fed with cholesterol free and cholesterol-enriched diets. *J Ethnopharmacol* 72: 331–336.

Kar, A. Choudhary, B.K. Bandyopadhyay, N.G. 2003. Comparative evaluation of hypoglycaemic activity of some Indian medicinal plants in alloxan diabetic rats. *J Ethnopharmacol* 84: 105–108.

Key, T.J. 2011. Fruit and vegetables and cancer risk. *Br J Cancer* 104(1): 6–11.

Khan, M.R. Omoloso, A.D. Khan, M.R. 1998. Momordica charantia and Allium sativum: broadspectrum antibacterial activity. *Korean J Pharmacognosy* 29: 155–158.

Lee-Huang, S. Huang, P.L. Nara, P.L. et al. 1990. MAP 30: a new inhibitor of HIV-1 infection and replication. *FEBS Lett* 272: 12–8.

Lee-Huang, S. Huang, P.L. Sun, Y. et al. 2000. Inhibition of MDA-MB-231 human breast tumor xenografts and HER2 expression by anti-tumor agents GAP31 and MAP30. *Anticancer Res* 20(2A): 653–659.

Li, M. Chen, Y. Liu, Z. et al. 2009. Anti-tumor activity and immunological modification of ribosome-inactivating protein (RIP) from Momordica charantia by covalent attachment of polyethylene glycol. *Acta Biochim Biophys Sin (Shanghai)* 41(9): 792–799.

Miura, T. Itoh, C. Iwamoto, N. et al. 2001. Hypoglycemic activity of the fruit of the Momordica charantia in type 2 diabetic mice. *J Nutr Sci Vitaminol* (Tokyo) 47: 340–344.

Mukhopadhyay, I. Sausville, E.A. Doroshow, J.H. et al. 2006. Molecular mechanism of adaphostin-mediated G1 arrest in prostate cancer (PC-3) cells: signaling events mediated by hepatocyte growth factor receptor, c-Met, and p38 MAPK pathways. *J Biol Chem* 281: 37330–37344.

Nelson, W.G., De Marzo, A.M. Isaacs, W.B. 2003. Prostate cancer. *N Engl J Med* 349: 366–381.

Nerurkar, P., Ray, R.B. 2010. Bitter melon: antagonist to cancer. *Pharm Res.* 27: 1049–1053.

Pitchakarn, P. Ogawa, K., Suzuki, S. et al. 2010. Momordica charantia leaf extract suppresses rat prostate cancer progression in vitro and in vivo. *Cancer Sci* 101(10): 2234–2240.

Pitchakarn, P. Suzuki, S. Ogawa, K. et al. 2011. Induction of G1 arrest and apoptosis in androgen-dependent human prostate cancer by Kuguacin J, a triterpenoid from Momordica charantia leaf. *Cancer Lett* 306: 142–150.

Pitchakarn, P. Suzuki, S. Ogawa, K. et al. 2012. A triterpeniod from Momordica charantia leaf, modulates the progression of androgen-independent human prostate cancer cell line, PC3. *Food Chem Toxicol* 50: 840–847.

Rajamoorthi, A. Shrivastava, S. Steele, R. et al. 2013. Bitter melon reduces head and neck squamous cell carcinoma growth by targeting c-Met signaling. *PLoS One.* 8: e78006. doi: 10.1371/journal.pone.0078006.

Rathi, S.S. Grover, J.K. and Vats, V. 2002. The effect of Momordica charantia and Mucuna pruriens in experimental diabetes and their effect on key metabolic enzymes involved in carbohydrate metabolism. *Phytother Res* 16: 236–243.

Ray, R.B. Raychoudhuri, A. Steele, R. et al. 2010. Bitter melon (*Momordica charantia*) extract inhibits breast cancer cell proliferation by modulating cell cycle regulatory genes and promotes apoptosis. *Cancer Res* 70: 1925–1931.

Robertson, B.W. Bonsal, L. Chellaiah, M.A. 2010. Regulation of Erk1/2 activation by osteopontin in PC3 human prostate cancer cells. *Mol Cancer* 9: 260.

Ru, P. Steele, R. Nerurkar, P.V. et al. 2011. Bitter melon extract impairs prostate cancer cell-cycle progression and delays prostatic intraepithelial neoplasia in TRAMP model. *Cancer Prev Res (Phila).* 4: 2122–2130.

Ryan, C.J. Tindall, D.J. 2011. Androgen receptor rediscovered: the new biology and targeting the androgen receptor therapeutically. *J Clin Oncol* 29(27): 3651–3658.

Sarkar, S. Pranava, M. Marita, R. 1996. Demonstration of the hypoglycemic action of Momordica charantia in a validated animal model of diabetes. *Pharmacol Res* 33: 1–4.

Singh, N. Chakraborty, R. Bhullar, R.P. et al. 2014. Differential expression of bitter taste receptors in noncancerous breast epithelial and breast cancer cells. *Biochem Biophys Res Commun* 446: 499–503.

Tsuzuki, T. Tokuyama, Y. Igarashi, M. Miyazawa, T. 2004. Tumor growth suppression by alpha-eleostearic acid, a linolenic acid isomer with a conjugated triene system, via lipid peroxidation. *Carcinogenesis* 25(8): 1417–1425.

Wu, S.J. Ng, L.T. 2008. Antioxidant and free radical scavenging activities of wild bitter melon (Momordica charantia Linn. var. abbreviata Ser.) in Taiwan. *LWT-Food Sci Technol* 41: 323–330.

Xia, W. Spector, S. Hardy, L. et al. 2000. Tumor selective G2/M cell cycle arrest and apoptosis of epithelial and hematological malignancies by BBL22, a benzazepine. *Proc Natl Acad Sci U S A* 97: 7494–7499.

Xiong, S.D. Yu, K. Liu, X.H. et al. 2009. Ribosome-inactivating proteins isolated from dietary bitter melon induce apoptosis and inhibit histone deacetylase-1 selectively in premalignant and malignant prostate cancer cells. *Int J Cancer* 125(4): 774–782.

CHAPTER 10

Prostate Cancer and the Therapeutic Potential of Pomegranate

Omran Karmach and Manuela Martins-Green

CONTENTS

10.1 PROSTATE CANCER AND TREATMENT OPTIONS

Prostate cancer cases are dramatically on the rise, primarily because of increased life expectancy. More and more men are living long enough to be affected by this disease, with many dying from prostate cancer metastasis (Pienta et al., 1993). Prostate cancer appears to disproportionately affect African-American men (Pienta et al., 1993). This is likely because these men have an increased susceptibility to androgen receptor (AR) mutations. These mutations are often due to alternative splicing events that lead to constitutive activation of the receptor. Under these conditions the activated AR translocates to the nucleus and activates transcription independently of ligand binding (Harris et al., 2009). In 2012, there were approximately 2.8 million men living with prostate cancer in the United States alone[1] and by 2015, approximately 221,000 new cases were detected (www.seer.cancer.gov). Generally, the survival rate of prostate cancer within the first 5 years is very high (98.9%); during this time the cancer can be contained, preventing spreading/metastasis (www. seer.cancer.gov). However, metastasis cannot be stopped indefinitely. When it occurs, the survival rate is dramatically reduced (28%) (www.seer.cancer.gov). In 2015, prostate cancer accounted for 13.3% of all the new cancer cases, making it the third most common cancer in the United States (only 400 cases behind lung cancer) (www.seer.cancer.gov). These numbers are quite alarming, considering that prostate cancer only affects men.

Medically, prostate cancer development is divided into four stages. In stage I, the cancer is localized to the prostate, with prostate-specific antigen (PSA) levels lower than 10 and a Gleason score of 6 or less (www.cancer.gov). Stage II is subdivided into stages IIA and IIB (NCI database). To be considered stage IIA, the cancer can be in more or less than half of a prostate lobe but the patient has to have a PSA of less than 20 and a Gleason score of 7 (www.cancer.gov). In stage IIB, the cancer still cannot be felt on rectal examination, but PSA levels are higher than 20 with a Gleason score of 7 or higher (www.cancer.gov). In stage IIB, the cancer has spread beyond the prostate primarily to the seminal vesicles. During this stage, PSA levels and Gleason scores do not offer adequate insight into the severity of the disease because patients can have a range of scores. Therefore, patients are categorized in this stage if the cancer has spread beyond the prostate (www.cancer.gov). Finally, in stage IV, PSA levels and Gleason scores can vary greatly (as they can in stage III), but in stage IV the important characteristic is the spreading of the cancer beyond the seminal vesicles into the rectum, bladder, or bones through the lymphatic or the vascular system (www.cancer.gov).

Currently patients have many options for treatment, including surgery, radiation therapy, cryosurgery, hormone therapy, chemotherapy, vaccine treatment, and bone-directed treatment (Sountoulides and Rountos, 2013). The treatment used depends on the age of the patient, life expectancy, the aggressiveness of the cancer, the doctor, the side effects of the chosen treatment, and whether the patient is willing to accept the intervention (www.cancer.gov). At early stages of the disease surgical removal of the prostate is a very effective, curative treatment; the men can live free of the disease for the rest of their lives. However, the danger occurs when the cancer recurs and/or metastasizes. Recurrence of the cancer can be controlled with hormone ablation therapy (Leuprolide/Lupron®), which takes advantage of the growth dependence of prostate cancer on the androgen, testosterone (Table 10.1). Many of the current androgen ablation therapies focus on inhibiting androgen synthesis. The primary pathway for androgen production is directly linked to the production of gonadotropin-releasing hormone (GNRH) in the hypothalamus (Figure 10.1). GNRH then acts in the pituitary, stimulating the release of luteinizing hormone (LH). LH, in turn, binds receptors on the interstitial cells in the testes to stimulate the production of testosterone which, in the prostate, can be converted to the AR ligand, dihydrotestosterone (DHT). A second, less effective pathway to produce androgens also begins in the hypothalamus (Figure 10.1). This pathway starts with the secretion of corticotropin-releasing hormone (CRH) that activates adrenocorticotropic hormone (ACTH). ACTH then stimulates the adrenal glands to release several hormones, including androgens. This second pathway only contributes 10–20% of the androgen production and therefore is considered not to be an effective target on its own but is often targeted in combination with targeting the GNRH pathway (Sountoulides and Rountos, 2013).

Hormone ablation therapy has many side effects because it essentially eliminates the androgens in the body that in the adult man maintain energy, sex drive, muscle mass, and bone structure (Auchus, 2004). Over time, the cancer develops ways to bypass hormone dependence, becoming a highly aggressive, castration-resistant prostate cancer (CRPC) that metastasizes to the lung, liver, and bone (Stavridi et al., 2010; Chuu et al., 2011). In addition to the hormone ablation, chemotherapy using drugs such as docetaxel and cabazitaxel, which affect microtubule function, is available today to treat CRPC (Table 10.1). Unfortunately, it is not very effective because prostate cancer cells divide slowly and, as with prostatectomy and hormone ablation therapy, the treatments are aggressive and have many side effects (Hoffman-Censits and Fu, 2013). As a result, researchers are looking for novel strategies to treat prostate cancer.

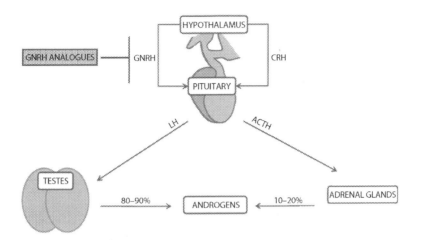

Figure 10.1   Androgen production pathways. In one pathway, GNRH released from the hypothalamus stimu-lates the production of LH in the pituitary. LH binds receptors on the interstitial cells in the testes and stimulates the production of testosterone which, in the prostate, can be converted to the AR ligand, dihydrotestosterone (DHT). In the other pathway androgen production begins with the release of CRH from the hypothalamus. CRH activates ACTH which then stimulates the adrenal glands to release several different hormones, including androgens.

Table 10.1   Drugs to Treat Prostate Cancer

How it Works	Drug Name(s)	Status
Hormone ablation	Leuprolide/Lupron®	Approved 1993 for prostate cancer
	Abiraterone/Zytiga®	Approved 2011 for prostate cancer
Chemotherapy drugs	Docetaxel	Approved 2004 for prostate cancer
	Cabazitaxel	Approved 2010 for prostate cancer
Blockers of the androgen receptor	Bicalutamide/Casodex→	Approved 1995 for prostate cancer
	MDV3100/enzalutamide/Xtandi®	Approved 2011 for prostate cancer
	ARN-509	Preparing for Phase III for prostate cancer
Cancer vaccines	Sipuleucel-T/Provenge®	Approved 2010 for prostate cancer
	PSA-TRICOM/ Prostvac→	Phase III for prostate cancer
	Ipilimumab/Yervoy→	Approved for late-stage melanoma Phase III for prostate cancer
Growth factors	Cabozantinib	Approved for thyroid cancer Phase III for prostate cancer
	Terazosin/Hytrin	Approved 2009 to relax muscles in enlarged prostates to improve urination
	Doxazosin/Cardura	Approved 2010 to relax muscles in enlarged prostates to improve urination
Bone-directed therapy	Denosumab/Xgeva→/Prolia→	Approved 2011 for prostate cancer patients at high risk for bone fracture due to androgen deprivation therapy
	Zoledronic acid/Zometa→	Approved 2002 for hypercalcemia of malignancy and bone metastasis in prostate cancer
Epigenetic modification	Vorinostat/Zolinza→	Approved for cutaneous T-cell lymphoma, proposed for prostate cancer clinical trials
DNA repair enzymes	Olaparib/Lynparza→	Approved for ovarian cancer Phase I/II for prostate cancer

Abnormalities in androgen–AR interactions are well recognized in promoting prostate cancer growth and metastasis (Lee et al., 2014). Many therapies target these abnormalities to inhibit the AR in an attempt to fight prostate cancer. There are currently a number of drugs that inhibit the action of the androgen by blocking AR (Tan et al., 2015; Mateo et al., 2014). The most commonly used drug for this purpose is the first generation of AR inhibitors, bicalutamide (Casodex→) (Table 10.1) (Osguthorpe and Hagler, 2011). Bicalutamide works by binding to the AR, inhibiting ligand-binding and therefore receptor activation and the downstream gene targeting (Furr and Tucker, 1996). Two more recently discovered drugs that work similarly are enzalutamide and ARN-509 (Table 10.1). Enzultamide, previously known as MDV3100, binds the AR with an affinity five times greater than bicalutamide. This drug has been FDA approved since 2011 for treatment of patients whose prostate cancer progressed after chemotherapy; this approval was extended in 2012 for men with CRPC (Guerrero et al., 2013; Quintela et al., 2015). ARN-509 is currently in preparation to enter FDA phase III of testing, and it is an analog of enzultamide that has shown greater potency in xenograft experiments (Rathkopf et al., 2013). Enzalutamide (Xtandi®), combined with androgen biosynthesis inhibitors such as abiraterone (Zytiga®), have shown great promise as androgen deprivation therapies to prolong overall survival rate among patients with metastatic prostate cancer (Sartor and Pal, 2013; Ryan et al., 2013) (Table 10.1).

More recently, the FDA approved sipuleucel-T (Provenge®), which is an autologous cellular immunotherapy to treat metastatic prostate cancer (Provenge, 2014) (Table 10.1). Sipuleucel-T utilizes the immune system of the patient to attack cells expressing prostatic acid phosphatase (PAP), which is produced by more than 95% of prostate cancer cells (Provenge, 2014). The treatment begins with the extraction of immature antigen-presenting cells (APCs) from a patient via leukapheresis (Provenge, 2014). These immune cells are taken to a sipuleucel-T–producing laboratory where they are cultured with a recombinant antigen PAP-GM-CSF (Provenge, 2014). PAP is the antigen the APCs will be processing, while granulocyte macrophage colony–stimulating factor (GM-CSF) is an immune cell activator that supports APC maturation. APCs are cultured outside of the patient to remove them from the immunosuppressant environment created by the prostate cancer cells. The APCs engulf the recombinant antigen, and then mature and express the antigen on their surface. Mature APCs are the constituents of the sipuleucel-T immunotherapy and are then infused into the patient. In the body, the APCs activate resting T-cells and induce their proliferation and maturation (Provenge, 2014). These T-cells then recognize and attack the PAP expressing prostate cancer cells, creating an immune response against the cancer. In the clinical trial on which this approval was granted, the median overall survival rate of patients who received sipuleucel-T improved by only 4.5 months (Provenge, 2014). However, subsequent studies with a more targeted selection of patients reported that sipuleucel-T extended median overall survival of patients with metastatic CRPC from 17.3 months in the control group to 23.4 months in the treated group. This treatment is costly, but has shown a great promise for some patients (Higano et al., 2010).

Another vaccine, PSA-TRICOM, (Prostvac→), has recently entered FDA-approved phase III testing (Singh et al., 2015) (Table 10.1). Prostvac is a poxviral vector–based vaccine that works by initiating an immune response against PSA. The viral vector has the gene for PSA that has been modified, making it more immunogenic, as well as the genes for three human T-cell costimulatory molecules, CD80, LFA-3, and ICAM-1, which enhance the patient's immune response (Gulley et al., 2013). Once introduced into the body, PSA is taken up by dendritic cells and anti-PSA T-cells are activated. These T-cells will attack and lyse prostate cancer cells that are producing PSA, and take up components from the lysed cells to use as a guide to better target other cancer cells. This creates a cancer therapy that will adjust to the patient (Gulley et al., 2013). A similar drug, ipilimumab (Yervoy→) is now being tested for use in prostate cancer. It is already approved for the treatment of melanoma (Wei et al., 2016) (Table 10.1). Yervoy is a monoclonal antibody that, like Prostvac, augments T-cell activation and proliferation by blocking the T-cell negative regulator CTLA-4 (Fong et al., 2008). In essence, these two drugs enhance innate mechanisms in the immune system to kill the cancer cells.

Growth factors control the balance between cell growth, proliferation and apoptosis, which are fundamental to the regulation of prostate growth (Reynolds and Kyprianou, 2006). Any disruption in this balance often leads to the loss of apoptosis and increase in the ability to promote cell survival and proliferation, unavoidably leading to tumorigenesis and cancer progression (Reynolds and Kyprianou, 2006). By targeting the growth factors controlling these pathways, researchers hope to control cancer cells and prevent them from entering the metastatic phase characteristic of later stage cancers. For example, cabozantinib is a potent dual inhibitor of the tyrosine kinases c-MET and vascular endothelial growth factor receptor 2 (VEGFR2), and has been shown to reduce or stabilize metastatic bone lesions in CRPC patients (Yakes et al., 2011; Smith et al., 2013) (Table 10.1). Although there are many challenges due to the complicated, multidimensional nature of these pathways, inhibiting growth factor signaling has its benefits regarding prostate cancer therapy. Currently, there are ongoing studies focusing on dissecting the molecular mechanism underlying the anti-growth action of quinazoline-based compounds such as doxazosin and terazosin (Garrison et al., 2007) (Table 10.1). Other pathways are also being studied. For example, SENP1 has been shown to regulate cyclin D1, a cell cycle regulator, emerging as an important therapeutic target (Bawa-Khalfe et al., 2010).

A more recent approach in treating prostate cancer targets the bone. Bone-directed therapies are important because prostate cancer is very likely to spread to the bone. Drugs such as denosumab (Xgeva→, Prolia→) or bisphosphonates (zoledronic acid [Zometa→]) focus on preventing/slowing down the spread of the cancer to the bones (Table 10.1). The mechanism focuses on deactivation of osteoclasts, which are bone cells that break down the hard mineral structure of bones to allow for bone growth and healing (Väänänen et al., 2000) These cells become overly active when cancer cells spread to the bone, causing acceleration in bone decay.

Some prostate cancer therapies target epigenetic modifications, which can be used to detect phenotypes that are known to lead to cancer. These therapies attempt to reverse the cancer phenotype using DNA demethylating drugs such as DZNep or DNA deacetylase inhibitors such as vorinostat (Kleb et al., 2016) (Table 10.1). Epigenetic modifications affect the expression of specific genes and play essential roles in tumor initiation and progression (Li et al., 2005). Abnormal epigenetic events such as DNA hypo- and hypermethylation and altered histone acetylation have been observed in prostate cancer (Li et al., 2005). Although the list of aberrant epigenetically regulated genes continues to grow, only a few have shown promising results as potential targets for treatment (Li et al., 2005). Prostate cancer development involves many mutations in the prostate epithelial cells, usually causing developmental changes such as resistance to apoptotic death, constitutive proliferation, and occasionally differentiation into androgen-independent cells leading to CRPC (Li et al., 2005). Researchers are attempting to pinpoint the mutations that are most common in the pathways involved in prostate cancer. Mutations can be offset by either inhibiting constitutively active mutants or activating inhibited ones.

Recent studies involving DNA repair targets have produced results showing the possibility of selective targeting of DNA repair enzymes to enhance and/or augment chemotherapy and radiation therapies as well as overcoming drug resistance (Kelley and Fishel, 2008). Although counterintuitive, inhibition of DNA repair enzymes seems to be a feasible way to kill cancer cells. Many cancers arise from mutations that render specific genes or proteins more active or less active (Kelly and Fishel, 2008). However, regardless of the mutation, cancer cells have to have a degree of DNA repair to keep their functionality. If those enzymes are specifically targeted, then the cancer cells suffer excessive DNA damage leading to cell death. For example, olaparib is FDA approved for the treatment of ovarian cancer and works by inhibiting the DNA repair enzyme poly ADP ribose polymerase (PARP) (Taneja, 2016) (Table 10.1). This inhibition targets cancer cells that rely on PARP to repair their DNA, eventually stopping their proliferation due to overwhelming DNA damage. This is now being studied for prostate cancer.

10.2 POMEGRANATE IN THE TREATMENT OF PROSTATE CANCER

Despite the plethora of therapies available to treat prostate cancer, all have adverse side effects; therefore, there has been an impetus to identify natural remedies to fight this cancer. Among these natural remedies are pomegranate juice (PJ) and/or pomegranate extracts (PE). Pomegranate is the fruit of the tree *Punica granatum*; it is cultivated in Mediterranean countries, Afghanistan, India, China, Japan, Russia, and some parts of the United States (Longtin, 2003; Langley, 2000). Pomegranates have been used in folk medicine for centuries. They have strong antioxidant, anti-inflammatory, anti-angiogenic, and pro-apoptotic effects and inhibit cell migration and chemotaxis while increasing cell adhesion (Figure 10.2), all processes involved in inhibition of tumor development, and metastasis (Khan et al., 2008; Gil et al., 2000; Lansky and Newman, 2007; Kim et al., 2002). Indeed, the antioxidant activity of pomegranates has been shown to be higher than that of red wine or green tea. These two dietary substances have shown promise in preclinical prostate cancer models and in patients with prostate cancer (Noda et al., 2002). Below we discuss data on the effects of PJ, PE, and specific components of the fruit on prostate cancer cells in culture, in animal models, and in clinical trials, and describe how they have been used to study the mechanisms involved in prostate cancer progression.

10.2.1 Pomegranate Extracts and Juice

Pomegranate juice and extracts have been shown to regulate several molecular pathways and often have many overlapping functions that alter processes involved in cancer progression and

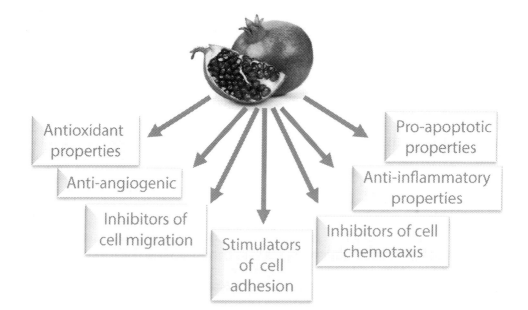

Figure 10.2 Components of pomegranate found in the peel, juice, and seed oil. They have antioxidant, anti-angiogenic, anti-migration, adhesion stimulating, anti-chemo taxis, anti-inflammatory, and pro-apoptotic properties.

metastasis. Extracts of pericarp polyphenols (EP), fermented juice polyphenols (W), and cold-pressed seed oil (oil) were studied on different prostate cancer cell lines as well as in a xenograft tumor model (Albrecht et al., 2004). Three cell lines were studied: PC3 cells, which are very aggressive, androgen independent, do not produce PSA, and are highly metastatic; DU145 cells, which are moderately aggressive, androgen independent, do not express PSA, and have a moderate potential of metastasis; and LNCaP cells, which are the least aggressive of the three, respond to androgens, produce PSA, and have very low metastatic potential. All extracts (EP, W, and oil) inhibit proliferation of the three cell lines in a dose-dependent manner. More interestingly, at lower doses EP and W had a significantly larger effect on the DU145 cells than on the LnCaP and PC3 cells, although the difference is significantly narrowed at higher doses. Oil, on the other hand, at lower doses had a significantly bigger effect on LnCaP cell proliferation than on PC3 and DU145 cells. At higher doses the oil stimulated the same levels of regulation on both LnCaP and DU145, whereas PC3 remained significantly less affected. All three extracts also increased apoptosis and reduced metastasis in PC3 xenograft mouse tumor models at very similar rates (Albrecht et al., 2004). These results suggest that different stages of prostate cancer respond differently to these treatments.

More recent studies have been performed with the commercially available pomegranate extract (POMx). The effects of POMx induce apoptosis in human LAPC4 cells, which were derived from a xenograft established from a lymph node metastasis and 22RV1 prostate cancer cells, which were derived from a xenograft that was serially propagated in mice after castration-induced regression and relapse of the parental, androgen-dependent CWR22 xenograft (Koyama et al., 2010; Rettig et al., 2008). POMx increased JNK phosphorylation and decreased Akt and mTOR activation in these cells, which is consistent with the pro-apoptotic function reported in previous studies. In 22RV1 prostate cancer cells, POMx treatment decreased insulin-like growth factor-1 (IGF-1) expression in a dose-dependent manner. Moreover, co-treatment with POMx in the presence of IGF-1 blocked the apoptotic effects of POMx. These results strongly suggest that POMx, at least in part, regulates cell cycle progression through inhibition of the IGF-1 signaling pathway (Koyama et al., 2010; Rettig et al., 2008).

Other studies with POMx were performed to determine the effects of these extracts on angiogenesis, a process that is critical for tumor growth. POMx extract inhibits angiogenesis *in vitro* and *in vivo* (Sartippour et al., 2008; 2007; Li et al., 2012). *In vitro* POMx reduced the proliferation of LnCaP cells and significantly reduced vascular endothelial growth factor (VEGF) secretion, as well as hypoxia-inducible factor 1-alpha (HIF-1α) in a dose-dependent manner. Both VEGF and HIF-1α are major driving factors of angiogenesis and are often upregulated in tumors. In addition, POMx reduced the size of xenograft LAPC4 tumors in SCID mice, reduced protein levels of HIF-1α, and decreased the overall vessel density in the tumors. It should be noted that LAPC4 cells are not very aggressive prostate cancer cells; they produce PSA and respond to androgens, but nonetheless can metastasize to the bone.

The AR is known to be a major driver of prostate cancer proliferation. In these studies, LNCaP–AR (a more aggressive androgen independent LNCaP) and DU-145 were treated with pomegranate polyphenols, PJ, and ellagitannin-rich extract to study the effects of these extracts on the expression of genes for key androgen-synthesizing enzymes and the AR (Hong et al., 2008). *In vitro* proliferation studies showed that PJ was the most effective among the three extracts in inhibiting cell proliferation for all three cell types. Whereas PJ and ellagic acid–rich extracts were the most effective at inducing apoptosis in LNCaP, ellagic acid alone was most effective in inducing apoptosis in DU145 cells. All treatments fared equally with LNCap-AR. Furthermore, both POMx and PJ treatments most consistently reduced the levels of key androgen-synthesizing enzymes and of AR in all the cell types examined in this study.

Shortly after these studies, it was found that PEs had antiproliferative as well as pro-apoptotic properties by regulating cyclin-dependent kinase (cdk) and the cdk inhibitor machinery in PC3 cells (Malik and Mukhtar, 2006). In these studies, the PE was shown to disrupt PC3 growth through regulation of cdks, molecules that disrupted the G1 phase in the cell cycle. More specifically, the investigators showed that the PE downregulated cyclin D1, D2 and E and cdk2, cdk4, and cdk6 and upregulated p21 and p27. It is well established that these cyclins will signal the cell for a G1-to-S–phase transition, while p21 and p27 inhibit the action of these cyclins (Sanchez and Dynlacht, 2005). Furthermore, the extract showed pro-apoptotic properties through the upregulation of pro-apoptotic proteins such as Bcl-2–associated X protein (Bax), and the downregulation of pro-survival proteins such as B-cell lymphoma 2 (Bcl-2) (Malik at al., 2005). Therefore, these results suggest that PEs attenuate proliferation through cell arrest in G1-to-S–phase transition and by stimulating apoptosis (Malik and Mukhtar, 2006; Sanchez and Dynlacht, 2005; Malik et al., 2005).

We have also shown that 1% or 5% PJ are very effective in inhibiting many of the processes involved in prostate cancer progression and metastasis. These studies were carried out *in vitro* using a very aggressive and metastatic prostate cell line (PC3). PC3 cells were treated with PJ for 24 h. The treated cells showed reduced growth, increased adhesion, and decreased migration and chemotaxis. Further analysis revealed that the increase in cell adhesion occurs through upregulation of genes such as CD44 and Laminin β-3 (LAMB3), while decreasing cell migration and chemotaxis through the attenuation of hyaluronan-mediated motility receptor (HMMR), anillin, and E-cadherin. In addition, cancer-related cytokines/chemokines such as interleukin-6 (IL-6), interleukin-1β (IL-1β), and regulated on activation, normal T-cell–expressed and secreted (RANTES) was also downregulated (Wang et al., 2011).

10.2.2 Pomegranate Components

The medicinal components of pomegranate can be found in different parts of the fruit: the seeds, the peel, and the juice (Table 10.2). The peel contains many molecules that protect the fruit from insects, UV, and parasites – in particular, luteolin – and it also has the potential to serve a similar function in mammals (Viuda-Martos et al., 2010). The juice is rich in vitamins, minerals, sugar, ellagitannins, and other polyphenols (Viuda-Martos et al., 2010). Lastly, the dried seeds are approximately 18% oils, with punicic acid comprising 65% of the total oil. This great diversity in the composition of the pomegranate fruit allows researchers to study individual components from different parts of the pomegranate to determine their effects on human health. The most important and frequently studied components are the flavonoids, ellagitanins, and the seed oil. These classes of molecules, found in different parts of the pomegranate, regulate reactive oxygen species (ROS), cell proliferation, cell migration, and chemotaxis, all of which are important in inflammation and metastasis and are crucial in prostate cancer development and progression. Here we focus on three molecules that come from different parts of the fruit to study and determine their synergistic effect on prostate cancer: luteolin from the peel, ellagic acid from the juice, and punicic acid from the seeds. These components have been previously studied individually and shown to have great promise in regulating functions and pathways that are known to be involved in prostate cancer progression and metastasis (Wang et al., 2011; 2012).

Table 10.2 Pomegranate Components

Pomegranate seed oil	Conjugated linolenic acid, linoleic, oleic, stearic, punicic, eleostearic, catalpic acids
Pomegranate peel	Luteolin, quercetin, kaempferol, gallagic, EA glycosides, EA, punicalagin, punicalin, pedunculagin
Pomegranate juice	Anthocyanins, glucose, organic acid, ascorbic acid, EA, ETs, gallic acid, caffeic acid, catechin, quercetin, rutin, minerals

10.2.2.1 Luteolin (3′,4′,5,7-tetrahydroxyflavone)

Luteolin is a flavonoid present primarily in the peel of pomegranates. It functions as a ROS scavenger through its own oxidation, by chelating transition metal ions responsible for the generation of ROS. In addition to this, luteolin inhibits ROS-generating oxidases. For example, luteolin suppresses $O2•^-$ formation by inhibiting xanthine oxidase activity and suppressing lipoxygenase, cyclooxygenase, and ascorbic acid–stimulated malonaldehyde formation in lipids (Zhang et al., 2014). Luteolin has also been shown to act as an anti-inflammatory agent. Pretreating murine macrophages with luteolin inhibited LPS-stimulated TNFα and IL-6 release, and blocked the activation NF-κB and the mitogen-activated protein kinase (MAPK) family members ERK, p38, and JNK (Zhang et al., 2014). Finally, luteolin has been shown to bind to the ATP-binding pocket of several kinases, inhibiting their activity. These kinases include protein kinase C (PKC), proto-oncogene tyrosine-protein kinase Src, (c-Src), vaccinia-related kinase, phosphatidylinositide 3-kinases (PI3), c-Jun N-terminal kinases (JNK) and p90 ribosomal S6 kinase (Zhang et al., 2014; Hassoun et al., 2006; Bellik et al., 2013; Rosillo et al., 2011) (Figure 10.3A in color insert). Luteolin is therefore able to suppress several of the pathways mentioned above.

10.2.2.2 Ellagic Acid

Ellagic acid is a natural antioxidant found in many fruits and vegetables. It has been shown to have antiproliferative activity in prostate cancer (Marín et al., 2013). The primary antioxidant mechanism of action of ellagic acid has been attributed to the direct scavenging of free radicals (Marín et al., 2013). Ellagic acid can replenish glutathione (GSH) levels and can chelate transition metal ions responsible for the generation of ROS (Vanella et al., 2013). Furthermore, ellagic acid has DNA protection properties. One of the mechanisms by which it inhibits mutagenesis and carcinogenesis is protecting the DNA by masking the binding sites from mutagens or carcinogens (Marín et al., 2013). Ellagic acid also plays a large role as an anti-inflammatory agent. It has been shown to reduce the effects of pro-inflammatory nitric oxide (NO), melanoma differentiation-associated protein (MDA), IL-1β, tumor necrosis factor alpha (TNF-α), cyclooxygenase-2 (COX-2) and decrease expression of nuclear factor kappa (NF-κB), while increasing production of the anti-inflammatory molecules GSH and interleukin-10 (IL-10) (Edderkaoui et al., 2008; 2013; Zhao et al., 2013) (Figure 10.3B in color insert). Ellagic acid is also a potent antiproliferative and pro-apoptotic molecule both *in vitro* and *in vivo* in many types of cancer, including prostate, breast, pancreas, and ovarian (Chung et al., 2013; Huang et al., 2009; Mishra and Vinayak, 2013; 2014; Aiyer et al., 2010; 2012; Gasmi and Sanderson, 2010; Boussetta et al., 2009; Narayanan et al., 1999; Oltersdorf et al., 2005). It also inhibits LNCaP cell growth through activation of rapamycin and reducing intracellular levels of β-catenin (Marín et al., 2013). Ellagic acid also downregulates anti-apoptotic proteins and silences information regulator 1, human antigen R, and hemeoxygenase-1. This polyphenol also increases the expression of the tumor suppressor protein p21 (Chung et al., 2013). Therefore, ellagic acid, much like luteolin, suppresses many of the pathways involved in prostate cancer progression.

10.2.2.3 Punicic Acid

Punicic acid is a polyunsaturated fatty acid found in pomegranate seed oil. Punicic acid has anticarcinogenic properties as well as antidiabetic properties (Wang et al., 2012; 2014). Specifically, punicic acid inhibits AR transfer and accumulation in the nucleus, and reduces the levels of prostate-specific antigen and steroid 5α-reductase type 1 (Wang et al., 2012) (Figure 10.3C in color insert). Punicic acid has also been shown to activate apoptosis through caspase-dependent pathways, as well as inhibit TNFα-induced neutrophil hyperactivation (Kito et al., 2001). These properties make punicic acid a very interesting molecule with a high potential to be used in prostate cancer specific treatments.

Despite the fact that luteolin, ellagic acid, and punicic acid individually have potential for treatment of prostate cancer, their combined effect has only recently been determined by us. Indeed, when used in combination, they are more potent than the individual components.

We have shown that L+E+P (luteolin [L], ellagic acid [E], and punicic acid [P]) in combination mimic the effects of the 5% PJ *in vitro*. They regulate cell-cycle regulators including Ras association domain-containing protein 1 (RASSF1), protein 53 (P53) (and its main regulator mouse double minute 2 homolog [MDM2]), cyclin-dependent kinase inhibitor 2A (CDKN2A), enhancer of zeste homolog 2 (EZH2) and PTEN (Sathyanarayana et al., 2003). In addition, cancer cells usually proliferate rapidly, thus an influx of angiogenesis is almost always observed because the cancer cells need the extra nutrition and oxygen to support their rapid expansion. L+E+P downregulated VEGF and significantly reduced new blood vessel development (Sathyanarayana et al., 2003). We have also shown that L+E+P treatment upregulates extracellular matrix receptor III (CD44) and LAMB3 (Sathyanarayana et al., 2003; Wang et al., 2014), both of which have been shown to be essential proteins for maintaining the integrity of cell adhesion in epithelial tissue, and both known to be downregulated in prostate cancer (Pantuck et al., 2006; Paller et al., 2013). *In vitro* adhesion assays showed that L+E+P increase cell adhesion of PC3 cells, and in scratch assays these components reduced PC3 cell migration (Stenner-Liewen et al., 2013). We also showed, using assays performed in chemotaxis chambers, that these components inhibit chemotaxis of PC3 cells towards stromal cell–derived factor 1α (SDF1α), a chemokine important in attraction of prostate cancer cells to the bone (Sathyanarayana, 2003; Wang et al., 2014). Therefore, the combination of these components inhibits crucial pathways for reducing prostate cancer metastasis.

In vivo, our studies showed that treatment of PC3 xenograft tumors in severe combined immune deficiency (SCID) mice with L+E+P significantly decreased tumor size, metastasis, and blood vessel density (Stenner-Liewen et al., 2013). SCID mice were used in these studies because they are immune-deficient, which allows us to grow these tumors *in vivo*. The mice were treated with L+E+P from the time of injection of the PC3 cells and then 5 days a week. The tumors were allowed to grow for 8 weeks before they were excised for measurements and further analysis. Because the PC3 cells contained luciferase, we were able to perform weekly images by injecting the mice with D-luciferin, the substrate for luciferase. Only the tumor cells were able to cleave D-luciferin and emit light, allowing us to follow tumor growth in the same animal over the 8 weeks by performing bioluminescence imaging. Treated mice showed reduced tumor growth as well as reduced number of metastases (Stenner-Liewen et al., 2013). Furthermore, qPCR analysis confirmed the regulation of several genes we had shown to be regulated *in vitro*. These genes include PTEN, GPX, and CDKN2A. We are currently using L+E+P to test their cancer preventative capabilities.

10.3 CLINICAL RELEVANCE

The ability to transition from experimental/bench studies to clinical studies is a crucial step in developing new therapeutic methods. Three major clinical trials with PJ have been carried out, two of which have shown very promising results. The first trial was published in 2006, showing that men who were treated with 8 ounces of PJ daily, following surgery or radiotherapy, had a statistically significant increase in PSA-doubling time. Mean PSA-doubling time significantly increased with treatment from a mean of 15 months at baseline to 54 months post-treatment (Luo et al., 2006). The second trial was a double blind randomized trial in which the patients were given 1 or 3 g of POMx (Freedland et al., 2013) The overall PSA-doubling time was lengthened from 11.9 months at baseline to 18.5 months after treatment. More specifically, the PSA doubling time increased from

11.9 to 18.8 months in the low-dose groups, and 12.2 to 17.5 months in the high-dose group, with no significant difference between dose groups (Freedland et al., 2013). No significant side effects were observed in either group, aside from diarrhea in 1.9% and 13.5% of patients in the 1- and 3-g dose groups, respectively. However, the third clinical trial, published in 2013, claimed that daily PJ intake has no effect on PSA-doubling time in patients with advanced prostate cancer (Stenner-Liewen et al., 2013). In this study, only patients with a PSA value ≥ 5 ng/mL were included. The patients were given 500 mL of PJ for 4 weeks and then 250 mL for 4 more weeks. Results showed no significant difference of PSA doubling time in treated and non-treated individuals. Unfortunately, the results of the first and second trials cannot be compared with the results in the third trial because the design of the trials was not the same. Indeed, the third trial selected individuals with high PSA, whereas the first trial opted for patients with lower PSA, and the second trial did not use initial PSA levels as a selection factor. Moreover, the time of treatment was much shorter in the third trial (8 weeks vs 18 months) and, in the first 4 weeks, the amount of juice consumed was double that of the first and second trials. Taken together, these data indicate that longer treatments need to be administered before positive results can be seen and significant conclusions can be drawn. These discrepancies in methodology make drawing reliable conclusions difficult. However, from these trials and the experimental work, POMx, PJ, or any other PEs/components appear to be most effective when used at earlier stages of cancer development.

10.4 PERSPECTIVES

The problems facing the scientific and medical communities today can be divided into three categories: (1) lack of dependable, noninvasive, and affordable methods of detecting prostate cancer; (2) lack of knowledge of the initiation mechanisms, and (3) lack of a comprehensive noninvasive treatment with minimal side effects.

10.4.1 Lack of Dependable, Noninvasive, and Affordable Methods of Detecting Prostate Cancer

To date, the American Cancer Society still suggests monitoring PSA levels for early cancer detection. While this is a good practice, PSA levels do not always correspond to the cancer stage; the levels of this molecule will only rise after the AR has become very active, meaning that the prostate already contains cancer cells, or will in short order develop malignant cells, leaving no room for prevention. That being said, PSA measurements are still advisable because of the accessibility, noninvasiveness, and affordability of testing. PSA readings will then prompt a biopsy if deemed necessary, which is an invasive procedure that yields limited information about the stage of cancer. The same is true with Gleason scores, which do not always reflect the cancer stage. One patient may have stage I cancer with a Gleason score of 6, while another may be at stage II with a Gleason score of 2. Therefore, even biopsies are not sufficient on their own to determine the stage of the cancer. Other early detection methods such as genetic testing for predisposition to prostate cancer, or detecting biomarkers other than PSA, such as kallikrein 11 from seminal plasma (Veveris-Lowe et al., 2007; Diamandis et al., 2002), are in the development stages. Any types of sequencing-based approaches are at the moment prohibitively expensive. In addition, if these tests are being used as a means to detect early signs of cancer, then they will need to be performed multiple times throughout the individual's life, which only compounds the cost per patient. Therefore, new, reliable, reproducible, noninvasive, and cost-effective detection tests need to be developed to detect prostate cancer in a stage that is still curable without major side effects.

10.4.2   Lack of Knowledge of the Initiation Mechanisms

The processes involved in prostate cancer initiation are not well known. What we have now is limited knowledge that leads us to speculate on potential mechanisms rather than having well-delineated mechanisms of initiation. Current mouse models of prostate cancer all rely on single or multiple knockouts of tumor suppressor genes. There are no current models that specifically address the other altered processes that lead to prostate cancer. This leaves a gap in the field and in our ability to study how deregulating these different systems will lead to or stimulate normal prostate epithelial cells to transform and progress to prostate cancer cells. Therefore, more studies and more diverse animal models are needed before we can make meaningful and significant contributions in understanding the underlying mechanism(s) of prostate cancer initiation.

10.4.3   Lack of a Comprehensive Noninvasive Treatment with Minimal Side Effects

As stated above, there are many different treatments currently on the market that target a specific protein, process, or stage of prostate cancer. However, none of these offer a cure, and they are often accompanied by a combination of difficult-to-tolerate and challenging side effects that may drive patients away from the treatments. Therefore, we are in great need of treatments that are effective and noninvasive, and that can be tolerated with minimal side effects. Although such a groundbreaking treatment has yet to be developed, we can speculate as to what possible mechanisms this novel treatment would utilize. Whereas hormone ablation, chemotherapy, or AR inhibition have offered a good starting point in the past several decades, their associated side effects along with the high relapse potential cannot be overlooked. The next-generation treatments need to take advantage of new diagnostic tools and new biomarkers that give insight into the specific problems of each patient, because prostate cancer can be caused by a variety of pathways and will require different care depending on its stage. Therefore, it is important to take advantage of the current tools used to personalize medicine. Prevention is another avenue that should be taken, by focusing on rebalancing the prostate proliferation mechanisms, and protecting the DNA from mutation by keeping the repair enzymes at homeostatic levels and functionally active. We are still a long way from prevention and personalized treatments, but the field is slowly and steadily moving towards individualized treatments.

10.5   CONCLUSION

Pomegranate juice, pomegranate extract, and/or individual components, have remarkable abilities to control prostate cancer growth and metastasis. They reduce proliferation *in vitro* and tumor size *in vivo*, while increasing cell adhesion and inhibiting cell migration, thereby reducing metastasis. Such qualities make these components promising candidates for further testing as potential alternative treatments. Their ability to reduce the growth of androgen-independent prostate cancer cells makes studying these components key in possibly treating relapsed patients. More importantly, PEs have shown great potential as a preventive or defensive measure against potential cancer initiators. The ability to regulate ROS and inflammation as well as protect DNA from damage could be key for the development of novel prostate cancer inhibitors.

REFERENCES

Aiyer, H.S. Gupta, R.C. 2010. Berries and ellagic acid prevent estrogen-induced mammary tumorigenesis by modulating enzymes of estrogen metabolism. *Cancer Prev Res* 3(6): 727–737.

Aiyer, H.S. Warri, A.M. Wood, D.R.E. et al. 2012. Influence of berry polyphenols on receptor signaling and cell-death pathways: implications for breast cancer prevention. *J Agric Food Chem* 60(23): 5693–5708.

Albrecht, M. Jiang, W. Kumi-Diaka, J. et al. 2004. Pomegranate extracts potently suppress proliferation, xenograft growth, and invasion of human prostate cancer cells. *J Med Food* 7(3): 274–283.

Auchus, R.J. 2004. The backdoor pathway to dihydrotestosterone. *Trends Endocrinol Metab* 15(9): 432–438.

Bawa-Khalfe, T. Cheng, J. Lin, S.H. et al. 2010. SENP1 induces prostatic intraepithelial neoplasia through multiple mechanisms. *J Biol Chem* 285(33): 25859–25866.

Bellik, Y. Boukraâ, L. Alzahrani, H.A. et al. 2013. Molecular mechanism underlying anti-inflammatory and anti-allergic activities of phytochemicals: an update. *Molecules* 18(1): 322–353.

Boussetta, T. Raad, H. Lettéron, P. et al. 2009. Punicic acid a conjugated linolenic acid inhibits TNFalpha-induced neutrophil hyperactivation and protects from experimental colon inflammation in rats. *PLoS One* 4(7): e6458.

Chung, Y.C, Lu, L.C. Tsai, M.H. et al. 2013. The inhibitory effect of ellagic acid on cell growth of ovarian carcinoma cells. *Evid Based Complement Alternat Med* 2013: 306705.

Chuu, C.P. Kokontis, J.M. Hiipakka, R.A. 2011. Androgens as therapy for androgen receptor-positive castration-resistant prostate cancer. *J Biomed Sci* 18: 63.

Diamandis, E.P. Okui, A. Mitsui, S. et al., 2002. Human kallikrein 11: a new biomarker of prostate and ovarian carcinoma. *Cancer Res* 62(1): 295–300.

Edderkaoui, M. Lugea, A. Hui, H. Eibl, G. Lu, Q.Y. Moro, A. et al. 2013. Ellagic acid and embelin affect key cellular components of pancreatic adenocarcinoma, cancer, and stellate cells. *Nutr Cancer* 65(8): 1232–1244.

Edderkaoui, M. Odinokova, I. Ohno, I. et al. 2008. Ellagic acid induces apoptosis through inhibition of nuclear factor kappa B in pancreatic cancer cells. *World J Gastroenterol* 14(23): 3672–3680.

Fong, L. Small, E.J. 2008. Anti-cytotoxic T-lymphocyte antigen-4 antibody: the first in an emerging class of immunomodulatory antibodies for cancer treatment. *J Clin Oncol* 26(32): 5275–5283.

Freedland, S.J. Carducci, M. Kroeger, N. et al. 2013. A double-blind, randomized, neoadjuvant study of the tissue effects of POMx pills in men with prostate cancer before radical prostatectomy. *Cancer Prev Res* (Phila) 6(10): 1120–1127.

Furr, B.J. Tucker, H. 1996. The preclinical development of bicalutamide: pharmacodynamics and mechanism of action. *Urology* 47(1A Suppl): 13–25; discussion 29–32.

Garrison, J.B. Shaw, Y.J. Chen, C.S. et al. 2007. Novel quinazoline-based compounds impair prostate tumorigenesis by targeting tumor vascularity. *Cancer Res* 67(23): 11344–11352.

Gasmi, J. Sanderson, J.T. 2010. Growth inhibitory, antiandrogenic, and pro-apoptotic effects of punicic acid in LNCaP human prostate cancer cells. *J Agric Food Chem* 58(23): 12149–12156.

Gil, M.I. Tomas-Barberan, F.A. Hess-Pierce, B. et al. 2000. Antioxidant activity of pomegranate juice and its relationship with phenolic composition and processing. *J Agric Food Chem* 48: 4581–4589.

Guerrero, J. Alfaro, I.E. Gómez, F. et al. 2013. Enzalutamide, an androgen receptor signaling inhibitor, induces tumor regression in a mouse model of castration-resistant prostate cancer. *The Prostate* 73(12): 1291–1305.

Gulley, J.L. Madan, R.A. Tsang, K.Y. et al. 2013. Immune impact induced by PROSTVAC (PSA-TRICOM), a therapeutic vaccine for prostate cancer. *Cancer Immunol Res* 2(2): 133–141.

Harris, W.P. Mostaghel, E.A. Nelson, P.S. Montgomery, B. 2009. Androgen deprivation therapy: progress in understanding mechanisms of resistance and optimizing androgen depletion. *Nat Clin Pract Urol* 6(2): 76–85.

Hassoun, E.A. Vodhanel, J. Holden, B. Abushaban, A. 2006. The effects of ellagic acid and vitamin E succinate on antioxidant enzymes activities and glutathione levels in different brain regions of rats after subchronic exposure to TCDD. *J Toxicol Environ Health A* 9(5): 381–393.

Higano, C.S. Small, E.J. Schellhammer, P. et al. 2010. Sipuleucel-T. *Nat Rev Drug Discov* 9(7): 513–514.

Hoffman-Censits, J. Fu, M. 2013. Chemotherapy and targeted therapies: are we making progress in castrate-resistant prostate cancer? *Semin Oncol* 40(3): 361–374.

Hong, M.Y. Seeram, N.P. Heber, D. 2008. Pomegranate polyphenols downregulate expression of androgen synthesizing genes in human prostate cancer cells overexpressing the androgen receptor. *J Nutr Biochem* 19(12): 848–855.

Huang, S.T. Wang, C.Y. Yang, R.C. et al. 2009. Phyllanthus urinaria increases apoptosis and reduces telomerase activity in human nasopharyngeal carcinoma cells. *Forsch Komplementmed* 16(1): 34–40.

Kelley, M. Fishel, M. 2008. DNA repair proteins as molecular targets for cancer therapeutics. *Anticancer Agents Med Chem* 8(4): 417–425.

Khan, N. Afaq, F. Mukhtar, H. 2008. Cancer chemoprevention through dietary antioxidants: progress and promise. *Antioxid Redox Signal* (10): 475–510.

Kim, N.D. Mehta, R. Yu, W. et al. 2002. Chemopreventive and adjuvant therapeutic potential of pomegranate (punica granatum) for human breast cancer. *Breast Cancer Res Treat* 71: 203–217.

Kito, H. Suzuki, H. Ichikawa, T. et al. 2001. Hypermethylation of the CD44 gene is associated with progression and metastasis of human prostate cancer. *Prostate* 49(2): 110–115.

Kleb, B. Estécio, M.R. Zhang, J. et al. 2016. Differentially methylated genes and androgen receptor re-expression in small cell prostate carcinomas. *Epigenetics* 18: 1–10.

Koyama, S. Cobb, L.J. Mehta, H.H. et al. 2010. Pomegranate extract induces apoptosis in human prostate cancer cells by modulation of the IGF-IGFBP axis. *Growth Horm IGF Res* 20(1): 55–62.

Langley, P. 2000. Why a pomegranate? *BMJ* (321): 1153–1154.

Lansky, E.P. Newman, R.A. 2007. Punica granatum (pomegranate) and its potential for prevention and treatment of inflammation and cancer. *J Ethnopharmacol* 109: 177–206.

Lee, J.H. Isayeva,T. Larson, M. et al. 2014. Endostatin is a novel inhibitor of androgen receptor function in prostate cancer. *Cancer Res* 74(19): 612.

Li, L.-C. Carroll, P.R. Dahiya, R. 2005. Epigenetic changes in prostate cancer: implication for diagnosis and treatment. *J Natl Cancer Inst* 97(2): 103–115.

Li, W.W. Li, V.W. Hutnik, M. et al. 2012. Tumor angiogenesis as a target for dietary cancer prevention. *J Oncol* 2012: 879623.

Longtin, R. 2003. The pomegranate: nature's power fruit? *J Natl Cancer Inst* 95: 346–348.

Luo, L.Y. Shan, S.J. Elliott, M.B. et al. 2006. Purification and characterization of human kallikrein 11, a candidate prostate and ovarian cancer biomarker, from seminal plasma. *Clin Cancer Res* 12: 742–750.

Malik, A. Afaq, F. Sarfaraz, S. et al. 2005. Pomegranate fruit juice for chemoprevention and chemotherapy of prostate cancer. *Proc Natl Acad Sci U S A* 102(41): 14813–14818.

Malik, A. Mukhtar, H. 2006. Prostate cancer prevention through pomegranate fruit. *Cell Cycle* 5(4): 371–373.

Marín, M. María Giner, R. Ríos, J.L. Carmen, R.M. 2013. Intestinal anti-inflammatory activity of ellagic acid in the acute and chronic dextrane sulfate sodium models of mice colitis. *J Ethnopharmacol* 150(3): 925–934.

Mateo, J. Smith, A. Ong, M. De Bono, J.S. 2014. Novel drugs targeting the androgen receptor pathway in prostate cancer. *Cancer Metastasis Rev* 33: 567–579.

Mishra, S. Vinayak, M. 2013. Ellagic acid checks lymphoma promotion via regulation of PKC signaling pathway. *Mol Biol Rep* 40(2): 1417–1428.

Mishra, S. Vinayak, M. 2014. Ellagic acid induces novel and atypical PKC isoforms and promotes caspase-3 dependent apoptosis by blocking energy metabolism. *Nutr Cancer* 66(4): 675–681.

Narayanan, B.A. Geoffroy, O. Willingham, M.C. et al. 1999. P53/p21 (WAF1/CIP1) expression and its possible role in G1 arrest and apoptosis in ellagic acid treated cancer cells. *Cancer Lett* 136(2): 215–221.

Noda, Y. Kaneyuki, T. Mori, A. Packer, L. 2002. Antioxidant activities of pomegranate fruit extract and its anthocyanidins: delphinidin, cyanidin, and pelargonidin. *J Agric Food Chem* 50: 166–171.

Oltersdorf, T. Elmore, S.W. Shoemaker, A.R. et al. 2005. An inhibitor of bcl-2 family proteins induces regression of solid tumours. *Nature* 435(7042): 677–681.

Osguthorpe, D.J. Hagler, A.T. 2011. Mechanism of androgen receptor antagonism by bicalutamide in the treatment of prostate cancer. *Biochemistry* 50(19): 4105–4113.

Paller, C. Ye, X. Wozniak, P. et al. 2013. A randomized phase II study of pomegranate extract for men with rising PSA following initial therapy for localized prostate cancer. *Prostate Cancer Prostatic Dis* 16(1): 50–55.

Pantuck, A. Leppert, J. Zomorodian, N. et al. 2006. Phase II study of pomegranate juice for men with rising prostate-specific antigen following surgery or radiation for prostate cancer. *Clin Cancer Res* 12(13): 4018–4026.

Pienta, K.J. Esper, P.S. 1993. Risk factors for prostate cancer. *Ann Intern Med* 118(10): 793–803.

Prostate Cancer Treatment. National Cancer Institute. http://www.cancer.gov/types/prostate/patient/prostate-treatment-pdq#section/_120 (accessed on 8 April 2016).

Provenge [prescribing information]. 2014. Seattle, WA: Dendreon Corporation.

Quintela, M.L. Mateos, L.L. Estévez, S.V. et al. 2015. Enzalutamide: a new prostate cancer targeted therapy against the androgen receptor. *Cancer Treatment Rev* 41(3): 247–253.

Rathkopf, D.E. Morris, M.J. Fox, J.J. et al. 2013. Phase I study of ARN-509, a novel antiandrogen, in the treatment of castration-resistant prostate cancer. *J Clin Oncol* 31(29): 3525–3530.

Rettig, M.B. Heber, D. An, J. et al. 2008. Pomegranate extract inhibits androgen-independent prostate cancer growth through a nuclear factor-κB-dependent mechanism. *Mol Cancer Ther* 7(9): 2662–2671.

Reynolds, A.R. Kyprianou, N. 2006. Growth factor signalling in prostatic growth: significance in tumour development and therapeutic targeting. *Br J Pharmacol* 147 Suppl 2: S144–152.

Rosillo, M. Sanchez-Hidalgo, M. de la Lastra, C. 2011. Protective effect of ellagic acid, a natural polyphenolic compound, in a murine model of Crohn's disease. *Biochem Pharmacol* 82(7): 737–745.

Ryan, C.J. Smith, M.R. de Bono, J.S. et al. 2013. Abiraterone in metastatic prostate cancer without previous chemotherapy. *N Engl J Med* 368(2): 138–148.

Sanchez, I. Dynlacht, B.D. 2005. New insights into cyclins, cdks, and cell cycle control. *Semin Cell Dev Biol* (16): 311–321.

Sartippour, M.R. Seeram, N.P. Rao, J.Y. et al. 2008. Ellagitannin-rich pomegranate extract inhibits angiogenesis in prostate cancer in vitro and in vivo. *Int J Oncol* 32(2): 475–480.

Sartor, O. Pal, S.K. 2013. Abiraterone and its place in the treatment of metastatic CRPC. *Nat Rev Clin Oncol.* 10(1): 6–8.

Sathyanarayana, U.G. Padar, A. Suzuki, M. et al. 2003. Aberrant promoter methylation of laminin-5-encoding genes in prostate cancers and its relationship to clinicopathological features. *Clin Cancer Res* 9(17): 6395–6400.

SEER Stat Fact Sheets: Prostate Cancer Surveillance, Epidemiology, and End Results Program. Cancer of the Prostate. http://seer.cancer.gov/statfacts/html/prost.html (accessed on 8 April 2016).

Singh, P. Pal, S.K. Alex, A. et al. 2015. Development of PROSTVAC immunotherapy in prostate cancer. *Future Oncol* 11(15): 2137–2148.

Smith, D.C. Smith, M.R. Sweeney, C. et al. 2013. Cabozantinib in patients with advanced prostate cancer: results of a phase II randomized discontinuation trial. *J Clin Oncol* 31(4): 412–419.

Sountoulides, P. Rountos, T. 2013. Adverse effects of androgen deprivation therapy for prostate cancer: prevention and management. *ISRN Urol* 2013: 240108.

Stavridi, F. Karapanagiotou, E.M. Syrigos, K.N. 2010. Targeted therapeutic approaches for hormone-refractory prostate cancer. *Cancer Treat Rev* 36(2): 122–130.

Stenner-Liewen, F. Liewen, H. Cathomas, R. et al. 2013. Daily pomegranate intake has no impact on PSA levels in patients with advanced prostate cancer – results of a phase IIb randomized controlled trial. *J Cancer* 4(7): 597–605.

Tan, M.H. Li, J. Xu, H.E. et al. 2015. Androgen receptor: structure, role in prostate cancer and drug discovery. *Acta Pharmacol Sin* 36(1): 3–23.

Taneja, S.S. 2016. Re: DNA-repair defects and olaparib in metastatic prostate cancer. *J Urol* 195: 925–928.

Väänänen, H.K. Zhao, H. Mulari, M. Halleen, J.M. 2000. The cell biology of osteoclast function. *J Cell Sci* 113: 377–381.

Vanella, L. Di Giacomo, C. Acquaviva, R. et al. 2013. Apoptotic markers in a prostate cancer cell line: effect of ellagic acid. *Oncol Rep* 30(6): 2804–2810.

Veveris-Lowe, T.L. Kruger, S.J. Walsh, T. et al. 2007. Seminal fluid characterization for male fertility and prostate cancer: kallikrein-related serine proteases and whole proteome approaches. *Semin Thromb Hemost* 33(1): 87–99.

Viuda-Martos, M. Fernández-López, J. Pérez-Álvarez, J.A. 2010. Pomegranate and its many functional components as related to human health: a review. *Compr Rev Food Sci Food Saf* 9: 635–654.

Wang, L. Alcon, A. Yuan, H. et al. 2011. Cellular and molecular mechanisms of pomegranate juice-induced anti-metastatic effect on prostate cancer cells. *Integr Biol* 3(7): 742–754.

Wang, L. Ho, J. Glackin, C. Martins-Green, M. 2012. Specific pomegranate juice components as potential inhibitors of prostate cancer metastasis. *Transl Oncol* 5(5): 344–355.

Wang, L. Li, W. Lin, M. et al. 2014. Luteolin, ellagic acid and punicic acid are natural products that inhibit prostate cancer metastasis. *Carcinogenesis* 35(10): 2321–2330.

Wang, L. Martins-Green, M. 2014. Pomegranate and its components as alternative treatment for prostate cancer. *Int J Mol Sci* 15(9): 14949–14966.

Wei, X.X. Fong, L. Small, E.J. 2016. Prospects for the use of ipilimumab in treating advanced prostate cancer. *Expert Opin Biol Ther* 16(3): 421–432.

Yakes, F.M. Chen, J. Tan, J. et al. 2011. Cabozantinib (XL184), a novel MET and VEGFR2 inhibitor, simultaneously suppresses metastasis, angiogenesis, and tumor growth. *Mol Cancer Ther* 10(12): 2298–2308.

Zhang, H-M. Zhao, L. et al. 2014. Research progress on the anticarcinogenic actions and mechanisms of ellagic acid. *Cancer Biol Med* 11(2): 92–100.

Zhao, M. Tang, S.N. Marsh, J.L. et al. 2013. Ellagic acid inhibits human pancreatic cancer growth in Balb/C nude mice. *Cancer Lett* 337: 210–217.

CHAPTER **11**

Zyflamend and Prostate Cancer Therapy

Jay Whelan, Yi Zhao, E-Chu Huang, Amber MacDonald, and Dallas Donohoe

CONTENTS

11.1 REVIEW OF ZYFLAMEND

Herbs and spices have been used to enhance the flavor of food, and their bioactive constituents are known for their antioxidant and anti-inflammatory properties (Viuda-Martos et al., 2011; Srinivasan, 2014). A variety of mechanisms and molecular targets have been identified to explain

Table 11.1 Specifications for Active Ingredients in Zyflamend

Botanical	Representative Bioactive Compounds	Part Used	Method of Extraction	Marker/Component Specifications
Rosemary (19.2%) (*Rosmarinus officinalis*)	Rosmarinic acid	Leaf	Supercritical CO_2	Diterpene phenols (22–24%), Essential oils (3–5%)
	Ursolic acid	Leaf	Water and alcohol	Diterpene phenols (24–26%)
	Carnosol			
Ginger (12.8%) (*Zingiber officinale*)	Gingerol	Rhizome	Supercritical CO_2	Pungent compounds (24–35%), Zingiberene ($\geq$8%)
	Shogaol	Rhizome	Water and alcohol	Pungent compounds ($\geq$3%)
	Paradol			
Turmeric (14.1%) (*Curcuma longa*)	Curcumoids	Rhizome	Water and alcohol	Curcuminoids ($\geq$11%)
	Turmerones	Rhizome	Supercritical CO_2, water	Curcumin ($\geq$0.5%), total essential oil with α- and β-turmerone 70–90%)
Holy Basil (12.8%) (*Ocimum sanctum*)	Ursolic acid	Leaves	Water and alcohol	Ursolic acid (2–3%)
Green Tea (12.8%) (*Camellia sinensis*)	Epigallocatechin	Leaves	Water	Polyphenols ($\geq$45%)
	Epigallocatechin gallate			
	Epicatechin gallate			
Hu Zhang (10.2%) (*Polygonum cuspidatum*)	Resveratrol	Radix/ rhizome	Water and alcohol	Resveratrol ($\geq$8%)
Chinese Goldthread (5.1%) (*Coptis chinensis*)	Berberine	Root	Water and alcohol	Berberine ($\geq$6%)
	Coptisine			
Barberry (5.1%) (*Berberis vulgaris*)	Berberine	Root bark	Water and alcohol	Berberine ($\geq$6%)
Oregano (5.1%) (*Origanum vulgare*)	Carvacrol	Leaf	Supercritical CO_2, water	Essential oils (8–12%), phenolic antioxidants ($\geq$4.5%)
	Linalool			
	Rosmarinic acid			
	Thymol			
Baikal Skullcap (2.5%) (*Scutellaria baicalensis*)	Baicalin	Root	Water and alcohol	Baicalin ($\geq$17%)
	Baicalein			Baicalein ($\geq$1.5%)
	Wogonin			Wogonin ($\geq$0.4%)

Data summarized from Huang et al., 2012.

some of their health-promoting effects (Manson, 2005; Howells et al., 2007). Increasingly, research exploring the impact of natural products, in particular botanicals, on chronic diseases such as cancer has generated new interest not only in prevention, but also in conjunction with standard treatments for those individuals with existing disease.

Zyflamend® (New Chapter, Brattleboro, VT) is a commercial preparation comprised of the extracts of 10 herbs (w/w): holy basil (*Ocimum sanctum*), turmeric (*Curcuma longa*), ginger (*Zingiber officinale*), green tea (*Camellia sinensis*), rosemary (*Rosmarinus officinalis*), hu zhang (*Polygonum cuspidatum*), barberry (*Berberis vulgaris*), oregano (*Origanum vulgare*), baikal skullcap (*Scutellaria baicalensis*), and Chinese goldthread (*Coptis chinensis*) (Table 11.1). A detailed description of

Zyflamend and the quality assurance of the mixture has been described previously in detail (Huang E-C et al., 2012). Individual herbs are subjected to supercritical CO_2 and hydroethanolic extraction procedures to achieve the specific ranges of select bioactive compounds (as described in Table 11.1).

Zyflamend was originally designed by combining herbs reported to have antioxidant and inflammatory properties. For example, Zyflamend reduces the production of proinflammatory eicosanoids (Yang et al., 2007; 2008), inhibits the activities of both isoforms of cyclooxygenase (COX-1 and COX-2), as well as 12- and 5-lipoxygenases (Yang et al., 2007; 2008), and inhibits the activation of nuclear factor kappa-light-chain-enhancer of activated B cells (NF-κB) (Burke et al., 2015; Kunnumakkara et al., 2012; Sandur et al., 2007) and the subsequent production of cytokine-inducible nitric oxide (iNOS) (Ekmekcioglu et al., 2011). Furthermore, Zyflamend has been reported to reduce C-reactive protein (CRP) levels in humans (Capodice et al., 2009). CRP is an acute-phase reaction protein produced in response to inflammation (Thiele et al., 2015).

To date, there have been 18 research articles using Zyflamend, most of which have focused on the anticancer effects of this blend, covering *in vitro*, preclinical, and clinical studies involving the prostate, bone, skin, kidney, breast, and pancreas (Huang E-C et al., 2012; Yang et al., 2007; 2008; Burke et al., 2015; Kunnumakkara et al., 2012; Sandur et al., 2007; Ekmecioglu et al., 2011; Capodice et al., 2009; Huang E-C et al., 2011; 2014; Zhao et al., 2015; Bemis et al., 2005; Bilen et al., 2015; Kim et al., 2012; Mohebati et al., 2012; Rafailov et al., 2007; Yan et al., 2012; Subbaramaiah et al., 2013), with prostate being the most studied.

The overall objective of this review is to outline how Zyflamend may be of use as an adjuvant to prostate cancer therapy by reviewing preclinical and clinical data as it relates to prostate cancer progression from an androgen-dependent to more advanced androgen-independent phases.

11.2 PROSTATE CANCER

Prostate cancer (PrC) is the most commonly diagnosed solid malignancy and has become the second leading cause of cancer-related deaths in men in most Western developed countries (American Cancer Society: http://www.cancer.org/acs/groups/content/@editorial/documents/document/acspc-044552.pdf).

The survivability of PrC is high if diagnosis is early (5-year survival rates >98%) and confined to the tissue of origin (American Cancer Society: http://www.cancer.org/cancer/prostatecancer/detailedguide/prostate-cancer-survival-rates). However, if the disease migrates to other tissues, such as bone and lung, prognosis becomes dramatically less positive. Once tumors become metastatic (i.e., bone and lung), they are very difficult to treat and prognosis is poor, with a 5-year survival rate of 28% (American Cancer Society: http://www.cancer.org/cancer/prostatecancer/detailedguide/prostate-cancer-survival-rates). For the most part, PrC is temporarily responsive to hormone ablative therapy, as prostate epithelial cells are dependent on androgens for growth. Although more than 95% of patients will respond to hormone ablative therapy (also referred to as androgen deprivation therapy [ADT]), most find their PrC will eventually relapse and become hormone refractory. Secondary treatments are commonly used when hormone ablation fails to control disease progression (Bilen et al., 2015). These include radiation, immunotherapy, and chemotherapy; however, metastatic castrate-resistant PrC, particularly in bone, is for many invariably fatal.

11.3 HISTORICAL USE OF ZYFLAMEND

The first reported clinical case study involving Zyflamend occurred in 2007 (Rafailov et al., 2007). A 70-year-old African-American male with high-grade prostatic intraepithelial neoplasia

(HGPIN; a potentially precancerous form of the disease) with a prostate-specific antigen (PSA) level of 9.7 ng/mL was treated orally with Zyflamend (3 pills/day). PSA is a common biomarker to monitor PrC progression. After 18 months of treatment, the patient was reportedly PIN and cancer free. This study was followed up by a larger Phase I trial involving 29 subjects diagnosed with HGPIN who were treated orally with Zyflamend (3 pills/day) using an open-labeled escalation design where the subjects were their own controls (Capodice et al., 2009). Of the 15 patients who were biopsied at the end of the study (18 months), PSA levels were reduced by 20 to 50% in 48% of the subjects, 60% had benign tissue (no HGPIN), 27% had HGPIN in one lobe, and 13% were diagnosed with PrC. Unfortunately, there was not a control arm associated with this study. In 2015, a more recent case study performed at MD Anderson Cancer Center reported a patient with advanced castrate-resistant PrC who was treated with Zyflamend (two pills/day) (Bilen et al., 2015). This was an 81-year-old African-American male whose PSA levels were exponentially increasing despite previously undergoing radical prostatectomy, radiation therapy, and hormone ablative therapy. After a year's treatment with Zyflamend, his PSA levels dropped from 4.5 ng/mL to 0.4 ng/mL and remained stable 2 years thereafter. Importantly, no serious side effects from Zyflamend were reported in any of these studies.

11.4 PROSTATE CANCER MODELS USED IN THESE STUDIES

Based in part on these previous results, this chapter investigates potential molecular mechanisms that could reveal a rationale for using this polyherbal mixture with standard therapies in the treatment of PrC. The studies in this chapter used cell lines derived from the CWR22 lineage (human) (Pretlow et al., 1993; Wainstein et al., 1994; Cheng et al., 1996; Nagabhushan et al., 1996). These cells were chosen because they can mimic the progression of human PrC *in vivo*, progressing from androgen dependent (CWR22) to androgen independent (castrate resistant) (CWR22R) growth following hormone deprivation in preclinical experimental models (Nagabhushan et al., 1996; McEntee et al., 2008). Unlike androgen-independent PC3 and DU145 PrC cells, the castrate-resistant cells derived from the CWR22 lineage (i.e., CWR22R, CWR22Rv1) have a functional androgen receptor and produce PSA, characteristics shared by castrate-resistant tumors in humans.

11.5 ZYFLAMEND AND *IN VIVO* MODELS OF PROSTATE CANCER

11.5.1 Human Equivalent Doses

As surrogates for human inquisition, animal models reside at the core of medical innovation. Through careful environmental control, these genetically similar models facilitate therapeutic advancements in the magnitude of human disease. Preclinical animal models are not intended to replace humans, but be a substitute that is often better controlled and better able to answer narrow research questions that could not be done, on a practical basis, with humans. Rodent dietary composition is of particular interest as it provides a way to assess the translational ability of individual dietary constituents, through appropriate dosing of nutrients, with physiological effects observed in humans consuming similar levels. A common challenge faced by researchers who are interested in interspecies comparisons is identifying a scientifically validated background diet and appropriate doses for supplemented nutrients.

In order to maximize translatability, studies presented here have used formulated diets that mimic the Western diet using supplemented doses that are commonly recommended for humans by appropriately allometrically scaling them to rodents. The rationale for this is simple. Rodent experiments are typically performed using inbred models that are genetically identical, are fed identical diets, have identical circadian rhythms (light:dark cycles), experience similar exercise patterns, and are housed under identical conditions. If you can't get a desired response in rodents using human equivalent doses (not pharmacological doses), you cannot expect to see positive responses in humans using human equivalent doses if humans are genetically diverse, with a composition of diet as varied as the people who eat them, all having heterogeneous lifestyles, under different living environments and exercise patterns. Thus, the use of a human background diet with human equivalent doses is critical if the data from preclinical research models are to have any application to humans. Consistent with this approach, all data presented here are based on human equivalent dosing (as described in detail elsewhere: Huang E-C., 2012; Rucker et al., 2002; Blanchard et al., 2015; Weldon and Whelan, 2011).

11.5.2   Zyflamend and Androgen-Dependent Tumor Growth

To mimic androgen-dependent growth, CWR22 PrC cells were seeded and grown subcutaneously in castrated, male nude (*nu/nu*) mice, supplemented with a slow-releasing testosterone pellet (growth of the PrC cells is dependent upon androgens). The animals were then fed diets with and without Zyflamend (at human equivalent doses). Zyflamend supplementation significantly inhibited tumor growth by ~50% within 2 weeks (Figure 11.1). These results mimic the effects of Zyflamend using the human PrC cell line LNCaP *in vitro*, a cell line dependent upon androgens for proliferation (Yan et al., 2012).

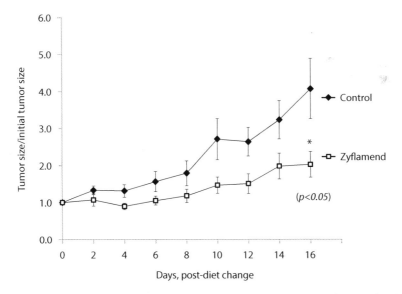

Figure 11.1   Growth of androgen-dependent CWR22-derived tumors in castrated male athymic nude mice co-inserted subcutaneously with a slow-releasing testosterone pellet following dietary treatment with and without Zyflamend relative to the initial size of the tumors (Huang E-C et al., 2012). Following 1 week on a control diet that mimicked a Western diet (Day 0), animals remained on the control diet (closed diamonds) or were placed on a diet supplemented with Zyflamend (0.06% w/w, human equivalent dose of 2 capsules) (open squares). *Tumor size is significantly different between groups at p<0.05. The data (n=9/control group; n=8/Zyflamend group) are presented as means ± SEM.

11.5.3   Zyflamend and Androgen-Dependent Tumor Regression

When androgen-dependent LNCaP cells were treated in combination with Zyflamend and bicalu-timide (an androgen receptor inhibitor that is used in standard-of-care for ADT), they inhibited cell proliferation (*in vitro*) synergistically (Yan et al., 2012). To interrogate any synergistic/additive effects of Zyflamend when combined with ADT *in vivo*, testosterone pellets were removed from castrated animals bearing full CWR22-derived tumors (to mimic ADT) and then fed diets with and without Zyflamend (Huang E-C et al., 2012). Within 4 days, the tumors from the Zyflamend-treated group regressed (Figures 11.2 and 11.3), but regression of the tumors from the control animals was delayed (Figure 11.3A). The variability in response to ADT treatment was significantly less with Zyflamend treatment compared to animals not supplemented with Zyflamend (Figures 11.2 and 11.3B). Furthermore, while all tumors eventually regressed following ADT, the time needed to regress tumors to 50% of their original size was almost cut in half with Zyflamend treatment (11 days vs 19 days) (Huang E-C et al., 2012). These data suggest that the interaction of Zyflamend with ADT enhanced the effectiveness of treatment and reduced the variability of response.

11.5.4   Zyflamend and Androgen-Independent (Castrate-Resistant) Tumor Growth

While one of the treatments for advanced forms of PrC is ADT, tumors eventually relapse, as evidenced by changes in circulating PSA levels. Zyflamend has been shown to inhibit proliferation *in vitro* of androgen-independent (i.e., PC3) (Yang et al., 2007; Huang E-C et al., 2014) and castrate-resistant (i.e., CWR22Rv1) (Huang E-C et al., 2011; 2014) PrC cells and to reduce gene expression of PSA (CWR22Rv1, PC3) (Huang E-C et al., 2011; Yan et al., 2012). Studies *in vivo* show that Zyflamend fed to mice at human equivalent doses inhibited tumor growth of CWR22Rv1-derived

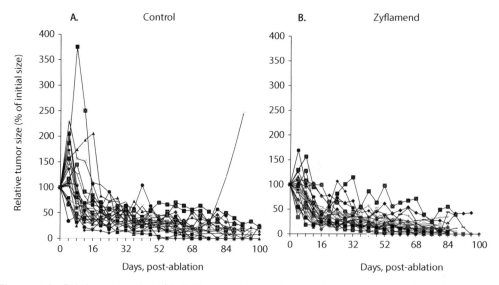

Figure 11.2   Relative tumor size of individual castrated athymic male nude mice inserted with androgen-dependent CWR22 PrC cells following the removal of a subcutaneously inserted testosterone pellet (post-ablation 0–100 days) (Huang E-C et al., 2012). Each line represents tumor regression from an individual mouse. (A) Mice fed a control diet (n=22) that mimics a human equivalent background diet. (B) Mice fed a control diet supplemented with Zyflamend (0.06% w/w, human equivalent dose of 2 capsules) (n=28).

tumors by 46% within 2 weeks (Figure 11.4) (Huang E-C et al., 2012). Circulating PSA levels were detected in only 1 of 14 animals tested in the Zyflamend group as compared to almost half of the animals from the control group (6 out of 13) (Huang E-C et al., 2012). Similar results (reductions in PSA) were observed in clinical trials and case studies of individuals provided oral doses of Zyflamend (Capodice et al., 2009; Bilen et al., 2015).

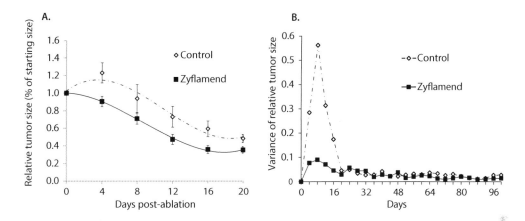

Figure 11.3 (A) Relative tumor size of androgen-dependent CWR22-derived tumors in castrated athymic male nude mice following the removal of a subcutaneously inserted testosterone pellet (post-ablation 0–20 days) (Huang E-C et al., 2012). These figures represent a summary of the data presented in Figure 11.2. Following hormone ablation, the tumors in the control group (dotted line) continued to increase in size prior to regression (after Day 8), while those from the Zyflamend group (solid line) began to shrink almost immediately (see Day 4). (Data presented as means ± SEM). (B) Mean variance of tumor size from animals on each diet following hormone ablation (control, dotted line; Zyflamend, solid line). The inter-animal variability of tumor response was significantly reduced in the Zyflamend-supplemented group (p<0.001). These data suggest that Zyflamend enhances the effect of ADT and reduces the variability of the response.

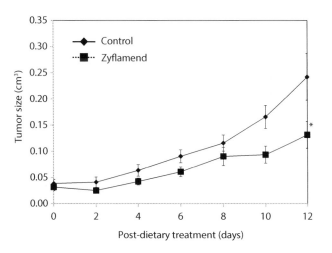

Figure 11.4 The growth of castrate-resistant CWR22Rv1-derived tumors when orally treated with and without Zyflamend at human equivalent doses (Huang E-C et al., 2012). CWR22Rv1 cells were inserted subcutaneously in castrated male athymic nude mice on control (diamonds) or Zyflamend-supplemented (squares) diets (0.06% w/w, human equivalent dose of 2 capsules). *Tumor size is significantly different between groups at p<0.05. The data (n=10/group) are presented as means ± SEM.

11.6   MECHANISMS OF ACTION

11.6.1   Tumor Suppressor Proteins P21 and P27

Cyclin-dependent kinases (CDKs) are important components that positively regulate the cell cycle. Tumor suppressor proteins like p21 (also referred to as p21^{Cip1} or p21^{Waf1}) and p27 (also referred to as p27^{Kip1}) are CDK inhibitors, blocking the cell cycle at various points. Thus, increased expression of p21 and p27 are important targets for the treatment of cancer. In CWR22Rv1 castrate-resistant PrC cells, Zyflamend upregulated the expression of p21 and p27 (mRNA and protein) in a dose-dependent manner and increased nuclear localization (p21) (Figure 11.5 in color insert) (Huang E-C et al., 2014). Inhibition of cell proliferation was directly related in part to these changes. When Zyflamend was combined with overexpression of p21, cell proliferation was further inhibited, suggesting Zyflamend's effects are not solely dependent upon p21, but involve multiple mechanisms. Similar results were observed with PC3 cells, with an increased expression of p21 in the presence of Zyflamend (Yang et al., 2007). In a variety of melanoma cell lines, Zyflamend induced G2/M cell cycle arrest, results that would be consistent with upregulation of p21 and p27 (Ekmekcioglu et al., 2011) as a general mechanism related to antiproliferative effects. In addition, Zyflamend regulates the cell cycle by decreasing cyclin D1, and via the reduction in the phosphorylation of retinoblastoma (Rb) (Yang et al., 2007).

11.6.2   Histone Acetylation

The expression of p21 is in part regulated by histone acetylation. Acetylation of N-terminal tails of histones relaxes the chromatin, allowing for easier access of transcriptional coactivators to DNA, increasing gene expression. If this hyperacetylation occurs at tumor suppressor genes, upregulation of gene expression occurs. For example, hyperacetylation near Sp1-binding sites of the proximal promotor is a key regulator of p21 expression (Ocker and Schneider-Stock, 2007). Histone acetyl-transferases are mediators of histone acetylation and are important in posttranslational modification of histones (Das et al., 2009; Marmorstein, 2001; Marmorstein and Trievel, 2009). CBP/p300 is one of three major subtypes (Marmorstein, 2001; Marmorstein and Trievel, 2009).

Regulation of acetylation is a balance between acetylators and deacetylators (Verdone et al., 2006). Deacetylation of histones results in compacted DNA or non-accessible DNA that is wrapped around the chromatin, inhibiting gene expression (Khan and Thangue, 2012). Histone deacetylases (HDACs) are a family of enzymes that are important in deacetylation of a variety of proteins with anticancer properties. Acetylated histones are a primary substrate for class I and II HDACs (particularly HDACs 1–7; HDAC8 does not appear to be expressed in PrC epithelial cells) (Khan and Thangue, 2012; Waltregny et al., 2004), and are a new target for chemotherapeutic drugs (Marks et al., 2001). HDACs, particularly 1–4, are known inhibitors of p21 expression (Ocker and Schneider-Stock, 2007; Gui et al., 2004; Lagger et al., 2003; Zupkovitz et al., 2010; Mottet et al., 2009; Wilson et al., 2006), and HDAC4 has been linked to p21 expression through its effects on Sp1 binding sites (Mottet et al., 2009). HDACs are involved in all aspects of promoting cancer, including proliferation, cell cycle, DNA repair, angiogenesis, migration, resistance to chemotherapy, and inhibition of differentiation and apoptosis (as reviewed in Khan and Thangue, 2012; Witt et al., 2009).

Zyflamend was shown to increase acetylation of histone 3 in CWR22Rv1 cells (Huang E-C et al., 2014). To investigate the mechanism, upstream modulators were evaluated. Zyflamend downregulated the gene expression of all class I and II HDACs (Viuda-Martos et al., 2011; Srinivasan, 2014; Manson, 2005; Howells et al., 2007; Huang E-C et al., 2012; Yang et al., 2007; 2008). Of those HDACs tested, Zyflamend downregulated protein levels of HDACs 1, 2, 4, and 7, results duplicated by trichostatin A (TSA), a universal HDAC inhibitor (Huang E-C et al., 2014). When Zyflamend was provided in the diets of mice with CWR22Rv1-derived tumors, tumor growth was inhibited by almost 50% and protein levels of HDAC1 and 4 (the only HDACs evaluated *in vivo*) were reduced when compared to tumors of animals on the control diet (Huang E-C et al., 2012). These results are particularly important for castrate-resistant PrC where there is enhanced nuclear localization of HDAC4 coupled with its relationship with histone acetylation near Sp1 binding sites (Mottet et al., 2009). HDAC1 is also important in advanced PrC, as it has been reported that its expression is higher in castrate-resistant PrC cells compared with androgen dependent cells (Waltregny et al., 2004). Furthermore, overexpression of HDAC2 is associated with shorter relapse times (Weichert et al., 2008).

With regard to histone acetylation, Zyflamend increased overall acetylation of histone 3 (Huang E-C et al., 2014) and increased the activation of CBP/p300, an important histone acetyltransferase that mediates the acetylation of histone 3 (Das et al., 2009) and has been linked to p21 expression (Owen et al., 1998; Xiao et al., 2000). Consistent with histone acetylation, cellular levels of acetyl CoA increased following Zyflamend treatment.

In summary, it appears that Zyflamend epigenetically increases the expression of p21 by enhancing histone acetyl transferase activity, and through the inhibition of histone deacetylases (Huang E-C et al., 2014).

11.6.3 Mitogen-Activated Protein Kinases

Mammalian cells have a number of well-characterized subfamilies of mitogen-activated protein kinases (MAPKs), including extracellular signal–related kinase 1/2 (Erk1/2), p38, and c-Jun NH2-terminal kinase (JNK). The histone acetyltransferase activity of CBP/p300 has been shown to be activated by these MAPKs (49, 50). This activation appears to be mediated in part via phosphorylation of Elk-1 (Li et al., 2003; Ilagan et al., 2006; Wagner and Nebreda, 2009; Bogoyevitch et al., 2004; Cuenda and Rousseau, 2007). Elk-1 is a transcription factor whose interaction with p300 following phosphorylation enhances histone acetyl transferase activity (Li et al., 2003; Ait-Si-Ali et al., 1999). CBP/p300 is involved in p21 transcription via Sp1 binding sites (Xiao et al., 2000). Enhanced expression of p21 has been shown to be mediated by JNK, p38 and Erk1/2 (Gan et al., 2011; Kim et al., 2014; Du and Wu, 2012).

Zyflamend enhances p21 expression (mRNA and protein) (Yang et al., 2007; Huang E-C et al., 2014), phosphorylation of Elk-1, and activation of CBP/p300 (Huang E-C et al., 2014). When cells were treated with inhibitors of Erk1/2, and then with Zyflamend, p21 expression was abrogated (Huang E-C et al., 2014). These results suggest that expression of p21 may be facilitated in part by activation of Erk1/2 through CBP/p300-mediated histone acetylation, coupled with downregulation of HDACs.

11.6.4 Androgen Receptor

The androgen receptor is a key mediator in the progression of PrC and an important target for ADT (androgen deprivation therapy) (Taplin and Balk, 2004; Chen et al., 2004). A key feature of castrate-resistant PrC is augmentation and/or reactivation of androgen receptor signaling in the absence of androgens (as reviewed in Pienta and Bradley, 2006). Part of this could be due to promiscuous receptors (i.e., point mutations) (Yang et al., 2011), intracellular levels of androgen receptor (i.e., increased expression) (Linja et al., 2001; Waltering et al., 2009), and outlaw pathways (activation via nonsteroids, such as insulin-like growth factor receptor, [IGF-R]) (Wu et al., 2006; Liao et al., 2005). It is known that androgens upregulate fatty acid and cholesterol biosynthesis in PrC cells for the generation of new membranes in rapidly dividing cells (Swinnen et al., 1998; Heemers et al., 2001).

Zyflamend decreased androgen receptor expression by 65% in CWR22Rv1 PrC cells *in vitro* (Huang E-C et al., 2011; Yan et al., 2012) and downregulated fatty acid synthesis (Zhao et al., 2015). These results were partially replicated *in vivo* (Huang E-C et al., 2012). Similar results were observed with LNCaP cells (Yan et al., 2012). Zyflamend also reduced cellular and nuclear localization of androgen receptor (Figure 11.6 in color insert) (Huang E-C et al., 2011). Interestingly, HDAC6 (whose expression is reduced by Zyflamend) has been reported to mediate the nuclear translocation of the androgen receptor (Ai et al., 2009). The effects of Zyflamend on protein levels of the androgen receptor were related to a reduction in synthesis with no effect on protein turnover (Huang E-C et al., 2011). Regarding the exploration of outlaw pathways, Zyflamend reduced the expression of insulin-like growth factor-1 receptor (IGF-1R) and antagonized IGF-1-stimulated cell proliferation (Huang E-C et al., 2011). While reducing the expression of IGF-1R did not appear to affect androgen receptor expression (Huang E-C et al., 2011), downstream signaling of the androgen receptor was inhibited by Zyflamend (Yan et al., 2012).

11.6.5 5′ Adenosine Monophosphate-Activated Protein Kinase

5′ Adenosine monophosphate-activated protein kinase (AMPK) is a key regulator of energy homeostasis in the cell and is considered an important tumor suppressor. AMPK is a multimeric protein consisting of a catalytic subunit (α) and two regulatory subunits (β and γ) (Hardie et al., 2012). Activation occurs following phosphorylation of Thr172 on the α-subunit by potentially four kinases, LKB1 (Hawley et al., 1996), CaMKKβ (Hawley et al., 2005), TAK1 (Herrero-Martin et al., 2009; Momcilovic et al., 2006), and MLK3 (Luo et al., 2015). CaMKKβ is activated via changes in intracellular calcium concentrations. Inactive LKB1 is found in the nucleus and is translocated to the cytosol following phosphorylation, where it interacts with two accessory proteins STRAD and MO25 (Hawley et al., 2003), enhancing its ability to phosphorylate AMPK (Xie et al., 2008). LKB1 is considered a tumor suppressor protein because inactivation is associated with a variety of cancers (Gan and Li., 2014).

Upon phosphorylation, AMPK downregulates lipogenesis by inhibiting acetyl CoA carboxylase, fatty acid synthase, sterol regulatory-element binding protein-1C (SREBP-1C), and HMG CoA reductase, as well as protein synthesis via the inhibition of the mTORC pathway (as reviewed in Hardie and Alessi, 2013). To support rapid proliferation, PrC cells require an upregulation of the biosynthesis of fatty acids and cholesterol. The growth inhibitory effects of AMPK are directly associated with inhibition of the lipogenic pathways, as the carbons from acetyl CoA are preferentially incorporated into new membrane phospholipids (Zadra et al., 2014). Concomitantly, AMPK upregulates a variety of catabolic pathways, including fatty acid oxidation.

AMPK activation can be upregulated by exogenous application of 5-aminoimidazole-4-carboxamide ribonucleotide (AICAR). AICAR is a compound commonly used as a "positive" control with *in vitro* assays, as it is converted to 5-aminoimidazole-4-carboxamide-1-b-D-ribofura nosyl monophosphate (ZMP), an analogue of AMP that allosterically activates AMPK. AICAR is also an intermediate in *de novo* purine biosynthesis and has recently been shown to have the ability to activate AMPK *in vivo* (Asby et al., 2015). Similarly, metformin is an antidiabetic drug with anticancer properties (Hadad et al., 2013) that activates AMPK (Rena et al., 2013). Metformin, like Zyflamend, has been shown to significantly reduce PSA levels when used in combination with other therapies (Bilen et al., 2015). For example, in a reported case study a patient exhibited recurrence of PrC despite radical prostatectomy, bilateral orchiectomy, and chemotherapy. However, following treatment with Zyflamend plus metformin, PSA levels decreased from 15.1 ng/mL to <0.1 ng/mL (Bilen et al., 2015). In addition, AMPK has been reported to downregulate androgen receptor and PSA expression (Zadra et al., 2014), effects shared by Zyflamend treatment. Recent research has suggested a relationship exists between AMPK activation, MAP kinases, p21, and cyclin D1 (cell cycle regulator) (Kim et al., 2014; Du et al., 2012; Zhao Z. et al., 2014; Cai et al., 2013; Li et al., 2015). New pharmacologic agents that selectively target AMPK activation, such as MT (Waltering et al., 2009; Wu et al., 2006; Liao et al., 2005; Swinnen and Verhoeven, 1998; Heemers et al., 2001; Ai et al., 2009; Hardie et al., 2012; Hawley et al., 1996; 2005; Herrero-Martin et al., 2009; Momcilovic et al., 2006; Luo et al., 2015; Hawley et al., 2003; Xie et al., 2008; Gan and Li, 2014; Hardie and Alessi, 2013), confirms the strategic role of AMPK in treating PrC (Zadra et al., 2014).

Zyflamend, like AICAR, increases the phosphorylation of Thr172 of the α-subunit of AMPK (Figure 11.7) (Zhao et al., 2015). Our preliminary results clearly show that Zyflamend also increases phosphorylation of LKB1 and subsequent AMPK, and treatment with an inhibitor of LKB1 attenuates this response (unpublished data). Zyflamend's activation of AMPK downregulated expression of SREBP-1C, fatty acid synthase, and inhibited acetyl CoA carboxylase (via phosphorylation) (Figure 11.8), thus inhibiting fatty acid synthesis in castrate-resistant CWR22Rv1 cells (Zhao et al., 2015). This is important because *de novo* fatty acid synthesis is required for completion of the cell cycle (Scaglia et al., 2014). To further demonstrate downstream signaling through AMPK activation, Zyflamend inhibited the mTORC signaling pathway in part via phosphorylation of raptor and downregulation of GβL and p-S6K (Figure 11.8) (Zhao et al., 2015).

It has been proposed that the primary source of acetyl CoAs for histone acetylation is derived from cytosolic citrate (as catalyzed by ATP-citrate lyase) (Fan et al., 2015). Inhibiting acetyl CoA carboxylase by Zyflamend expands the intracellular pool of acetyl CoA (Zhao et al., 2015), and in doing so would reduce cellular levels of malonyl CoA. Malonyl CoA is an inhibitor of carnitine palmitoyl transferase-1, a key regulator of mitochondrial fatty acid oxidation. Consistent with this scenario, fatty acid oxidation is significantly increased by Zyflamend (Figure 11.9 in color insert) (Zhao et al., 2015). A summary of these effects is presented in Figure 11.10.

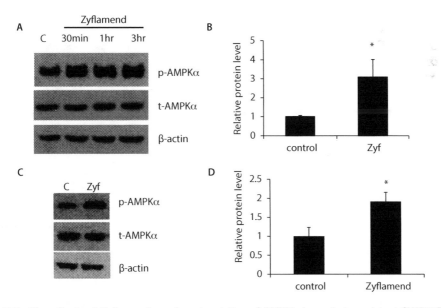

Figure 11.7 The effects of Zyflamend on phosphorylation of AMPKα in castrate-resistant CWR22Rv1 and androgen-independent PC3 prostate cancer cell lines (Zhao et al., 2015). Protein levels of p-AMPKα were determined in CWR22Rv1 cells treated ± Zyflamend (200 μg/ml, 0–3 hr) with data summarized at the 30 min time point (bar graph) (A, B). Protein levels of p-AMPKα were determined in PC3 cells treated ± Zyflamend (200 μg/ml, 30 min) (C, D). Data is presented as mean±SD, n=3. Group comparisons, Zyflamend versus control, * p<0.05.

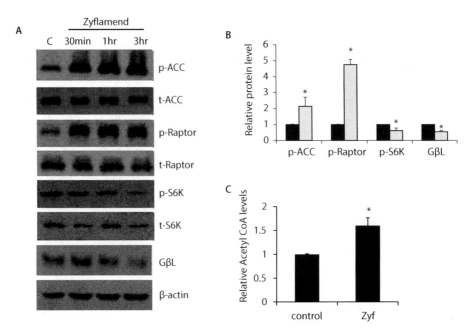

Figure 11.8 Regulation of downstream targets of AMPK ±Zyflamend in castrate-resistant CWR22Rv1 cells (Zhao et al., 2015). The effects of Zyflamend treatment (0.5–3 hr) on phosphorylation of acetyl CoA carboxylase (ACC), raptor and S6K and protein levels of GβL (A, B). Data is presented as mean ± SD, n=3. Group comparisons, Zyflamend versus control, * p<0.05. Effects of Zyflamend on total cellular levels of acetyl CoA (C). Data is presented as mean±SD, n=3. Group comparisons, Zyflamend versus control, * p<0.05.

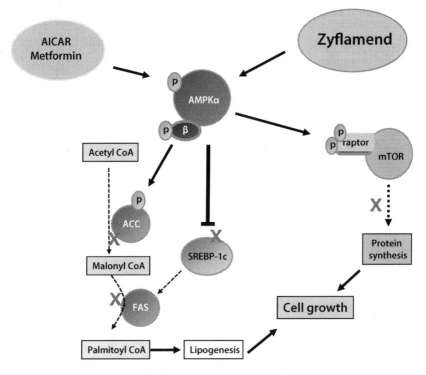

Figure 11.10 Summary of the effects of Zyflamend on AMPK and its downstream signaling.

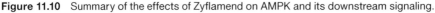

11.7   ZYFLAMEND AND OXIDATION OF GLUCOSE

The preferential utilization of glucose by cancer cells is well known (Liberti and Locasale, 2016). Dependency upon glucose for PrC cell proliferation appears to be higher for androgen-independent PrC cells as compared to androgen-dependent cells (Vaz et al., 2012), and inhibition of glucose utilization or the pentose phosphate pathway inhibits proliferation (Li et al., 2015). Utilization of glucose can provide needed ATPs, carbons for fatty acid synthesis, and when shuttled through the pentose phosphate pathway can enhance nucleotide biosynthesis and produce the reducing equivalence (i.e., NADPH) for lipogenesis and combat increases in reactive oxygen species. Recent evidence also suggests that intermediates in the pentose phosphate pathway may inhibit the activation of AMPK via LKB1 (Lin et al., 2015). Interestingly, when CWR22Rv1 cells were treated with Zyflamend, glucose oxidation was significantly inhibited (Figure 11.11).

11.8   SYNERGY OF COMPONENTS: BIOCHEMICAL AND MOLECULAR CONVERGENCE

Bioactives from plant sources (i.e., botanicals, fruits, vegetables) or foods are typically tested using the "reductionist" approach. That is, cells are treated with individually purified compounds (i.e., phytonutrients, vitamins) derived from those sources at increasing doses (dose response) and a concentration is identified where cell growth is inhibited by 50% (IC_{50}). The assumption is that the major effect of the food or botanical can be explained by the prominent bioactive. Each unique compound has a distinctive IC_{50} for a particular cancer cell line, and relative biological activities of the bioactives can be ascertained by comparing the IC_{50} values across a variety of cells. For example, the average IC_{50} for curcumin (a bioactive in turmeric) across a variety of cell lines is 21 μM (Table 11.2). This can be compared to the IC_{50} values for berberine, ar-turmerone, and coptisine of 41 μM, >257 μM, and 29 μM, respectively (Zhao et al., 2014). Unfortunately, the levels of these

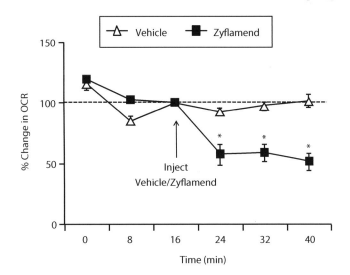

Figure 11.11   Effect of Zyflamend on glucose oxidation. The percentage change in the oxygen consumption rate (OCR) in castrate-resistant CWR22Rv1 cells treated with vehicle (olive oil) or Zyflamend (solubilized in olive oil) in KHB media containing only 2.5 mM glucose was measured with the Seahorse XF24 Extracellular Analyzer (for experimental details see Zhao et al., 2015). Data are presented as the mean ± SEM, n=6/time point, * $p<0.05$.

compounds found in human tissues are in the low nanomolar range, if detectable at all (as reviewed in Zhao et al., 2014), due to their low bioavailability. This questions the translatability of this type of result (the use of suprapharmacological doses) (Table 11.2).

Consistent with the goal of translatability, the level of Zyflamend used in the diets of athymic nude mice (*nu/nu*) bearing-CWR22(R) tumors (Figures 11.1 and 11.4) was equivalent to humans consuming 3 capsules/d (Huang E-C et al., 2012) – an easily achievable dose. To better understand how this preparation could be biologically active at such low doses, we investigated the synergy of action of individual extracts as they compared to isolated bioactives derived from their parent sources. For example, if curcumin was the only compound with bioactivity in the extract of turmeric, then the effects of turmeric would be identical to pure curcumin at the same levels of curcumin. If turmeric was more biologically active than curcumin at equivalent levels of curcumin, then there must be other bioactive compounds in turmeric producing additive or synergistic effects.

Table 11.2 *In Vitro* Antiproliferative Effects of Berberine, Curcumin, *ar*-Turmerone and Coptisine in a Variety of Cell Lines Based on IC_{50} Concentrations (µM)

Berberine		Curcumin		*ar*-Turmerone		Coptisine	
Cell Line	IC_{50}	Cell Line	IC_{50}	Cell Line	IC_{50}	Cell Line	IC_{50}
HeLa	20	KBM-5	3.8	MDA-MB-231	>100	MDA-MB-231	78
L1210	10	Jurkat	4.3		50	Hela	35
A431	75	U266	7.6		>462	MDA-MB-468	63
DU145	100	A549	17	MCF-7	>100	HepG2	203
U937	15	U87	15		>50		3.5
MCF7	20	T98G	31		>462	Hep3B	5.4
CL1-5	7.5	PC3	32	HepG2	>100	SK-Hep1	1.4
Colo205	80	LNCaP	53		300	PLC/PRF/5	6.6
C6	10	DU-145	30		>462	K562	7.2
U-87	20	MCF-7	20	Hep3B	564	U937	1.5
VSMC	200	MCF7/LCC2	20	Huh-7	472	Raji	0.6
B16	3	MCF7/LCC9	20	U937	185	P3H1	11
RPMI 8226	5	Mean	21	K562	185	LoVo	2.7
MDA-MB231	25			L1210	116	LoVo/Dx	12.5
NPC-HK1	200			U937	111	HT29	1.5
EAC	2			RB1-2H3	162	Mean	29
YES-6	3			Mean	>243		
NIH-3T3	30						
A7r5	23						
HepG2	39						
Hep3B	45						
Sk-Hepl	10						
PLC/PRF/5	40						
K562	43						
U937	28						
P3H1	24						
Raji	1.8						
L929	120						
Mean	41						

Derived from Zhao Y et al., 2014. With permission.

To test this hypothesis, we examined two of the extracts found in Zyflamend that are commonly used together in traditional Chinese medicine, turmeric and Chinese goldthread (Zhao et al., 2014). The experimental design is presented in Figure 11.12. We tested whether turmeric and Chinese goldthread were more effective than their major bioactives in isolation (curcumin and berberine, respectively), and if this were the case, whether these results could be due to the interaction of "companion" compounds; i.e., other bioactives contained in the extracts of origin, such as *ar*-turmerone (from turmeric) and coptisine (from Chinese goldthread). We also tested whether turmeric and Chinese goldthread would act synergistically, and if so, if that could be due to the interaction of bioactives unique to each of those extracts (i.e., curcumin combined with berberine). Proliferation of CWR22Rv1 cells was inhibited to a greater extent with either turmeric or Chinese goldthread when compared to equivalent concentrations of curcumin or berberine, respectively (Zhao et al., 2014), suggesting companion compounds might be responsible for these enhanced effects (Figure 11.13). *ar*-Turmerone is a bioactive found in turmeric, but not Chinese goldthread, and coptisine is a bioactive found in Chinese goldthread, but not turmeric. When curcumin was combined with its companion compound *ar*-turmerone, their capacity to inhibit cell proliferation was highly synergistic, where their minimum effective doses were reduced from micromolar concentrations to physiologically relevant nanomolar concentrations. Similar results were observed when berberine was combined with its companion compound coptisine. This helps to explain why the extracts are so much more effective than the isolated bioactives – it is more than just an additive effect (Figure 11.13).

The synergism between the two extracts yielded similar results on inhibition of cell proliferation using CWR22Rv1 PrC cells (Table 11.3). When turmeric was combined with Chinese goldthread, each extract enhanced the effectiveness of the other 52-fold (Zhao et al., 2014). This effect on proliferation was explained in part due to the synergism between curcumin and berberine, where the minimum effective doses of these bioactives were reduced from micromolar concentrations to nanomolar concentrations. These results clearly demonstrate that there is enhanced effectiveness

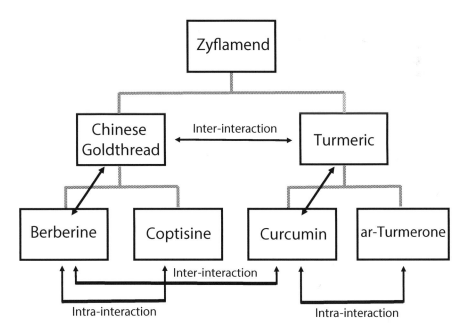

Figure 11.12 Experimental design. Comparisons were made between herbs and their major bioactives, among combinations of herbs (inter-interaction of herbs) and combinations of bioactives from the same herb (intra-interaction of isolated bioactives) or different herbs (inter-interactions of isolated bioactives) (Zhao et al., 2014).

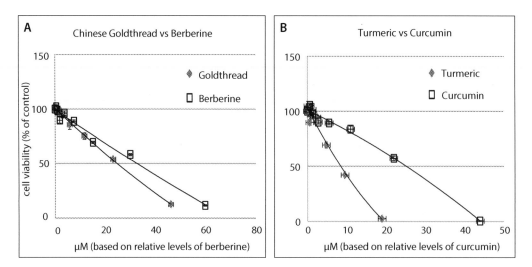

Figure 11.13 The comparison of berberine and curcumin on cell proliferation compared to their herbal extracts of origin, Chinese goldthread and turmeric, respectively, in castrate-resistant CWR22Rv1 cells. Following normalization based on the relative amount of berberine in Chinese goldthread and the relative amount of curcumin in turmeric, dose-response curves were compared between Chinese goldthread (diamonds) and berberine (open squares) in (A) and between turmeric (diamonds) and curcumin (open squares) in (B). The graphs are plotted based on the relative levels of berberine (graph A) or curcumin (graph B). Compared to individual compounds, herbal extracts had a more pronounced effect on reducing cell proliferation compared to their isolated bioactives (shifts in IC_{50} values to the left) (Zhao et al., 2014).

of combinations as compared to individual bioactives, or even individual extracts, used in isolation (Table 11.3).

To demonstrate that these synergistic effects can also be observed at the molecular level, we tested the synergy of these bioactives on inhibiting TNFα-mediated NF-κB promoter activation (Table 11.4). NF-κB is a transcription factor important in inflammation and cancer. The minimum effective doses of curcumin and *ar*-turmerone in inhibiting NF-κB promoter activation were 20 μM and 275 μM, respectively. When curcumin was combined with *ar*-turmerone, these levels dropped to nanomolar concentrations (630 nM and 160 nM, respectively), and more importantly, curcumin enhanced the effectiveness of *ar*-turmerone 3,563-fold (dose reduction index). These results indicate that even compounds with poor efficacy can become highly biologically active in the presence of companion compounds. If we judged each compound only in isolation, the synergy between compounds would be overlooked.

11.9 SUMMARY AND CONCLUSIONS

11.9.1 Summary

Zyflamend is composed of the extracts of 10 herbs, each of which has been reported to exhibit anticancer properties individually under a variety of conditions. Many of these effects have been attributed to major bioactive compounds found naturally in each plant or preparation (Table 11.1). However, these compounds have yet to reveal bioactivity at human equivalent doses when used in isolation. Recent studies suggest that when these compounds are combined with other bioactives their efficacy is significantly enhanced and they may in turn enhance the action of other natural

Table 11.3 Dose-Effect Relationships of Berberine and Coptisine (from Chinese Goldthread), Curcumin and *ar*-Turmerone (from Turmeric), Chinese Goldthread and Turmeric and Their Combinations on Proliferation of CWR22Rv1 PrC Cells*

Isolated Compounds or Extracts and Combinations	Minimum Effective Dose (µM or ug/ml)[a]	Combination Index (CI)	Dose Reduction Index (DRI)
Berberine	7.5		
Coptisine	21		
Ber + Cop[b]	0.47 + 0.09	0.16	Berberine: 7 Coptisine: 15
Curcumin	5.5		
ar-turmerone	9.4		
Cur + *ar*-tur[c]	0.34 + 0.09	0.06	Curcumin: 18 *ar*-turmerone: 87
Berberine	7.5		
Curcumin	5.5		
Ber + Cur[d]	0.24 + 0.17	0.16	Berberine: 24 Curcumin: 24
Goldthread	65		
Turmeric	35		
GT + Tur[d]	1.10 + 0.51	0.14	Chinese GT: 52 Turmeric: 52

[a] Concentration derived from the dose-response curves where growth inhibition was significantly inhibited (p<0.05) (isolated bioactives, µM; extracts, ug/ml).
[b] Ratio based on relative amounts in Chinese goldthread.
[c] Ratio based on relative amounts in turmeric.
[d] Ratio based on IC_{50} values.

Note: Synergy was determined using the Chou-Talalay method (Chou et al., 2010) and presented in more detail in reference (Zhao et al., 2014). If the CI is <1, the interaction of two components is synergistic. DRI is a parameter that indicates the degree to which the concentration of a component can be reduced when used in combination with another component to maintain an equivalent effect. Abbreviations: *ar*-tur, *ar*-turmerone; Cop, coptisine; Cur, curcumin; GT, Chinese Goldthread; Tur, turmeric.

*Zhao et al., 2014.

bioactives that would otherwise be functionally inactive if evaluated in isolation. To underscore the importance of this kind of approach, there is an initiative designed to develop new therapeutic strategies that involve multiple targets and mechanisms, The Halifax Project (Block et al., 2015). The Halifax Project is a consortium of scientists and clinicians interested in improving therapeutic outcomes, i.e., resistance to treatment and disease relapse, through multitargeted therapeutic strategies.

Consistent with the goal of the The Halifax Project, the strength of Zyflamend to inhibit tumorigenesis at human equivalent levels appears to be related to its multiple mechanisms of action, summarized in Figure 11.14. Zyflamend has been shown to modify PrC cell tumorigenesis by modifying key regulators of cell survival and apoptosis. Zyflamend enhances the expression of tumor suppressor genes (i.e., p21 and p27), and these effects are related to its ability to increase histone acetylation. The pursuit of HDAC inhibitors as a novel treatment for cancer is of great interest to cancer researchers due to their multiple targets. Zyflamend has been shown to modify other regulators of the cell cycle, such as inhibition of Rb phosphorylation and downregulation of cyclin D1, in addition to inhibiting anti-apoptotic signaling molecules (i.e., Bcl-2, Bcl-xL).

Cancer cells utilize glucose for energy. This in turn generates reducing equivalents (i.e., NADPH) to combat oxidative stress and sugars for nucleotide formation (i.e., ribose-5-phospahate) via the pentose phosphate pathway, and carbon skeletons for fatty acid synthesis (via acetyl CoA), all of which promote cancer (Figure 11.14). Cancer cells preferentially utilize glucose, and coordinately,

Table 11.4   Dose-Effect Relationships of Curcumin and *ar*-Turmerone (from Turmeric), Curcumin (from Turmeric) and Coptisine (from Chinese Goldthread), and Chinese Goldthread and Turmeric and Their Combinations on NF-κB Promoter Activity

Isolated Compounds or Extracts and Combinations	Minimum Effective Dose (μM or ug/ml)[a]	Combination Index (CI)	Dose Reduction Index (DRI)
Curcumin	20		
ar-turmerone	275		
Cur + *ar*-tur[b]	0.63 + 0.16	0.04	Curcumin: 23 *ar*-turmerone: 3563
Curcumin	20		
Coptisine	80		
Cur + Cop[c]	0.31+1.25	0.03	Curcumin: 70 Coptisine: 42
Goldthread	ND[d]		ND
Turmeric	70		ND
GT + Tur[e]	200 + 8.75	ND	

[a] Concentration derived from the dose-response curves where NF-κB transcription was significantly inhibited (p<0.05) (isolated bioactives, μM; extracts, ug/ml).
[b] Ratio based on relative amounts in turmeric.
[c] Ratio based on IC_{50} values.
[d] Chinese goldthread did not inhibit NF-κB transcriptional activation, as such, a minimum effective dose, CI or DRI could not be determined (ND).
[e] Therefore, an arbitrary level of Chinese goldthread was used in combination with turmeric.

Note: Synergy was determined using the Chou-Talalay method (Zhao et al., 2014) and presented in more detail in Zhao et al., 2014. If the CI is <1, the interaction of two components is synergistic. DRI is a parameter that indicates the degree to which the concentration of a component can be reduced when used in combination with another component to maintain an equivalent effect. Abbreviations: *ar*-tur, *ar*-turmerone; Cop, coptisine; Cur, curcumin; GT, Chinese goldthread; Tur, turmeric.

Zhao et al., 2014.

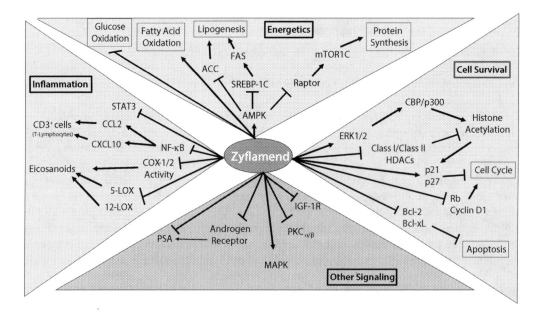

Figure 11.14   Summary of the effects of Zyflamend on prostate cancer based on the data in the literature. Zyflamend's effects at human relevant doses could be due to the fact that it has multiple targets and multiple mechanisms, including pathways involving energetics, inflammation, cell survival, and other targeted cell-signaling pathways.

lipogenesis is upregulated as newly formed fatty acids are earmarked for the generation of new membranes in the form of phospholipids. Zyflamend downregulates glucose oxidation and lipogenesis and redirects those fatty acids for mitochondrial β-oxidation by upregulating the tumor suppressor protein AMPK. In doing so, it coordinately inhibits the downstream signaling of mTOR1 complex, negatively affecting cell proliferation.

Inflammation and pro-inflammatory mediators, such as NF-κB, COX1/2, STAT3, cytokines, and eicosanoids, are in part at the heart of many cancers, including prostate cancer (as reviewed in Grivennikov et al., 2010; Izumi et al., 2014; and De et al., 2011). The interaction of NF-κB and STAT3 and the cytokines they mediate are a recurring theme in the relationship between inflammation and cancer (Grivennikov and Karin, 2010). As summarized in Figure 11.14, Zyflamend inhibits inflammation via multiple targets. It can downregulate NF-κB promoter activation, reduce STAT3 activation, inhibit chemokines that can attract CD3+ cells (T-lymphocytes) (Burke et al., 2015; Izumi et al., 2014; De et al., 2011), and can inhibit the formation of a variety of proinflammatory eicosanoids.

Many of these effects could be related to androgen receptor signaling (Izumi et al., 2014). Zyflamend has been shown to downregulate the androgen receptor and associated signaling molecules, such as IGF-1R and PSA. Its effects on upregulating MAP kinases appear to be in part related to histone acetylation. Importantly, these effects may be allied with ADT in the treatment of castrate-resistant PrC.

11.9.2 Conclusions

Zyflamend is a preparation derived from naturally occurring herbs. This review focused on the impact of Zyflamend on PrC following ADT and the castrate-resistant form of the disease. The current research provides hope that the use of these kinds of natural products may enhance the effectiveness of treatment. Their health-promoting properties should not be confused with or substitute for accepted medical treatment of cancer. Rather, the benefits may be complementary when used in conjunction with standard therapies as outlined in this review.

ACKNOWLEDGEMENT

This work was supported in part by a HATCH grant (#TEN00441) through the Tennessee Agricultural Experiment Station, (JW), University of Tennessee, Knoxville, TN 37996.

CONFLICTS OF INTEREST

The authors have no conflicts of interest. The University of Tennessee Agricultural Experiment Station and anyone affiliated with it have not been associated in the collection, analysis, or interpretation of data; in the writing or review of the report; or in the decision to submit the paper for publication.

REFERENCES

Ai, J. Wang, Y. Dar, J.A. et al. 2009. HDAC6 regulates androgen receptor hypersensitivity and nuclear local-ization via modulating Hsp90 acetylation in castration-resistant prostate cancer. *Mol Endocrinol* 23: 1963–72.

Ait-Si-Ali, S. Carlisi, D. Ramirez, S. et al. 1999. Phosphorylation by p44 MAP Kinase/ERK1 stimulates CBP histone acetyl transferase activity in vitro. *Biochem Biophys Res Commun* 262: 157–62.

Asby, D.J. Cuda, F. Beyaert, M. et al. 2015. AMPK activation via modulation of de novo purine biosynthesis with an inhibitor of ATIC homodimerization. *Chem Biol* 22: 838–48.

Bemis, D.L. Capodice, J.L. Anastasiadis, A.G. et al. 2005. Zyflamend, a unique herbal preparation with non-selective COX inhibitory activity, induces apoptosis of prostate cancer cells that lack COX-2 expression. *Nutr Cancer* 52: 202–12.

Bilen, M.A. Lin, S.H. Tang, D.G. et al. 2015. Maintenance therapy containing metformin and/or zyflamend for advanced prostate cancer: a case series. *Case Rep Oncol Med* 2015: 471861.

Blanchard, O.L. Smoliga, J.M. 2015. Translating dosages from animal models to human clinical trials – revis-iting body surface area scaling. *FASEB J* 29: 1629–34.

Block, K.I. Gyllenhaal, C. Lowe, L. et al. 2015. Designing a broad-spectrum integrative approach for cancer prevention and treatment. *Semin Cancer Biol* (35) Suppl: S276–S304.

Bogoyevitch, M.A. Boehm, I. Oakley, A. et al. 2004. Targeting the JNK MAPK cascade for inhibition: basic science and therapeutic potential. *Biochim Biophys Acta* 1697: 89–101.

Burke, S.J. Karlstad, M.D. Conley, C.P. et al. 2015. Dietary polyherbal supplementation decreases CD3(+) cell infiltration into pancreatic islets and prevents hyperglycemia in nonobese diabetic mice. *Nutr Res* 35: 328–36.

Cai, X. Hu, X. Cai, B. et al. 2013. Metformin suppresses hepatocellular carcinoma cell growth through induc-tion of cell cycle G1/G0 phase arrest and p21CIP and p27KIP expression and downregulation of cyclin D1 in vitro and in vivo. *Oncol Rep* 30: 2449–57.

Capodice, J.L. Gorroochurn, P. Cammack, A.S. et al. 2009. Zyflamend in men with high-grade prostatic intraepithelial neoplasia: results of a phase I clinical trial. *J Soc Integr Oncol* 7: 43–51.

Chen, C.D. Welsbie, D.S. Tran, C. et al. 2004. Molecular determinants of resistance to antiandrogen therapy. *Nat Med* 10: 33–9.

Cheng, L. Sun, J. Pretlow, T.G. et al. 1996. CWR22 xenograft as an *ex vivo* human tumor model for prostate cancer gene therapy. *J Natl Cancer Inst* 88: 607–11.

Chou, T.C. 2010. Drug combination studies and their synergy quantification using the Chou-Talalay method. *Cancer Res* 70: 440–6.

Cuenda, A. Rousseau, S. 2007. p38 MAP-kinases pathway regulation, function and role in human diseases. *Biochim Biophys Acta* 1773: 1358–75.

Das, C. Lucia, M.S. Hansen, K.C. et al. 2009. CBP/p300-mediated acetylation of histone H3 on lysine 56. *Nature* 459: 113–7.

De, N.C. Kramer, G. Marberger, M. et al. 2011. The controversial relationship between benign prostatic hyper-plasia and prostate cancer: the role of inflammation. *Eur Urol* 60: 106–17.

Du, L. Wu, W. 2012. A mimic of phosphorylated prolactin induces apoptosis by activating AP-1 and upregu-lating p21/waf1 in human prostate cancer PC3 cells. *Oncol Lett* 4: 1064–8.

Ekmekcioglu, S. Chattopadhyay, C. Akar, U. et al. 2011. Zyflamend mediates therapeutic induction of autoph-agy to apoptosis in melanoma cells. *Nutr Cancer* 63: 940–9.

Fan, J. Krautkramer, K.A. Feldman, J.L. et al. 2015. Metabolic regulation of histone post-translational modifi-cations. *ACS Chem Biol* (10): 95–108.

Gan, L. Wang, J. Xu, H. et al. 2011. Resistance to docetaxel-induced apoptosis in prostate cancer cells by p38/p53/p21 signaling. *Prostate* 71: 1158–66.

Gan, R.Y. Li, H.B. 2014. Recent progress on liver kinase B1 (LKB1): expression, regulation, downstream sig-naling and cancer suppressive function. *Int J Mol Sci* 15: 16698–718.

Grivennikov, S.I. Greten, F.R. Karin, M. 2010. Immunity, inflammation, and cancer. *Cell* 140: 883–99.

Grivennikov, S.I. Karin, M. 2010. Dangerous liaisons: STAT3 and NF-kappaB collaboration and crosstalk in cancer. *Cytokine Growth Factor Rev* 21: 11–9.

Gui, C.Y. Ngo, L. Xu, W.S. et al. 2004. Histone deacetylase (HDAC) inhibitor activation of p21WAF1 involves changes in promoter-associated proteins, including HDAC1. *Proc Natl Acad Sci U S A* 101: 1241–6.

Hadad, S.M. Hardie, D.G. Appleyard, V. et al. 2013. Effects of metformin on breast cancer cell proliferation, the AMPK pathway and the cell cycle. *Clin Transl Oncol* 16(8): 746–52.

Hardie, D.G. Alessi, D.R. 2013. LKB1 and AMPK and the cancer-metabolism link – ten years after. *BMC Biol* 11: 36.

Hardie, D.G. Ross, F.A. Hawley, S.A. 2012. AMPK: a nutrient and energy sensor that maintains energy homeostasis. *Nat Rev Mol Cell Biol* 13: 251–62.

Hawley, S.A. Boudeau, J. Reid, J.L. et al. 2003. Complexes between the LKB1 tumor suppressor, STRAD alpha/beta and MO25 alpha/beta are upstream kinases in the AMP-activated protein kinase cascade. *J Biol* 2: 28.

Hawley, S.A. Davison, M. Woods, A. et al. 1996. Characterization of the AMP-activated protein kinase kinase from rat liver and identification of threonine 172 as the major site at which it phosphorylates AMP-activated protein kinase. *J Biol Chem* 271: 27879–87.

Hawley, S.A. Pan, D.A. Mustard, K.J. et al. 2005. Calmodulin-dependent protein kinase kinase-beta is an alternative upstream kinase for AMP-activated protein kinase. *Cell Metab* 2: 9–19.

Heemers, H. Maes, B. Foufelle, F. et al. 2001. Androgens stimulate lipogenic gene expression in prostate cancer cells by activation of the sterol regulatory element-binding protein cleavage activating protein/sterol regulatory element-binding protein pathway. *Mol Endocrinol* 15: 1817–28.

Herrero-Martin, G. Hoyer-Hansen, M. Garcia-Garcia, C. et al. 2009. TAK1 activates AMPK-dependent cytoprotective autophagy in TRAIL-treated epithelial cells. *EMBO J* 28: 677–85.

Howells, L.M. Moiseeva, E.P. Neal, C.P. et al. 2007. Predicting the physiological relevance of in vitro cancer preventive activities of phytochemicals. *Acta Pharmacol Sin* 28: 1274–304.

Huang, E-C. Chen, G. Baek, S.J. et al. 2011. Zyflamend reduces the expression of androgen receptor in a model of castrate-resistant prostate cancer. *Nutr Cancer* 63: 1287–96.

Huang, E-C. McEntee, M.F. Whelan, J. 2012. Zyflamend, a combination of herbal extracts, attenuates tumor growth in murine xenograph models of prostate cancer. *Nutr Cancer* 64: 749–60.

Huang, E-C. Zhao, Y.C.G. Baek, S.J. et al. 2014. Zyflamend, a polyherbal mixture, down regulates class I and class II histone deacetylases and increases p21 levels in castrate-resistant prostate cancer cells. *BMC Complement Altern Med* 14: 68.

Ilagan, R. Pottratz, J. Le, K. et al. 2006. Imaging mitogen-activated protein kinase function in xenograft models of prostate cancer. *Cancer Res* 66: 10778–85.

Izumi, K. Li, L. Chang, C. 2014. Androgen receptor and immune inflammation in benign prostatic hyperplasia and prostate cancer. *Clin Investig (Lond)* 4: 935–50.

Khan, O. La Thangue, N.B. 2012. HDAC inhibitors in cancer biology: emerging mechanisms and clinical applications. *Immunol Cell Biol* 90: 85–94.

Kim, J.H. Park, B. Gupta, S.C. et al. 2012. Zyflamend sensitizes tumor cells to TRAIL-induced apoptosis through up-regulation of death receptors and down-regulation of survival proteins: role of ROS-dependent CCAAT/enhancer-binding protein-homologous protein pathway. *Antioxid Redox Signal* 16: 413–27.

Kim, W.G. Choi, H.J. Kim, T.Y. et al. 2014. The effect of 5-aminoimidazole-4-carboxamide-ribonucleoside was mediated by p38 mitogen activated protein kinase signaling pathway in FRO thyroid cancer cells. *Korean J Intern Med* 29: 474–81.

Kunnumakkara, A.B. Sung, B. Ravindran, J. et al. 2012. Zyflamend suppresses growth and sensitizes human pancreatic tumors to gemcitabine in an orthotopic mouse model through modulation of multiple targets. *Int J Cancer* 131: E292–E303.

Lagger, G. Doetzlhofer, A. Schuettengruber, B. et al. 2003. The tumor suppressor p53 and histone deacetylase 1 are antagonistic regulators of the cyclin-dependent kinase inhibitor p21/WAF1/CIP1 gene. *Mol Cell Biol* 23: 2669–79.

Li, L. Fath, M.A. Scarbrough, P.M. 2015. Combined inhibition of glycolysis, the pentose cycle, and thioredoxin metabolism selectively increases cytotoxicity and oxidative stress in human breast and prostate cancer. *Redox Biol* 4: 127–35.

Li, P. Zhao, M. Parris, A.B. et al. 2015. p53 is required for metformin-induced growth inhibition, senescence and apoptosis in breast cancer cells. *Biochem Biophys Res Commun* 464: 1267–74.

Li, Q.J. Yang, S.H. Maeda, Y. et al. 2003. MAP kinase phosphorylation-dependent activation of Elk-1 leads to activation of the co-activator p300. *EMBO J* 22: 281–91.

Liao, Y. Abel, U. Grobholz, R. et al. 2005. Up-regulation of insulin-like growth factor axis components in human primary prostate cancer correlates with tumor grade. *Hum Pathol* 36: 1186–96.

Liberti, M.V. Locasale, J.W. 2016. The Warburg effect: how does it benefit cancer cells? *Trends Biochem Sci* 41(3): 211–8.

Lin, R. Elf, S. Shan, C. et al. 2015. 6-Phosphogluconate dehydrogenase links oxidative PPP, lipogenesis and tumour growth by inhibiting LKB1-AMPK signalling. *Nat Cell Biol* 17: 1484–96.

Linja, M.J. Savinainen, K.J. Saramaki, O.R. et al. 2001. Amplification and overexpression of androgen receptor gene in hormone-refractory prostate cancer. *Cancer Res* 61: 3550–5.

Luo, L. Jiang, S. Huang, D. et al. 2015. MLK3 phophorylates AMPK independently of LKB1. *PLoS One* 10: e0123927.

Manson, M.M. 2005. Inhibition of survival signalling by dietary polyphenols and indole-3-carbinol. *Eur J Cancer* 41: 1842–53.

Marks, P. Rifkind, R.A. Richon, V.M. et al. 2001. Histone deacetylases and cancer: causes and therapies. *Nat Rev Cancer* 1: 194–202.

Marmorstein, R. 2001. Structure and function of histone acetyltransferases. *Cell Mol Life Sci* 58: 693–703.

Marmorstein, R. Trievel, R.C. 2009. Histone modifying enzymes: structures, mechanisms, and specificities. *Biochim Biophys Acta* 1789: 58–68.

McEntee, M.F. Ziegler, C. Reel, D. et al. 2008. Dietary n-3 polyunsaturated fatty acids enhance hormone ablation therapy in androgen-dependent prostate cancer. *Am J Pathol* 173: 229–41.

Mohebati, A. Guttenplan, J.B. Kochhar, A. et al. 2012. Carnosol, a constituent of Zyflamend, inhibits aryl hydrocarbon receptor-mediated activation of CYP1A1 and CYP1B1 transcription and mutagenesis. *Cancer Prev Res* 5: 593–602.

Momcilovic, M. Hong, S.P. Carlson, M. 2006. Mammalian TAK1 activates Snf1 protein kinase in yeast and phosphorylates AMP-activated protein kinase in vitro. *J Biol Chem* 281: 25336–43.

Mottet, D. Pirotte, S. Lamour, V. et al. 2009. HDAC4 represses p21(WAF1/Cip1) expression in human cancer cells through a Sp1-dependent, p53-independent mechanism. *Oncogene* 28: 243–56.

Nagabhushan, M. Miller, C.M. Pretlow, T.P. et al. 1996. CWR22: The first human prostate cancer xenograft with strongly androgen-dependent and relapsed strains both *in vivo* and in soft agar. *Cancer Res* 56: 3042–6.

Ocker, M. Schneider-Stock, R. 2007. Histone deacetylase inhibitors: signalling towards p21cip1/waf1. *Int J Biochem Cell Biol* 39: 1367–74.

Owen, G.I. Richer, J.K. Tung, L. et al. 1998. Progesterone regulates transcription of the p21(WAF1) cyclin-dependent kinase inhibitor gene through Sp1 and CBP/p300. *J Biol Chem* 273: 10696–701.

Pienta, K.J. Bradley, D. 2006. Mechanisms underlying the development of androgen-independent prostate cancer. *Clin Cancer Res* 12: 1665–71.

Pretlow, T.G. Wolman, S.R. Micale, M.A. et al. 1993. Xenografts of primary human prostatic carcinoma. *J Natl Cancer Inst* 85: 394–8.

Rafailov, S. Cammack, S. Stone, B.A. et al. 2007. The role of Zyflamend, an herbal anti-inflammatory, as a potential chemopreventive agent against prostate cancer: a case report. *Integr Cancer Ther* 6: 74–6.

Rena, G. Pearson, E.R. Sakamoto, K. 2013. Molecular mechanism of action of metformin: old or new insights? *Diabetologia* 56: 1898–906.

Rucker, R. Storms, D. 2002. Interspecies comparisons of micronutrient requirements: metabolic vs. absolute body size. *J Nutr* 132: 2999–3000.

Sandur, S.K. Ahn, K.S. Ichikawa, H. et al. 2007. Zyflamend, a polyherbal preparation, inhibits invasion, suppresses osteoclastogenesis, and potentiates apoptosis through down-regulation of NF-kappa B activation and NF-kappa B-regulated gene products. *Nutr Cancer* 57: 78–87.

Scaglia, N. Tyekucheva, S. Zadra, G. et al. 2014. De novo fatty acid synthesis at the mitotic exit is required to complete cellular division. *Cell Cycle* 13(5): 859–68.

Srinivasan, K. 2014. Antioxidant potential of spices and their active constituents. *Crit Rev Food Sci Nutr* 54: 352–72.

Subbaramaiah, K. Sue, E. Bhardwaj, P. et al. 2013. Dietary polyphenols suppress elevated levels of proinflammatory mediators and aromatase in the mammary gland of obese mice. *Cancer Prev Res (Phila)* 6: 886–97.

Swinnen, J.V. Verhoeven, G. 1998. Androgens and the control of lipid metabolism in human prostate cancer cells. *J Steroid Biochem Mol Biol* 65: 191–8.

Taplin, M.E. Balk, S.P. 2004. Androgen receptor: a key molecule in the progression of prostate cancer to hormone independence. *J Cell Biochem* 91: 483–90.

Thiele, J.R, Zeller, J. Bannasch, H. et al. 2015. Targeting C-reactive protein in inflammatory disease by preventing conformational changes. *Mediators Inflamm* 2015: 372432.

Vaz, C.V. Alves, M.G. Marques, R. et al. 2012. Androgen-responsive and nonresponsive prostate cancer cells present a distinct glycolytic metabolism profile. *Int J Biochem Cell Biol* 44: 2077–84.

Verdone, L. Agricola, E. Caserta, M. et al. 2006. Histone acetylation in gene regulation. *Brief Funct Genomic Proteomic* 5: 209–21.

Viuda-Martos, M. Ruiz-Navajas, Y. Fernandez-Lopez, J. et al. 2011. Spices as functional foods. *Crit Rev Food Sci Nutr* 51: 13–28.

Wagner, E.F. Nebreda, A.R. 2009. Signal integration by JNK and p38 MAPK pathways in cancer development. *Nat Rev Cancer* 9: 537–49.

Wainstein, M.A. He, F. Robinson, D. et al. 1994. CWR22: Androgen-dependent xenograft model derived from a primary human prostatic carcinoma. *Cancer Res* 54: 6049–52.

Waltering, K.K. Helenius, M.A. Sahu, B. et al. 2009. Increased expression of androgen receptor sensitizes prostate cancer cells to low levels of androgens. *Cancer Res* 69: 8141–9.

Waltregny, D. North, B. Van, M.F. et al. 2004. Screening of histone deacetylases (HDAC) expression in human prostate cancer reveals distinct class I HDAC profiles between epithelial and stromal cells. *Eur J Histochem* 48: 273–90.

Weichert, W. Roske, A. Gekeler, V. et al. 2008. Histone deacetylases 1, 2 and 3 are highly expressed in prostate cancer and HDAC2 expression is associated with shorter PSA relapse time after radical prostatectomy. *Br J Cancer* 98: 604–10.

Weldon, K.A. Whelan, J. 2011. Allometric scaling of dietary linoleic acid on changes in tissue arachidonic acid using human equivalent diets in mice. *Nutr Metab (Lond)* 8: 43.

Wilson, A.J. Byun, D.S. Popova, N. et al. 2006. Histone deacetylase 3 (HDAC3) and other class I HDACs regulate colon cell maturation and p21 expression and are deregulated in human colon cancer. *J Biol Chem* 281: 13548–58.

Witt, O. Deubzer, H.E. Milde, T. et al. 2009. HDAC family: what are the cancer relevant targets? *Cancer Lett* 277: 8–21.

Wu, J.D. Haugk, K. Woodke, L. et al. 2006. Interaction of IGF signaling and the androgen receptor in prostate cancer progression. *J Cell Biochem* 99: 392–401.

Xiao, H. Hasegawa, T. Isobe, K. 2000. p300 collaborates with Sp1 and Sp3 in p21(waf1/cip1) promoter activation induced by histone deacetylase inhibitor. *J Biol Chem* 275: 1371–6.

Xie, Z. Dong, Y. Scholz, R. et al. 2008. Phosphorylation of LKB1 at serine 428 by protein kinase C-zeta is required for metformin-enhanced activation of the AMP-activated protein kinase in endothelial cells. *Circulation* 117: 952–62.

Yan, J. Xie, B. Capodice, J.L. et al. 2012. Zyflamend inhibits the expression and function of androgen receptor and acts synergistically with bicalutimide to inhibit prostate cancer cell growth. *Prostate* 72: 244–52.

Yang, M. Xie, W. Mostaghel, E. et al. 2011. SLCO2B1 and SLCO1B3 may determine time to progression for patients receiving androgen deprivation therapy for prostate cancer. *J Clin Oncol* 29: 2565–73.

Yang, P. Cartwright, C. Chan, D. et al. 2007. Zyflamend-mediated inhibition of human prostate cancer PC3 cell proliferation: effects on 12-LOX and Rb protein phosphorylation. *Cancer Biol Ther* 6: 228–36.

Yang, P. Sun, Z. Chan, D. et al. 2008. Zyflamend reduces LTB4 formation and prevents oral carcinogenesis in a 7,12-dimethylbenz[alpha]anthracene (DMBA)-induced hamster cheek pouch model. *Carcinogenesis* 29: 2182–9.

Zadra, G. Photopoulos, C. Tyekucheva, S. et al. 2014. A novel direct activator of AMPK inhibits prostate cancer growth by blocking lipogenesis. *EMBO Mol Med* 6: 518–38.

Zhao, Y. Collier, J.J. Huang, E-C. et al. 2014. Turmeric and Chinese goldthread synergistically inhibit prostate cancer cell proliferation and NF-kB signaling. *Functional Foods Health Dis* 4: 312–39.

Zhao, Y. Donohoe, D. Huang, E.C. et al. 2015. Zyflamend, a polyherbal mixture, inhibits lipogenesisa and mTORC1 signalling via activation of AMPK. *J Funct Foods* 18: 147–58.

Zhao, Z. Yin, J.Q. Wu, M.S. et al. 2014. Dihydromyricetin activates AMP-activated protein kinase and P38(MAPK) exerting antitumor potential in osteosarcoma. *Cancer Prev Res (Phila)* 7: 927–38.

Zupkovitz, G. Grausenburger, R. Brunmeir, R. et al. 2010. The cyclin-dependent kinase inhibitor p21 is a crucial target for histone deacetylase 1 as a regulator of cellular proliferation. *Mol Cell Biol* 30: 1171–81.

CHAPTER 12

Scientific Evaluation of the Polyphenol Rich Whole Food Supplement Pomi-T®

Robert Thomas

CONTENTS

12.1 OVERVIEW

Polyphenol-rich foods, such as pomegranate, green tea, turmeric, and broccoli have demonstrated anticancer effects in laboratory studies. In humans, observational studies have linked their intake with a lower risk of chronic disease, including cancer. Concentrating these foods into a capsule is a convenient way to boost an individual's polyphenol intake but hitherto adequately powered double blind randomized controlled trials have not firmly established that this benefits health or markers of cancer progression.

This UK government-adopted trial involved 203 men with prostate cancer. They either had early disease or were experiencing a significant progressive PSA relapse after radiotherapy or surgery. In both cases they were not taking any other anticancer medication and were being watched carefully. They were randomized to receive either Pomi-T or an identical placebo. The patient, doctor, or statistician who analyzed the data was blind to the intervention arm. After 6 months there was a 63% difference in the rate of rise in PSA between the two groups, which was highly statistically significant (ANOVA, p-value=0.0008).

A further 2-year prospective study correlated 346 paired serum PSA levels with 346 high resolution magnetic resonance images (MRIs) of 138 men who had at least two prostate MRI scans and were taking Pomi-T. Men with tumor progression on MRI had a significant increase in PSA, those with tumor shrinkage or no disease seen had a significant fall in PSA, and those with stable disease had a stable PSA. This strong correlation (ANOVA, P-value <0.0001) demonstrates that the PSA effect of Pomi-T is not independent of MRI-defined disease.

These findings have been of great interest and reassurance to the 50 to 60% of men with prostate cancer who are interested in over-the-counter remedies, as they suggest that regular intake of this low-cost, well-tolerated polyphenol supplement prevents or delays progression to interventions with considerably more toxicities. Although these initial trials had no commercial funding, the product has now been commercialized by Helsinn Integrative Care (Lugano, Switzerland) who are collaborating with our academic unit for further research investigating its role for other cancer types and treatment-related symptoms.

12.2 INTRODUCTION

12.2.1 The Benefits of Polyphenols

Diets rich in polyphenols, the natural plant-based phytochemicals found in healthy foods, have been linked with lower risks of chronic illnesses such as dementia, high cholesterol, arthritis, heart disease, skin aging, and macular degeneration (Denny and Buttriss, 2007; Elmets et al., 2001; Karppi et al., 2012, Rezai-Zadeh et al., 2005; Porrini and Riso, 2008). Well-conducted population studies have also linked regular intake of polyphenols with lower risks of many cancers including breast (Hu et al, 2012), pancreatic (Banim et al., 2013), esophageal (Sun et al., 2007), ovarian (Wu and Yu, 2006; Tung et al., 2005), prostate (Giovannucci et al., 2002, Li et al., 2011; Joseph et al., 2004), and skin cancer (Heinen et al., 2007).

The anticancer effects of polyphenols, however, do not stop after a cancer diagnosis. Breast cancer survivors eating polyphenol-rich fruit, vegetables, soy, and green tea were found to have lower relapse rates (Pierce et al., 2007; Buck et al., 2011; Boyapati et al., 2005; Ogunleye et al., 2010). Individuals with skin cancer who had a high intake of leafy green vegetables and broccoli had lower rates of new cancer formation (Heinen et al., 2007). A healthy lifestyle including a polyphenol-rich diet has been linked to a slower rate of PSA among men with indolent prostate cancer (Ornish et al., 2008).

12.2.2   How Do Polyphenols Exert Their Anticancer Effects?

The most commonly cited anticancer effect of polyphenols is via their antioxidant properties, protecting the DNA from oxidative damage resulting from ingested or environmental carcinogens (Porrini and Riso, 2008; Parada and Aguilera, 2007, McLarty et al., 2009, Sonn et al., 2005). Polyphenols have, however, numerous other important properties, depending on their plant sources.

Green and black tea is rich in epigallocatechin gallate (EGCG), shown to block ornithine decarboxylase, an enzyme that signals cells to proliferate faster and bypass apoptosis (McLarty et al., 2009; Porrini and Riso, 2008; Liao et al., 2004). Green tea inhibits growth factors that promote breast and prostate cancer cell line proliferation, as well as blocking de-differentiation and preventing angiogenesis (Yang et al., 2002) (Figure 12.1A).

Curcumin gives turmeric its yellow color, slows down the growth of prostate cancer cells by blocking the cell cycle, increasing apoptosis, and preventing invasion and migration of cells (Somasundaram et al., 2002; Shah et al., 1999; Zhang et al., 2007; Iqbal et al., 2003). It inhibits tyrosine kinase activity of the EGFR (Dorai et al., 2000), has COX-I mediated antiinflammatory properties (Handler et al., 2007), and inhibits the growth of stem cells that give rise to breast cancer without harming normal breast cells (Kakarala et al., 2010) (Figure 12.1B).

Pomegranate, rich in ellagic acid, inhibits prostate cancer cell proliferation and induces apoptosis in laboratory studies (Rettig et al., 2008; Malik et al., 2005; Khan and Mukhtar, 2007; Barber et al., 2006; Choi et al., 2006). In breast cancer cell lines, it increases markers of cell adhesion and reduces migration, which are associated with metastasis (Rocha et al., 2012; Wang et al., 2011) (Figure 12.1C).

Broccoli is rich in isothiocyanate and sulforaphane, which inhibit growth and promote apoptosis of cancer cells (Sarkar et al., 2012). In humans, regular intake downregulates genes linked to cancer growth and upregulates genes linked to cancer suppression, particularly in the 50% of the population who carry a mutated glutathione S-transferase gene (Gasper et al., 2005; Joseph et al., 2004; Heinen et al., 2007) (Figure 12.1D).

12.3   BOOSTING THE DIET WITH A DAILY NUTRITIONAL SUPPLEMENT REDUCES CANCER RISK OR THE RATE OF ESTABLISHED CANCER PROGRESSION

Although diets deficient in minerals and vitamins have been associated with greater cancer risks and recurrence rates (Reichman et al., 1990; Leitzmann., 2003; Rock et al., 2005, Schenk et al., 2009), most studies of vitamin and mineral supplementation have shown little benefit, or have shown a slightly increased risk of cancer unless their use was limited to correcting a pre-existing micronutrient deficiency.

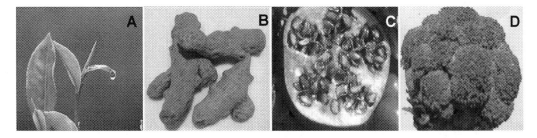

Figure 12.1   Representative images of (A): Green tea; (B) Turmeric; (C) Pomegranate; (D) Broccoli.

For example, in the EPIC study it was found that both patients on diets deficient in folate and patients taking the highest amounts of folate via supplements had higher cancer risks (Chuang, 2011). In two other Scandinavian studies, higher cancer risks were observed following vitamin B supplementation versus a placebo (Ebbing et al., 2009; Figueiredo et al., 2009). In individuals at high risk for lung cancer, vitamin A supplementation has been linked with an elevated risk of both lung and prostate cancer (Klein et al., 2011). In another large study of beta-carotene and retinol, lower risks of prostate cancer were shown for patients with low pre-intervention plasma levels of beta-carotene. However, patients with high pre-intervention levels of beta-carotene had a higher risk of cancer, particularly if they were smokers (Omenn et al., 1996; Albanes et al., 1994). In another double-blind randomized controlled trial (RCT) involving men with progressive prostate cancer, no difference was found between consumption of salicylate alone versus salicylate plus vitamin C, copper, and manganese gluconate (Thomas et al., 2009). In the well-known Health Professionals Follow-up Study, men who took supplemental zinc in excess of 100 mg/day or for long durations were more than twice as likely to develop advanced prostate cancer compared with control patients (Leitzmann et al., 2003). In the Selenium and Vitamin E Cancer Prevention Trial (SELECT), no benefit was found in the consumption of selenium supplements, and an increased prostate cancer incidence was correlated if it was taken with vitamin E supplementation (Klein et al., 2011). In an Australian study, individuals who took beta-carotene and vitamin E in supplement form had higher rates of new skin cancer formation (Heinen et al., 2007). Not all studies of vitamins and minerals were negative. In the SU.VI.MAX study, French adults were randomized either to a supplement containing ascorbic acid, vitamin E, beta-carotene, selenium, and zinc, or a placebo. In this study, there was no reduction in mortality or cancer-specific mortality overall in the supplement group, although a further analysis in men showed a reduction in the risk of prostate cancer (Hercberg et al., 2004). Later authors postulated this sex difference was related to French men having a lower baseline micronutrient status (Meyer et al., 2005).

The links between polyphenol-rich diets and lower risks of cancer relapse (Pierce et al., 2007; Buck et al., 2011; Ogunleye et al., 2010; Heinen et al., 2007; Boyapati et al., 2005) are encouraging but interventional studies evaluating polyphenol-rich food supplements are scarce, often underpowered, nonrandomized, and have multiple overlapping interventions making the results difficult to interpret (Posadzki et al., 2013). Despite these drawbacks, there are some interesting data emerging from studies of polyphenol-rich supplements. In the largest cohort study, the VITamins and Lifestyle (VITAL) cohort, a link was found between the use of grape seed extract and lower prostate cancer incidence (Brasky et al., 2011). In a small study of American men with prostate cancer, consumption of a tea extract was linked with a significant reduction in the levels of several growth factors that promote cancer growth, and a beneficial effect on PSA was also noted (McLarty et al., 2009). An RCT of 93 men managed with AS that included nutritional counseling and exercise showed significantly lower PSA levels compared to men on standard active surveillance (Ornish et al., 2008). In this study, as a secondary endpoint, serum from the participants added to prostate cancer cell lines demonstrated an eightfold inhibition of cellular growth in the active group compared to the control group (Ornish et al., 2008). In a phase II study of men with prostate cancer, PSA doubling time was significantly prolonged and markers of oxidative stress improved upon regular consumption of pomegranate juice (Pantuck et al, 2006). In two further phase II studies, one from the United States and the other from Italy, men consumed pomegranate seed extract, and similar effects on PSA were observed (Paller et al., 2013). In a small RCT involving men with prostate cancer, a small effect on PSA occurred following intake of a pill containing isoflavones and antioxidants (Schröder et al., 2005). However, in a larger study of saw palmetto or genistein evaluated separately, no benefit was shown for either prostate cancer or benign prostatic hypertrophy (Brasky et al., 2011; Bent et al., 2006; Spentzos et al., 2003). Likewise, despite the initial enthusiasm for lycopene from cohort observations (Giovannucci et al., 2002), the two most recent RCTs in men found no difference in

PSA progression (Barber et al., 2006; Clark et al., 2006), and studies in women have shown no reduction in the risk of breast cancer with regular intake (Hu et al., 2012).

In summary, trials evaluating vitamin and mineral supplements suggest that their benefit is restricted to correcting an underlying deficiency. This has prompted organizations such as the National Cancer Institute to issue statements that long-term vitamin and mineral supplementation should be discouraged unless they are used for correcting a known deficiency, and future studies should include detailed micronutrient testing (Cancernet-UK). Although polyphenol-rich supplements are showing some promise, it is clear that not all polyphenols have anticancer effects, and those that do are likely to have different benefits in different combinations among different individuals (Parada and Aguilera 2007; Greenwald et al., 2002; Porrini and Riso, 2008). Further trials of polyphenol combinations are imperative if we are going to fully explore their therapeutic potential, hence the rationale for the Pomi-T trial.

12.4   STUDY ONE: THE UK NATIONAL CANCER RESEARCH NETWORK POMI-T STUDY

This was a double blind, placebo-controlled randomized trial (RCT) evaluating the effect of a polyphenol-rich whole food supplement on PSA progression in men with prostate cancer. The study received no commercial funding, and financial support was provided by the charity Prostate Action UK.

Men with prostate cancer, managed with active surveillance (AS) or watchful waiting for a PSA relapse after radical treatments, were chosen for this study. They are an ideal cohort to evaluate a lifestyle intervention as they have a useful serum marker (the PSA) of their disease. In addition, medical interventions are often not indicated initially upon relapse (Klotz, 2012). These men appear to have a great interest in self-help remedies, as reports indicate that 50 to 70% of men with prostate cancer admit to taking over-the-counter supplements (Bauer et al., 2012; Uzzo, 2004).

12.4.1   Why Choose the Specific Blend of Ingredients within Pomi-T?

The four ingredients were determined by a scientific review of the international laboratory and clinic data by a team of nationalists and oncologists from the National Cancer Research Institute (NCRI) Complementary Therapies Research (trial development) Committee. The team considered a wide spectrum of phytochemical-rich foods but narrowed the search to these four as each had demonstrated anticancer activity in previously published laboratory or phase II trials. The ingredients originate from separate food categories (spice, herb, fruit, and vegetable) and each has its own unique blend of polyphenols and antioxidants with different modes of action (see below). In addition, having lower concentrations of four different foods is likely to have less potential adverse effects, as it avoids overconsumption of one particular type of polyphenol.

12.4.2   Quality Assurance

As this was a UK government-backed study, Pomi-T was and still is manufactured to nationally approved Food Standard Agency standards and EU compliance regulations. Unlike many over-the-counter supplements, the manufacturers also perform their own laboratory analysis of each ingredient to ensure it is pure, free from toxic contaminants, and has been sourced correctly. Mass spectrometry of random trial samples took place via Hull University (Hull, UK) and confirmed no estrogenic or chemotherapeutic contamination. The trial was approved by the National Ethics Committee, peer-reviewed by other members of the NCRI Complementary Therapies Research

Committee, and adopted and independently audited by the National Cancer Research Network. The randomization process was outsourced and independently audited by an external agency to ensure adherence to European Good Clinical Practice Guidelines. At the end of the trial, the data was externally audited and validated before being analyzed independently at Cranfield University.

12.4.3 Methodology

Out of a total of 208 men who were reviewed for eligibility between November 2011 and July 2012, 203 men gave consent for the trial and were randomized at the Primrose Oncology Unit (Bedford Hospital NHS Trust, UK). Men had an average age of 74 years (range 53–89 years), histologically confirmed prostate cancer, 59% were being managed with primary AS, and 41% had a PSA relapse post radiotherapy or surgery and were being managed with watchful waiting (WW); see Table 12.1. No men were receiving other cancer therapies. Men were randomized to either receive Pomi-T or an identical blinded placebo for 6 months (Figure 12.2).

Table 12.1   Summary of Baseline Characteristics in the Randomly Assigned Groups

Baseline Characteristic	Pomi-T Group	Placebo Group
Age (mean years)	71.8	76.4
PSA (mean µg/L)	6.5	6.5
Gleason grade <7	127 (95%)	57 (88%)
Gleason grade >7	7 (5%)	8 (12%)
Gleason grade mean	6.5	6.2
BMI (mean kg/m²)	28.1	28.3
Cholesterol (mean mmol/L)	4.87	4.72
BP (mean systolic/diastolic mmHg)	146/83	150/82
Serum glucose (mean mmol/L)	5.15	5.30
C-reactive protein (mean mg/L)	1.51	1.74

BMI, body mass index; BP, blood pressure. There was no statistical difference in the group characteristics.

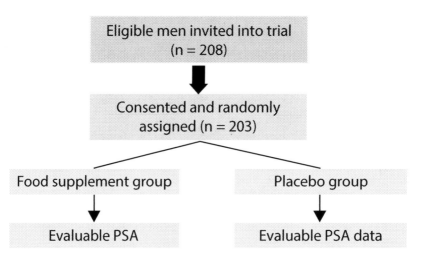

Figure 12.2 CONSORT diagram illustrating patient flow within the NCRN Pomi-T Trial.

12.4.4   Results

12.4.4.1   Percentage Rise in PSA

The median percentage change in PSA for patients in the Pomi-T group was a rise of 14.7% (95% confidence interval [CI] 3.4%–36.7%), compared to a rise of 78.5% (95% CI 48.1%–115.5%) for patients in the placebo group (Figure 12.3 in color insert). The median PSA increased at a significantly slower rate in the Pomi-T group compared to men taking placebo (difference of 63.8% ANCOVA, p=0.0008).

12.4.4.2   Percentage of Men in Whom Pomi-T Prevented a Change in Management

One hundred and fourteen (92.6%) men in the Pomi-T group continued surveillance or WW at the end of their involvement in the study, as opposed to 38 (74%) in the placebo group. This difference of 18.6% was statistically significant (p=0.01) (Figure 12.4).

12.4.4.3   Predetermined Subgroup Analysis

There was no significant difference in the median change in PSA from baseline to 6 months in the Pomi-T or placebo group between any of the predetermined subgroups (BMI, Gleason grade, age, or treatment category). There were no significant differences at the beginning or the end of the study between the subgroups for measures of cholesterol, blood pressure, serum glucose, or C-reactive protein.

12.4.4.4   Safety and Drug Interaction

No patients in either group reported central nervous system symptoms, such as agitation, insomnia, or tremors. In terms of drug interactions, none of the 20 men on warfarin reported any unexpected changes in their clotting parameters Likewise, none of the 38 men taking ramipril reported an unexpected change in their blood pressure.

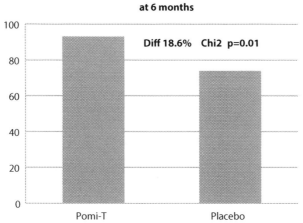

Figure 12.4   Percentage of men in whom Pomi-T prevented a change in management.

Table 12.2 Summary of the Adverse and Positive Events

	Pomi-T Group	Placebo Group	% Difference
Loose bowels	6 (4.5%)	0 (0%)	4.5 (ns)
Diarrhea	4 (3%)	1 (1.5%)	1.5 (ns)
Constipation	2 (1.5%)	0 (0%)	1.5 (ns)
Flatulence or bloating	9 (6.6%)	2 (3%)	3.6 (ns)
Rectal bleeding	0 (0%)	1 (1.5%)	1.5 (ns)
Nausea	0 (0%)	1 (1.5%)	1.5 (ns)
Worsening urinary flow	4 (3%)	2 (3%)	0 (ns)
Weight loss, feeling unwell	2 (1.5%)	6 (9%)	7.5% (ns)
Miscellaneous unrelated	7 (3.6%)	10 (13.4%)	9.8 (ns)
All adverse events	34 (24%)	23 (34%)	10 (ns)
Improved erectile function	1 (0.75%)	0 (0%)	0.75 (ns)
Improve urinary flow	4 (3%)	1 (1.5%)	1.5 (ns)
Reduced prostatic discomfort	1 (0.75%)	0 (0%)	0.75 (ns)
Improved bowel function	8 (6%)	0 (0%)	6 (ns)
Improved well-being	2 (1.5%)	2 (3%)	0 (ns)
All positive events	16 (12%)	3 (4.5%)	7.5 (ns)

ns, no significance.

12.4.4.5 Side Effects

Sixteen (12%) men in the Pomi-T group and 3 (4.6%) men in the placebo reported positive effects; however, the difference was not statistically significant (Table 12.2). Thirty-four (24%) men in the Pomi-T group and and 23 (34%) men in the placebo group reported adverse events, though this difference was also not statistically significant. Gastrointestinal events, considered separately, were reported by 21 (15.5%) men in the Pomi-T group as opposed to 5 (7.5%) men in the placebo group, but again this difference was not statistically significant.

12.4.4.6 Conclusions and Discussion of the Original Pomi-T Study

In this study, it was shown that men taking the whole food supplement Pomi-T had a significantly lower median percentage rise in PSA compared to men taking a placebo ($P<0.0001$). The difference in percentage rise in PSA between these groups from the start to end of the study was large (63.8%), and as the patient characteristics were well-balanced and the trial had sufficient numbers to ensure adequate statistical power, the results of this study offer clinically meaningful guidance for men contemplating nutritional supplements after prostate cancer.

Nevertheless, although the PSA measure has its shortcomings, men managed with AS or WW are greatly concerned with their serum levels, and a rise is often a determinant for changing management (Klotz, 2012). This was also highlighted in this trial cohort, as 47 men (8.4% in the Pomi-T group as opposed to 26% in the placebo group) opted to start a therapeutic intervention, particularly androgen deprivation therapy, when their PSA levels increased. While this was not a cost-effectiveness analysis, the tenfold price difference between Pomi-T and the LHRH agonists indicates a significant potential saving for men taking Pomi-T, and offers potential avoidance of the inevitable toxicities of androgen deprivation (Bourke et al., 2012).

The data reassuringly highlighted that Pomi-T was well tolerated with no overall statistical difference in side effects compared to a placebo. More men experienced non-significant bloating or diarrhea, but 15% of men reported beneficial effects, including better digestion and improvement of urinary symptoms. Previous studies have also shown turmeric to have an effect on symptoms of prostatitis, presumably via its anti-inflammatory properties [Shah, Handler]. One of the ingredients of Pomi-T, pomegranate seed, has been suggested to be a weak inhibitor of cytochrome P450 (CYP2C9). However, in the quantities used in this study, there were no unexpected changes in blood pressure or INR levels, which could have been related to interference of the metabolism of the popular blood pressure tablet ramipril or the anticoagulant warfarin.

The precise mechanism of action of the food combination was not investigated specifically in this clinical study, but as described in the background to the study, a review of previous laboratory studies suggested that the anticancer effects of these ingredients lie in their antiproliferative, antiangiogenic, proadhesion, antimetastatic and proapoptotic properties (Rettig et al., 2008; Malik et al., 2005; Khan and Mukhtar, 2007; Barber et al., 2006; Choi et al., 2006; Somasundaram et al., 2002; Shah et al., 1999; Zhang et al., 2007; Iqbal et al., 2003) rather than acting on the androgen receptors. The ingredients were intentionally selected to not have any phytoestrogenic or other hormonal effects (Wu and Yu, 2006; Choi et al., 2006). A subsequent analysis of serum testosterone in men who took Pomi-T after the study reported the mean levels to be completely normal, and this has been published separately (Thomas et al., 2014).

The results of this study were first provided as an oral presentation to the prestigious American Society of Clinical Oncology, then later published in the journal *Prostate Cancer and Prostatic Diseases* – both reflected in the scientific integrity of this study (Thomas et al., 2014). Nevertheless, a confirmatory larger national trial is planned as part of the second phase of the National Research Institute's PROVENT randomized trial run from the Institute of Preventative Medicine [PROVENT]. Some scientists have commented that the original Pomi-T study should have included analysis of other parameters of cancer progression, such as MRI or prostate biopsies. Formally incorporating MRI in the study design would have been cost prohibitive for a non-commercial study. In addition, although biopsy would have enhanced scientific competence, many men do not currently consent to repeat biopsies, and hence this inclusion would have reduced the rate of recruitment and increased the complexity and the cost. Fortunately, men in our institution managed with AS routinely have annual high resolution MRIs, so the issue of whether Pomi-T could have had a PSA effect only, without influencing underlying prostatic disease, was able to be addressed in a further prospective study.

12.5   STUDY TWO

This study involved MRI definition of cancer volume and its correlation with serum PSA in men undergoing lifestyle and nutritional interventions.

In this study, 346 paired serum PSA levels were correlated with 346 high resolution (diffusion weighted) MRIs of 138 men who had at least two prostate MRI scans over a 2-year period between 2013 and 2015. Men had histologically confirmed prostate cancer and were managed with active surveillance and were taking no other anticancer treatments apart from those taking Pomi-T.

Men with progression seen on MRI had a mean 39.78% rise in PSA (CI 28 to 52%), compared to those whose disease shrunk (−16.05%, CI 14 to −46%), remained stable (1.62% CI −3 to 5%), or was not visualized (−1.62%, CI −14 to 11%) (ANOVA, *P*-value <0.0001) (See Figure 12.5). This strong link between PSA dynamics and MRI-defined tumor progression provides reassurance to men on AS that their PSA dynamics reflect underlying tumor status as seen on MRI, especially in this group keen on lifestyle and nutritional self-help strategies such as Pomi-T (Thomas et al., 2015b).

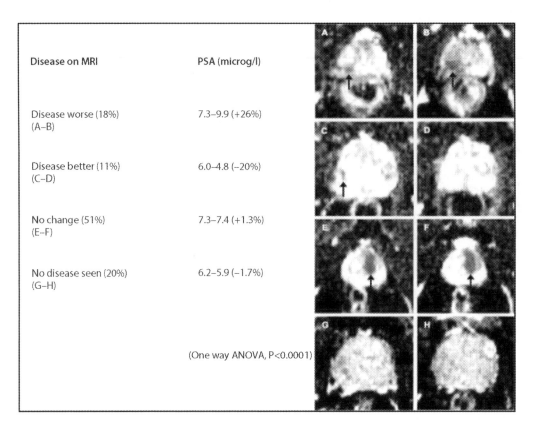

Disease on MRI	PSA (microg/l)
Disease worse (18%) (A–B)	7.3–9.9 (+26%)
Disease better (11%) (C–D)	6.0–4.8 (−20%)
No change (51%) (E–F)	7.3–7.4 (+1.3%)
No disease seen (20%) (G–H)	6.2–5.9 (−1.7%)
	(One way ANOVA, P<0.0001)

Figure 12.5 PSA changes over 1 year categorized by change of prostate cancer volume seen on diffusion weighted MRI.

12.6   CASE REPORTS

From a scientific perspective, case reports carry little credibility but for the individuals and their carers they are of utmost importance and their personal stories can help motivate others. Case reports also put lifestyle factors in perspective, as they show there is considerable overlap for different strategies. The first case report here relies only on diet, while the other two also include exercise and carcinogen avoidance.

12.6.1   Case One

A 69-year-old man presented in 2003 with urinary symptoms and was subsequently diagnosed with Gleason 8, stage 3 prostate cancer with a PSA of 150 g/dL. He received radiotherapy to his prostate and pelvic nodes and 2 years of adjuvant hormone therapies. Unfortunately, in 2006 his disease spread to his abdominal lymph nodes and he received further radiotherapy to these and further hormone therapy. In 2007 his PSA started increasing again and the nodes increased in size again, indicating hormone resistance. He received taxotere chemotherapy, which helped for a while, but by the end of 2008 his PSA increased again to 48 g/dL. At this stage, his wife started to make him broccoli soup then 2 years later started taking Pomi-T three times a day. Despite his previous intensive medical treatments and no other changes in his medication, his PSA started dropping.

Within 18 months it was 0.2 g/dL, the lowest it had been for many years. In addition, to the surprise of all involved in his care, the nodes seen on CT scan actually shrunk with 1 year and disappeared by 2015 (Figure 12.6 in color insert). At the time of writing this chapter he remained asymptomatic with a PSA <0.5 g/dl with no evidence of further metastatic disease.

12.6.2 Case Two

A 59-year-old woman presented with symptoms of anemia and rectal bleeding and was found to have cancer of the colon, which was subsequently surgically resected. In 2012, 2 years later, she was found to have a number of lung metastasis, confirmed histologically by the cardiothoracic surgeons but deemed inoperable. As she was asymptomatic, it was decided to embark on a series of lifestyle maneuvers while monitoring the disease carefully. As well as joining a walking group and gym, she changed her diet, reducing processed sugar and meat, significantly increasing legumes, colorful fruit and vegetables, and reducing carcinogenic foods. She also started taking three Pomi-T a day. Two years later, her metastases are smaller (Figure 12.7 in color insert) and she has none of the side effects of palliative chemotherapy, which still remains an option when she progresses in the future.

12.6.3 Case Three

A 60-year-old man presented with symptoms of intermittent abdominal obstruction and rectal bleeding, and was found to a have a cancer of the colon which was subsequently surgically resected. Despite adjuvant chemotherapy, he relapsed in his abdominal lymph nodes. These had grown on two consecutive CT scans over 3 months, corresponding to increasing blood markers of disease, cancer embryonic antigen (CEA) which increased from a normal of 4 to 1143 g/dL. Again, because he was asymptomatic and the disease could not be resected, palliative chemotherapy was put on hold, which allowed him to make some significant lifestyle changes. He started exercising 3 to 4 hours a week, stopped all processed sugar, stopped his intake of processed burnt meat and instead ate oily fish three times a week and legumes and pulses the other days, together with ample fruit, nuts, and vegetables. He continued a glass or two of good-quality red wine per week and started taking Pomi-T three times a day. Two years later his disease remained stable on CT, and his blood markers of bowel cancer reduced to 670 g/dL. The last time he was reviewed his CEA counts had started to rise again, indicating he may need chemotherapy in the near future. These lifestyle interventions have not cured him but during this time he has continued to work full time and enjoy a fulfilling lifestyle with his family, and hopefully after chemotherapy he can extend the period when he is disease stable (Figure 12.8 in color insert).

12.7 CONCLUSION

The significant effect on PSA after Pomi-T consumption is of great interest to the 700,000 men in the UK and 3.5 million men in the US living with prostate cancer, many of whom take self-help nutritional remedies (Bauer, Uzzo). Regular intake of this low-cost, well-tolerated polyphenol supplement is a particularly attractive option for men on AS or WW, as this trial suggests it could prevent progression to interventions with greater toxicities and stabilize PSA and tumor size seen on MRI. The further finding that Pomi-T intake does not affect serum testosterone and PSA monitoring correlated with underlying MRI-defined tumor volume provides additional reassurance.

12.8   FURTHER RESEARCH

A series of future trials is planned involving men with prostate cancer at different stages in their management, especially those taking androgen deprivation or managed with intermittent hormone therapy. The Institute of Preventative Medicine (London) is also planning to add Pomi-T to vitamin D and aspirin in the second phase of the PROVENT study involving men with early cancer, some of whom have a genetic risk of the disease. Likewise, further trials will evaluate the impact of Pomi-T for individuals with other cancers such as bowel, skin, and bladder. The anti-inflammatory benefits of polyphenols are going to be explored for other symptoms such as joint pain and hot flushes, and to increase male sperm count and improve exercise performance. Although the initial Pomi-T trial had no commercial funding, the product has now been commercialized by Helsinn Integrative (Switzerland) who are collaborating with our academic unit for financial support of these further research investigations, which is a welcome boost to the research program.

REFERENCES

Albanes, D. Heinonen, O.P. Huttunen, J.K. et al. 1994. The effect of vitamin E and beta carotene on the incidence of lung cancer and other cancers in male smokers. The Alpha-Tocopherol, Beta Carotene Cancer Prevention Study Group. *N Engl J Med* 330(15): 1029–1035.

Banim, P.J. Luben, R. McTaggart, A. et al. 2013. Dietary antioxidants and the aetiology of pancreatic cancer: a cohort study using data from food diaries and biomarkers. *Gut* 62(10): 1489–1496.

Barber, N.J. Zhang, X. Zhu, G.L. et al. 2006. Lycopene inhibits DNA synthesis in primary prostate epithelial cells in vitro and its administration is associated with a reduced prostate-specific antigen velocity in a phase II clinical study. *Prostate Cancer Prostatic Dis* 9(4): 407–413.

Bauer, C.M. Ishak, M.B. Johnson, E.K. et al. 2012. Prevalence and correlates of vitamin and supplement usage among men with a family history of prostate cancer. *Integr Cancer Ther* 11(2): 83–89.

Bent, S. Kane, C. Shinohara, K. et al. 2006. Saw palmetto for benign prostatic hyperplasia. *N Engl J Med.* 354(6): 557–566.

Bourke, L. Sohanpal, R. Nanton, V. et al. 2012. A qualitative study evaluating experiences of a lifestyle intervention in men with prostate cancer undergoing androgen suppression therapy. *Trials* 13: 208.

Boyapati, S.M. Shu, X.O. Ruan, Z.X. et al. 2005. Soy food intake and breast cancer survival: a follow up of the Shanghai Breast Cancer Study. *Breast Cancer Res Treat* 92: 11–17.

Brasky, T.M. Kristal, A.R. Navarro, S.L. et al. 2011. Specialty supplements and prostate cancer risk in the VITamins and Lifestyle (VITAL) cohort. *Nutr Cancer* 63(4): 573–582.

Buck, K. Vrieling, A. Zaineddin, A.K. et al. 2011. Serum enterolactone and prognosis of postmenopausal breast cancer. *J Clin Oncol* 29(28): 3730–3738.

Choi, C. Liao, Y. Wu, S. et al. 2006. The structure of pomegranate has no hormonal component. *Mass Spec Food Chem* 96; 562.

Chuang, S.C. Stolzenberg-Solomon, R. Ueland, P.M. et al. 2011. A U-shaped relationship between plasma folate and pancreatic cancer risk in the European Prospective Investigation into Cancer and Nutrition. *Eur J Cancer* 47(12): 1808–1816.

Clark, P.E. Hall, M.C. Borden, L.S Jr. et al. 2006. Phase I-II prospective dose-escalating trial of lycopene in patients with biochemical relapse of prostate cancer after definitive local therapy. *Urology* 67(6): 1257–1261.

Denny, A. Buttriss, J. Plant foods and health: focus on plant bioactives. 2007. EU Information Resource (EuroFIR) Consortium. Contract FOOD-CT-2005-513944.

Dorai, T. Gehani, N. Katz, A. 2000. Therapeutic potential of curcumin in human prostate cancer. II. Curcumin inhibits tyrosine kinase activity of epidermal growth factor receptor and depletes the protein. *Mol Urol* 4(1): 1–6.

Ebbing, M. Bønaa, K.H. Nygård, O. et al. 2009. Cancer incidence and mortality after treatment with folic acid and vitamin B12. *JAMA* 302(19): 2119–2126.

Elmets, C.A. Singh, D. Tubesing, K. et al. 2001. Cutaneous photoprotection from ultraviolet injury by green tea polyphenols. *J Am Acad Dermatol* 44(3): 425–432.

Figueiredo, J.C. Grau, M.V. Haile, R.W. et al. 2009. Folic acid and risk of prostate cancer: results from a randomized clinical trial. *J Natl Cancer Inst* 101(6): 432–435.

Gasper, A.V. Al-Janobi, A. Smith, J.A. et al. 2005. Glutathione S-transferase M1 polymorphism and metabolism of sulforaphane from standard and high-glucosinolate broccoli. *Am J Clin Nutr* 82(6): 1283–1291.

Giovannucci, E. Rimm, E.B. Liu, Y. et al. 2002. A prospective study of tomato products, lycopene, and prostate cancer risk. *J Natl Cancer Inst* 94: 391–398.

Greenwald, P. Milner, J.A. Anderson, D.E. et al. 2002. Micronutrients in cancer prevention. *Cancer Metastasis Rev* 21: 217–230.

Handler, N. Jaeger, W. Puschacher, H. et al. 2007. Synthesis of novel curcumin analogues and their evaluation as selective cyclooxygenase-1 (COX-1) inhibitors. *Chem Pharm Bull* 55(1): 64–71.

Heinen, M.M. Hughes, M.C. Ibiebele, T.I. et al. 2007. Intake of antioxidant nutrients and the risk of skin cancer. *Eur J Cancer* 43(18): 2707–2716.

Hercberg, S. Galan, P. Preziosi, P. et al. 2004. The SU.VI.MAX Study: a randomized, placebo-controlled trial of the health effects of antioxidant vitamins and minerals. *Arch Intern Med* 164(21): 2335–2342.

Hu, F. Wang, Yi. B. Zhang, W. et al. 2012. Carotenoids and breast cancer risk: a meta-analysis and meta-regression. *Breast Cancer Res Treat* 131(1): 239–253.

Iqbal, M. Sharma, S.D. Okazaki, Y. et al. 2003. Dietary supplementation of curcumin enhances antioxidant phase II metabolizing enzymes in mice. *Pharmacol Toxicol* 92: 33–38.

Joseph, M.A. Moysich, K.B. Freudenheim, J.L. et al. 2004. Cruciferous vegetables, genetic polymorphisms in glutathione S-transferases M1 and T1, and prostate cancer risk. *Nutr Cancer* 50(2): 206–213.

Kakarala, M. Brenner, D.E. Korkaya, H. et al. 2010. Targeting breast stem cells with the cancer preventive compounds curcumin and piperine. *Breast Cancer Res Treat* 122(3): 777–785.

Karppi, J. Laukkanen, J.A. Sivenius, J. et al. 2012. Serum lycopene decreases the risk of stroke in men: a population-based follow-up study. *Neurology* 79(15): 1540–1547.

Khan, N. Mukhtar, H. 2007. Pomegranate inhibits growth of primary lung tumors in mice. *Cancer Res* 67: 3475–3482.

Klein, E.A. Thompson, I.M Jr. Tangen, C.M. et al. 2011. Vitamin E and the risk of prostate cancer: the Selenium and Vitamin E Cancer Prevention Trial (SELECT). *JAMA* 306(14): 1549–1556.

Klotz, L. 2012. Active surveillance for favorable-risk prostate cancer: background, patient selection, triggers for intervention, and outcomes. *Curr Urol Rep* 13(2): 153–159.

Leitzmann, M.F. Stampfer, M.J. Wu, K. et al. 2003. Zinc supplementation and the risks of prostate cancer. *J Natl Cancer Inst* 95: 1004–1007.

Li, C. Ford, E.S. Zhao, G. et al. 2011. Serum α-carotene concentrations and risk of death among US Adults: the Third National Health and Nutrition Examination Survey Follow-up Study. *Arch Intern Med* 171(6): 507–515.

Liao, J. Yang, G.Y. Park, E.S. et al. 2004. Inhibition of lung carcinogenesis and effects on angiogenesis and apoptosis in A/J mice by oral administration of green tea. *Nutr Cancer* 48(1): 44–53.

Malik, A. Afaq, F. Sarfaraz, S. 2005. Pomegranate fruit juice for chemoprevention and chemotherapy of prostate cancer. *Proc Natl Acad Sci U S A* 102(41): 14813–14818.

McLarty, J. Bigelow, R.L. Smith, M. et al. 2009. Tea polyphenols decrease serum levels of prostate-specific antigen, hepatocyte growth factor, and vascular endothelial growth factor in prostate cancer patients and inhibit production of hepatocyte growth factor and vascular endothelial growth factor in vitro. *Cancer Prev Res (Phila)* 2(7): 673–682.

Meyer, F. Galan, P. Douville, P. 2005. Antioxidant vitamin and mineral supplementation and prostate cancer prevention in the SU.VI.MAX trial. *Int J Cancer* 116(2): 182–186.

Ogunleye, A.A. Xue, F. Michels, K.B. 2010. Green tea consumption and breast cancer risk or recurrence: a meta-analysis. *Breast Cancer Res Treat* 119(2): 477–484.

Omenn, G.S. Goodman, G.E. Thornquist, M.D. et al. 1996. Effects of a combination of beta carotene and vitamin A on lung cancer and cardiovascular disease. *N Engl J Med* 334(18): 1150–1155.

Ornish, D. Magbanua, M.J. Weidner, G. et al. 2008. Changes in prostate gene expression in men undergoing an intensive nutrition and lifestyle intervention. *Proc Natl Acad Sci U S A* 105(24): 8369–8374.

Paller, C.J. Ye, X. Wozniak, P.J. et al. 2013. A randomized phase II study of pomegranate extract for men with rising PSA following initial therapy for localized prostate cancer. *Prostate Cancer Prostatic Dis* 16(1): 50–55.

Pantuck, A.J. Leppert, J.T. Zomorodian, N. et al. 2006. Phase II study of pomegranate juice for men with rising prostate-specific antigen following surgery or radiation for prostate cancer. *Clin Cancer Res* 12(13): 4018–4026.

Parada, J. Aguilera, J.M. 2007. Food microstructure affects the bioavailability of several nutrients. *J Food Sci* 72(2): R21–32.

Pierce, J.P. Natarajan, L. Caan, B.J et al. 2007. Influence of a diet very high in vegetables, fruit, and fiber and low in fat on prognosis following treatment for breast cancer: the Women's Healthy Eating and Living (WHEL) randomized trial. *JAMA* 298(3): 289–298.

Porrini, M. Riso, P. 2008. Factors influencing the bioavailability of antioxidants in foods: a critical appraisal. *Nutr Metab Cardiovasc Dis* 80(4): 353–361.

Posadzki, P. Lee, M.S. Onakpoya, I. et al. 2013. Dietary supplements and prostate cancer: a systematic review of double-blind, placebo-controlled randomised clinical trials. *Maturitas* 75(2): 125–130.

PROVENT Study – Clinical effectiveness of aspirin and Vitamin D3 to prevent disease progression in men on Active Surveillance for men with Prostate cancer (Phase 1) ISCTN91422391 registration Doi: 10.1186/ISRCTN91422391.

Reichman, M.E. Hayes, R.B. Ziegler, R.G. et al. 1990. Serum vitamin A and subsequent development of prostate cancer in the first National Health and Nutrition Examination Survey Epidemiologic Follow-up Study. *Cancer Res* 50(8): 2311–2315.

Rettig, M.B. Heber, D. An, J. et al. 2008. Pomegranate extract inhibits androgen independent prostate cancer growth through a nuclear factor-kappaB-dependent mechanism. *Mol Cancer Ther* 7(9): 2662–2671.

Rezai-Zadeh, K. Shytle, D. Sun, N. et al. 2005. Green tea epigallocatechin-3-gallate (EGCG) modulates amyloid precursor protein cleavage and reduces cerebral amyloidosis in Alzheimer transgenic mice. *J Neurosci* 25(38): 8807–8814.

Rocha, A. Wang, L. Penichet, M. Martins-Green, M. 2012. Pomegranate juice and specific components inhibit cell and molecular processes critical for metastasis of breast cancer. *Breast Cancer Res Treat* 136(3): 647–658.

Rock, C.L. Flatt, S.W. Natarajan, L. et al. 2005. Plasma carotenoids and recurrence-free survival in women with a history of breast cancer. *J Clin Oncol* 23(27): 6631–6638.

Sarkar, R. Mukherjee, S. Biswas, J. et al. 2012. Sulphoraphane, a naturally occurring isothiocyanate induces apoptosis in breast cancer cells by targeting heat shock proteins. *Biochem Biophys Res Commun* 427(1): 80–85.

Schenk, J.M. Riboli, E. Chatterjee, N. et al. 2009. Serum retinol and prostate cancer risk: a nested case-control study in the prostate, lung, colorectal, and ovarian cancer screening trial. *Cancer Epidemiol Biomarkers Prev* 18(4): 1227–1231.

Schröder, F.H. Roobol, M.J. Boevé, E.R. et al. 2005. Randomized, double-blind, placebo-controlled crossover study in men with prostate cancer and rising PSA: effectiveness of a dietary supplement. *Eur Urol* 48(6): 922–930.

Shah, B.H. Nawaz, Z. Pertani, S.A. et al. 1999. Inhibitory effect of curcumin, a food spice from turmeric, on platelet-activating factor- and arachidonic acid-mediated platelet aggregation through inhibition of thromboxane formation and Ca2+ signaling. *Biochem Pharmacol* 58(7): 1167–1172.

Somasundaram, S. Edmund, N.A. Moore, D.T. et al. 2002. Curcumin inhibits chemotherapy-induced apoptosis in models of cancer. *Cancer Res* 62(13): 3868–3875.

Sonn, G.A. Aronson, W. Litwin, M.S. 2005. Impact of diet on prostate cancer: a review. *Prostate Cancer Prostatic Dis* 8: 304–310.

Spentzos, D. Mantzoros, C. Regan, M.M. et al. 2003. Minimal effect of a low-fat/high soy diet for asymptomatic, hormonally naive prostate cancer patients. *Clin Cancer Res* 9(9): 3282–3287.

Sun, C.L. Yuan, J.M. Koh, W.P. et al. 2007. Green tea and cancer risk: the Singapore Chinese Health Study. *Carcinogenesis* 28(10): 2143–2148.

Thomas, R. Butler, E. Macchi, F. et al. 2015a. Phytochemicals in cancer prevention and management? *BJMP* 8(2): 45–52.

Thomas, R. Oakes, R., Gordon, J. et al. 2009. A randomised double-blind phase II study of lifestyle counselling and salicylate compounds in patients with progressive prostate cancer. *Nut Food Science* 39(3): 295–305.

Thomas, R. Shaikh, M. Cauchi, M. et al. 2015b. Prostate cancer progression defined by MRI correlates with serum PSA in men undergoing lifestyle and nutritional interventions for low-risk disease. *J Lifestyle Disease Management* 1: 1–6.

Thomas, R. Williams, M. Sharma, H. et al. 2014. A double-blind, placebo-controlled randomised trial evaluating the effect of a polyphenol-rich whole food supplement on PSA progression in men with prostate cancer–the U.K. NCRN Pomi-T study. *Prostate Cancer Prostatic Dis* 17(2): 180–186.

Tung, K.H. Wilkens, L.R. Wu, A.H. 2005. Association of dietary vitamin A, carotenoids, and other antioxidants with the risk of ovarian cancer. *Cancer Epidemiol Biomarkers Prev* 14(3): 669–676.

Uzzo, R.G. Brown, J.G. Horwitz, E.M. et al. 2004. Prevalence and patterns of self-initiated nutritional supplementation in men at high risk of prostate cancer. *BJU Int* 93(7): 955–960.

Wang, L. Alcon, A. Yuan, H. et al. 2011. Cellular and molecular mechanisms of pomegranate juice-induced anti-metastatic effect on prostate cancer cells. *Integr Biol (Camb)* 3(7): 742–754.

Wu, A.H. Yu, M.C. 2006. Tea, hormone-related cancers and endogenous hormone levels. *Mol Nutr Food Res* 50(2): 160–169.

Yang, C.S. Maliakal, P. Meng, X. 2002. Inhibition of carcinogenesis by tea. *Annu Rev Pharmacol Toxicol* 42: 25–54.

Zhang, H.N. Yu, C.X. Chen, W.W et al. 2007. Curcumin down regulates gene NKX3.1 in prostate cancer cell lines (LNcaP). *Acta Pharmacologica Sinica* 28(3): 423–430.

CHAPTER 13

Approach of Ayurveda to Prostate Cancer

Vaishali Kuchewar

CONTENTS

13.1 CONCEPT OF CANCER IN AYURVEDA

Ayurvedic literature has no direct reference for the diagnosis of cancer, but detailed descriptions of various types of tumors such as gulma, granthi, utsedha, and arbuda are given. Specifically, arbuda can be correlated as malignant tumor because the clinical features of these two are similar (Sharma, 2007; Bhishagratha, 1991). Arbuda has been described as a round, large, muscular, immovable, deeply rooted, slowly growing swelling produced due to the aggravation of dosha vitiating the muscle, blood, and fatty tissues.

In Ayurvedic literature, pathophysiology as well as management of every disease is based on tridosha (functional unit of the body), sapta dhatu (structural unit), and agni (digestive fire). The three body-control systems are called tridosha, i.e. vata (governs flow and motion in the body). Vata is of prime importance in all homeostatic mechanisms and controls the other two principles, pitta and kapha. Pitta governs bodily functions concerned with heat and metabolism and directs all biochemical reactions and the process of energy exchange, and kapha governs the structure and cohesion of the organism and is responsible for biological strength, natural tissue resistance, and proper body structure. These two systems coordinate to perform the normal function of the body. Homeostasis depends on proper coordination of tridosha. Any imbalance in these body-control systems can result in the disease state. In any morbidity, one or two of the three bodily systems are out of control. This is not too harmful, as the body is still trying to coordinate among these systems. But if there is vitiation of tridosha, all three major bodily systems lose mutual coordination and thus cannot prevent tissue damage, resulting in a deadly morbid condition (Bhishagratha, 1991). It is said that the disease is difficult to cure or incurable if all the dosha are vitiated.

Dhatu (body tissue) is the structural unit of the body. Vitiated tridosha has a capacity to vitiate dhatu to cause disease. The type of disease depends on the involvement of dhatu. The seven dhatu (tissues) are rasa (plasma), rakta (blood), mamsa (muscle), meda (fat or lipids), asthi (bones and cartilage), majja (bone marrow and nerve tissue) and shukra (male reproductive tissue) or artava (female reproductive tissue). *Agni* is used in the sense of digestion and metabolism. Types of arbuda (malignant tumor) are described according to the involvement of dosha and dhatu.

13.1.1 Etiological Factors of Vitiation of Dosha and Dhatu

Ahara (diet) and vihara (daily routine, including behavior) are considered the major etiological factors for every disease. In most noncommunicable diseases like cancer, the etiological factor is not clear. Ahara and vihara might be responsible. Some causes are listed here for the derangement of dosha and dhatu involved in the pathogenesis of cancer (Sharma, 2007).

1. Vata aggravating factors: excessive intake of bitter, pungent, astringent, dry food, and stressful conditions.
2. Pitta aggravating factors: excessive intake of sour, salty, fried food, and excessive anger.
3. Kapha aggravating factors: excessive intake of sweet, oily food, and sedentary lifestyle.
4. Rakta aggravating factors: excessive intake of acidic food, fried and roasted food, alcoholic beverages, sour fruits are some examples. Excessive anger or severe emotional upset, working under scorching sun or near fire and hot conditions are some other causes (Sharma, 2007).
5. Mamsa aggravating factors: excessive use of exudative food like meat, fish, yoghurt, milk and cream, sleeping during the day, and overeating are some factors causing pathogenesis in the fatty tissues (Sharma, 2007)
6. Medo aggravating factors: excessive intake of oily food, sweets, alcohol, and sedentary lifestyle (Bhishagratha, 1991).

13.1.2 Etiological Factors of Arbuda (Tumor)

According to the Ayurvedic text *Madhav Nidan*, the following are the common etiological factors.

- Vidahi annapan (food having irritating properties)
- Tikshna aushadha (cytotoxic drugs)
- Viruddha ahara (incompatible food)
- Viruddha vihar (wrong lifestyle)
- Beeja dosha (genetic predisposition)
- Sukshma krimi (microorganisms)
- Vyavasaya (occupational hazards)
- Manovedana (psychological factors like stress, anxiety)
- Vardhakya (elderly)
- Paryavaranam (pollution)

13.1.3 Pathogenesis of Arbuda (Tumor)

In Ayurveda, pathogenesis of every disease is explained on the basis of tridosha, saptadhatu, and agni. The importance of agni is described by the sentence "Roga sarvepi mandegno" [all diseases are caused by derangement of metabolism]. Three types of agni are described: jatharagi (digestion at the level of gastrointestinal tract), bhutagni (metabolism in the liver) and dhatwagni (cellular metabolism). The decrease in agni is inversely proportional to the related tissue, and therefore in arbuda, a decreased state of dhatwagni (deranged metabolism) results in excessive tissue growth.

Undigested material is called ama (endotoxins). The theory states that the accumulation of undigested matter interferes with the normal function of dosha (disturbance in homeostasis).

13.1.4 Classical Features of Arbuda (Malignant Tumor)

Daurbalya (weakness)
Alpa poshan (malnourishment)
Balakshaya (extreme fatigue)
Ruja (pain)

13.2   PROSTATE CANCER IN AYURVEDA

There is no clear description of arbuda related to the prostate gland, but the disease *vatashthila* is described in Ayurvedic texts, which is correlated with prostate hypertrophy. The prostate gland is called *ashtila* (a small, stone-like structure). Another term, *mutraghata*, is also described in Ayurvedic text – Sushruta Samhita, an ancient Sanskrit text on medicine and surgery, believed to be written in the 6th century BCE and one of the foundation texts of the Ayurveda system. The word mutraghata comprises two different words: *mutra* and *aghata*, which stand for low urine output due to obstruction in the passage of urine. In the Ayurvedic perspective, vitiated tridosha causes abnormal growth of the prostate gland, which is a part of shukra dhatu (the male reproductive organ).

13.3 TREATMENT PRINCIPLE OF CANCER

Ayurveda is a medical system that deals not only with the body but with the mind and spirit as well. The fundamental aim of Ayurvedic therapy is to restore the balance between the three major body systems (Murthy, 2005a; 2005b). To balance tridosha, the following treatment principles are described.

13.3.1 Nidan Parivarjan (Abstinence from Root Cause)

The first step is to avoid the root cause of tridosha imbalance. The diet should be balanced, avoiding extremes that could further provoke the doshas. The diet should be easy to digest, nourish the body, and pacify tridosha. This is described as pathya and Apathya (do's and don'ts).

13.3.2 Samshodhan Chikitsa (Body Purifying Modalities)

This includes body purification measures to eliminate vitiated dosha. Both internal and external purification are achieved by five techniques known collectively as panchakarma chikitsa. These five techniques are as follows:

Vamana – Therapeutic emesis
Virechana – Therapeutic purging
Basti – Medicated enema
Nasya – Nasal administration of medicine
Rakta mokshana – Bloodletting

Selection of the procedure depends on the involvement of dosha and dhatu. In prostate cancer, according to the strength of the patient, virechana and basti can be advised.

13.3.3 Samshaman Chikitsa (Palliative Treatment)

This is useful to pacify the dosha. It is advised after shodhan chikitsa, or without shodhan chikitsa if dosha and dhatu involvement are minimal. It includes herbo-mineral preparations.

13.3.4 Treatment of Agni

It was previously discussed that jatharagni, bhutagni, and dhatvagni play an important role in homeostasis. Numerous medicines are available that act on different levels of agni. In prostate cancer, there is severe dysfunctioning of dhatvagni (tissue metabolism). As the disease spreads, jatharagni (digestion in gastrointestinal tract) and bhutagni (digestion in the liver) are also deranged. A herbal preparation, trikatu, which consists of equal amounts of three herbs – sunthi (*Zingiber officianalis*), maricha (*Piper nigrum*), and pippali (*Piper longum*) – is supposed to work on jatharagni. Bhringaraja (*Eclipta alba*), kutaki (*Picrorhiza kurroa*), and haridra (*Curcuma longa*) act at the level of bhutagni. There are multiple herbs that act on specific dhatvagni. These can be used according to the derangement of type of agni.

13.3.5 Satvavajaya Chikitsa

Ayurveda considers mind and body as one entity. Cancer patients are quite mentally unstable. Emotional support and psychotherapy are provided with yoga, meditation, prayers, and chanting. These are helpful in cultivating a positive attitude.

13.4 MEDICINAL TREATMENT

A holistic approach is the hallmark of treatment in Ayurveda. It demands that one herb or one drug will not cure the imbalance of dosha. Therefore, traditionally, in most cases, a combination of herbs is recommended for treatment (Garodia et al., 2007). Many herbs have been described for the treatment of cancer (Sastry, 2001; Balachandran and Govindarajan, 2005). These herbs are classified based on their rasa (taste) as katu (pungent), tikta (bitter), or kashaya (astringent), or other biophysical properties such as laghu (light), ruksha (dry), teekshna (sharp, penetrating), ushna (hot), ushna veerya (biopotency), and katu (pungent) vipaka (catabolic effects) (Singh, 2002).

In prostate cancer, some herbs can be used to support the healthy tissues of the prostate, reduce the growth of the tumor, and possibly prevent metastasis. The following single or combination drugs can be prescribed by considering their tumor-related properties.

13.4.1 Kanchanar (*Bauhinia variegata*)

This was widely used in traditional medicine to treat a wide range of complaints. According to an ancient Ayurvedic text, bhava prakash, the prabhava (special property) of kanchanar, is gandamalapaha (the ability to reduce swellings and growths). Another Ayurvedic text, Sharangadhara Samhita, written in the 13th century, describes different types of pulse in different disease conditions as:

Galagandam jayatyugram apachim arbudaani cha |
grantheen vranaani gulmaashcha kushtani cha bhagandharam ||

Kanchanar guggul is useful in any type of abnormal growth. Kanchanar has been used for millennia to clean and re-establish the tissues where abnormal growth or swelling occurs.

The common formulation is Kanchanar guggul.

Dose: 250–500 mg twice a day

13.4.2 Shilajit

This is an important drug of the ancient *materia medica*. It has a number of pharmacological activities and has been used for years as a rejuvenator and for treating a number of disease conditions (Acharya et al., 1988). Shilajit is a complex mixture of organic humic substances and humic nature, plant, and microbial metabolites occurring in rock rhizospheres (Ghosal, 1993; Agarwal et al., 2007; Agarwal et al., 2008a; 2008b). It is composed mainly of humic acid and fulvic acid. These two acids have been reported to possess cancer preventive properties (Peña-Méndez et al., 2005). Elderly patients (above 65 years old) are more at risk for development of cancer. DNA repair capacity decreases with increase in age mainly due to a decrease in endogenous antioxidants in the body, which might lead to the development of cancer. Therefore, intake of antioxidants with increasing age is suggested to arrest the oxidative damage (Borek, 2004). It has been shown that shilajit can delay the aging process and possibly lower the risk of cell impairment and damage (Meena et al., 2010; Murthy, 2005a; 2005b).

13.4.3 Gomutra (Cow Urine)

In the well-known Ayurvedic text Sushruta Samhita, gomutra (cow urine) has been described as having innumerable therapeutic values. In India, drinking of cow urine has been practiced for thousands of years. It can be used in the form of gomutra arka, which is prepared by distillation of the cow urine and is more palatable due to its lower ammonia content. Cow urine therapy is suggested to possess potent anticancer abilities due to the properties listed below (Dhama et al., 2005).

> DNA-repairing potential: Cow urine efficiently repairs damaged DNA. Damage of DNA by chemicals is the major cause for cancer. Cow urine reduces the spread of malignant cancers and helps fight tumors.
>
> Anti-free radicals: Free radicals cause cell damage, thereby inducing tumor cell growth or causing recurrence. Cow urine prevents free radicals.

13.4.4   Ashwagandha (*Withania somnifera*)

Withania somnifera Dunal, commonly known as ashwagandha, is reported to have antitumor, anti-stress, immunomodulatory, anti-inflammatory, and antibacterial effects (Chandrashekar et al., 1996; Devi et al., 1996; Archana and Namasivayam, 1999; Ziauddin et al., 1996; Umadevi, 1996). The roots of *W. somnifera* contain several alkaloids, withanolides, a few flavonoids, and reducing sugars (Ganzera et al., 2003; Jayaprakasam et al., 2003; Kaur et al., 2003; Matsuda et al., 2001). Several studies support the role of ashwagandha as an effective cancer chemopreventive agent; however, limited information is available regarding the mechanism of regulation of these chemopreventive effects (Spelman et al., 2006).

Based on its pro-apoptotic and immunomodulatory effects, ashwagandha can be useful as a complementary therapy for integrative oncology care.

Dose: Ashwagandha powder: 3–6 g twice a day
        Ashwagandha Ghana (extract): 250–500 mg per day

13.4.5   Dadima (*Punica granatum*)

This herb is mentioned in all ancient Sanskrit scriptures of Ayurveda. It has been commonly used as an edible fruit, as well as for medicinal purposes. It is known as tridoshaghna (i.e. normalizes vitiated dosha). Its effects on prostate cancer have been investigated in the cell culture system, animal models, and in a phase II clinical trial in humans. Various preparations, in the form of oils, fermented juice polyphenols, and pericarp polyphenols have been tested on human prostate cancer (PCa) cell growth both *in vitro* and *in vivo*. Each preparation inhibited growth of human prostate cancer cells, whereas normal prostate epithelial cells were significantly less affected (Albrecht et al., 2004; Lansky et al., 2005a; 2005b; Seeram et al., 2005; 2007; Sartippour et al, 2008; Malik and Mukhtar, 2006; Malik et al., 2005; Hong et al., 2008).

Antiproliferative and pro-apoptotic properties of pomegranate fruit extract (PFE) against human PCa cells have also been demonstrated both in the cell culture system and in a xenograft mouse model (Malik and Mukhtar, 2006; Malik et al., 2005). Oral infusion of PFE to mice resulted in a significant inhibition in tumor growth as observed by prolongation of tumor appearance. Tumor growth inhibition was accompanied with a concomitant decrease in serum prostate-specific antigen, and serum PSA levels were 70–85% lower in PFE-fed mice as compared to water-fed mice (Malik et al., 2005).

In a phase II clinical trial, Pantuck et al. (2006) recruited patients with rising PSA and gave them 8 ounces of pomegranate juice daily until disease progression. This study suggested that pomegranate consumption may retard PCa progression, which may prolong not only survival but also improve the quality of life of patients.

13.4.6 Haridra (*Curcuma longa*)

This is a bitter tasting tropical plant of the Zingiberaceae family cultivated extensively in Asia, India, China, and many other countries (Wickenberg et al., 2010). It has been traditionally used in Ayurvedic medicine to treat multiple symptoms and as a natural remedy for many ailments and afflictions. Now scientists from Ludwig-Maximilian University in Munich, led by Beatrice Bachmeier, have discovered how curcumin suppresses metastases of certain cancers (Bachmeier, 2012). The study was focused on the use of curcumin as a preventive agent in prostate cancer metastasis; breast cancer is also driven by the same type of latent or chronic inflammatory reactions, producing pro-inflammatory proteins known as cytokines. In the study, performed in animals, curcumin was able to decrease two of these cytokines, CXCL1 and CXCL2 (Killian et al., 2012).

13.4.7 Gokshura (*Tribulus terestris*)

This is one of the most important herbs for the urogenital system. The following properties mentioned in Ayurvedic literature balance the vitiated dosha.

- Rasa (taste based on activity): Madhura (sweet)
- Guna (properties): Guru (heavy to digest), Snigdha (unctuous)
- Veerya (potency): Sheeta (cooling)
- Vipaka (taste after digestion based on activity): Madhura (sweet)
- Karma (pharmacological action): Bruhana (nourishing), vatanut (pacifies vata dosha), vrusya (aphrodisiac), ashmarihara (removes urinary stone), vastishodhana (cures bladder ailments)

It is used in folk medicines as a tonic, aphrodisiac, palliative, astringent, stomachic, antihypertensive, diuretic, lithotriptic, and urinary disinfectant. The dried fruit of the herb is very effective in most genitourinary tract disorders. It is a vital constituent of gokshuradi guggul, a potent Ayurvedic medicine used to support proper functioning of the genitourinary tract (Khare, 2007).

13.4.8 Rasa Aushadhi (Metallic Preparation)

In the Ayurvedic description, several metallic preparations have been in clinical use since the twelfth century (Pattanaik et al., 2003). Rasa-Shastra is the Ayurvedic science that deals with the processing and different preparations of mercury and other metals. Mercury is used for its yoga-vahi or vehicular properties in a variety of preparations. Bhasma of different metals such as gold, silver, copper, and minerals such as sulfur, pearl, coral, and gems etc. are described in the ancient Ayurvedic literature. Metals are processed many times to result in a nontoxic, easily absorbable active compound.

13.4.8.1 Yashad Bhasma

This is a natural form of zinc offering tremendous therapeutic benefits for the genitourinary tract. Zinc plays an important role in the normal function and pathology of the prostate gland; reduced levels of tissue zinc and plasma zinc are associated with increased incidence of BPH and prostate carcinoma.

Dose: 250–500 mg twice a day

13.4.8.2 Tamra Bhasma

This is prepared from copper. It is used in Ayurvedic treatment for skin diseases, obesity, piles, asthma, tumor, etc. This medicine should be taken strictly under medical supervision.

Dose: 125–250 mg once or twice a day before or after food, or as directed by Ayurvedic physician. It is traditionally administered along with ghee, honey, milk, or sugar.

13.4.8.3 Vanga Bhasma

Vanga bhasma, an indigenous medicine prepared from tin metal, finds a place in the treatment of genitourinary tract diseases. The Ayurvedic literature shows that vanga bhasma has a specific role on sukravaha srotas (the male genital tract semen system).

Dose: 125–250 mg.

13.5 SUMMARY

Ayurvedic literature has no direct reference to the diagnosis of cancer, but detailed descriptions of various types of tumors such as gulma, granthi, utsedha, and arbuda are given. Specifically, arbuda is correlated with malignant tumor. In Ayurveda, the pathogenesis of every disease is explained on the basis of tridosha, saptadhatu, and agni. The importance of agni is described as "Roga sarvepi mandegno" [all diseases are caused by derangement of metabolism]. Ahara (diet) and vihara (daily routine including behavior) are considered to be the major etiological factors for every disease. The decrease in agni is inversely proportional to the related tissue, and therefore in arbuda, a decreased state of dhatwagni (deranged metabolism) results in excessive tissue growth. The terms vatashthila and mutraghata are both related to prostatomegaly

The fundamental aim of Ayurvedic therapy is to restore the balance between the three major body systems. The principles of treatment are nidan parivarjan (abstinence from root cause), samshodhan chikitsa (body purifying modalities), shaman chikitsa (palliative treatment), treatment of agni, and satvavajaya chikitsa. Many herbs are classified based on their rasa (taste) as katu (pungent), tikta (bitter), or kashaya (astringent) or other biophysical properties as laghu (light), ruksha (dry), teekshna (sharp, penetrating) and usna (hot), ushna veerya (biopotency), and katu (pungent) vipaka (catabolic effects). In prostate cancer, some herbs and metallic preparations can be used to support the healthy tissues of the prostate, reduce tumor growth, and possibly prevent metastasis.

Ayurveda can be helpful in the management of prostate cancer in the following ways:

1. As an adjuvant therapy
2. To minimize the side effects of chemotherapy
3. To slow the progress of the prostate cancer
4. To improve comfort and the quality of life of patient (via cell protective activity of drugs, described in rasayana therapy)

It can be concluded that integration of modern medicine and an Ayurvedic approach may be helpful to add years to the life and life to the years of prostate cancer sufferers.

REFERENCES

Acharya, S.B. Frotan, M.H. Goel, R.K. et al. 1988. Pharmacological actions of Shilajit. *Ind J Exp Biol* 26: 775–777.

Agarwal, S.P. Khanna, R. Karmarkar, R. et al. 2008a. Physico-chemical, spectral and thermal characterization of Shilajit, a humic substance with medicinal properties. *Asian J Chem* 20: 209–217.

Agarwal, S.P. Anwer, M.K. Aqil, M. 2008b. Complexation of furosemide with fulvic acid extracted from shilajit: a novel approach. *Drug Dev Ind Pharm* 34(5): 506–511.

Agarwal, S.P. Khanna, R. Karmarkar, R. et al. 2007. Shilajit: a review. *Phytotherapy Res* 21: 401–405.

Albrecht, M. Jiang, W. Kumi-Diaka, J. et al. 2004. Pomegranate extracts potently suppress proliferation, xenograft growth, and invasion of human prostate cancer cells. *J Med Food* 7: 274–283.

Archana, R. Namasivayam, A. 1999. Antistressor effect of Withania somnifera. *J Ethnopharmocol* 64: 91–93.

Bachmeier, B. Curcumin curbs metastases. Available at: https://www.en.uni-muenchen.de/news/news archiv/2012/bachmeier.html (accessed on 11 September 2014).

Balachandran, P. Govindarajan, R. 2005. Cancer: an Ayurvedic perspective. *Pharmacol Res* 51: 19–30.

Bhishagratha, K.L. 1991. Sushruta samhita. Vol. II. Nidan sthana. Chapter XI. Varanasi: Choukhamba Orientalia. p. 75–76.

Borek, C. 2004. Dietary antioxidants and human cancer. *Integr Cancer Ther* 3(4): 333–341.

Chandrashekar, A. Sharada, P. Solomon, E. et al. 1996. Antitumor and radiosensitizing effects of withaferin A on mouse Erhlich ascites carcinoma in vivo. *Acta Oncol* 35: 95–100.

Devi, P.U. Akagi, K. Ostapenko, V. 1996. Withaferin A. A new radiosensitizer from the Indian medicinal plant Withania somnifera. *Int J Radiat Biol* 69: 193–197.

Dhama, K. Chauhan, R.S. Singhal, L. 2005. Anti-cancer activity of cow urine: current status and future directions. *Int Jr Cow Sci* 1(2): 1–25.

Ganzera, M. Choudhary, M.I. Khan, I.A. 2003. Quantitative HPLC analysis of withanolides in Withania somnifera. *Fitoterapia* 74: 68–76.

Garodia, P. Ichikawa, H. Malani, N. et al, 2007. From ancient medicine to modern medicine: Ayurvedic concepts of health and their role in inflammation and cancer. *J Soc Integr Oncol* 5: 25–37.

Ghosal, S. 1993. *Shilajit: Its Origin and Vital Significance*. Traditional Medicine, Oxford – IBH, New Delhi; pp. 308–319.

Hong, M.Y. Seeram, N.P. Heber, D. 2008. Pomegranate polyphenols down-regulate expression of androgen-synthesizing genes in human prostate cancer cells overexpressing the androgen receptor. *J Nutr Biochem* 19: 848–855.

Jayaprakasam, B. Zhang, Y. Seeram, N.P. 2003. Growth inhibition of human tumor cell lines by withanolides from Withania somnifera leaves. *Life Sci* 74: 125–132.

Kaur, P. Sharma, M. Mathur, S. et al. 2003. Effect of 1-oxo-5beta, 6beta-epoxy-witha-2-ene-27-ethoxyolide isolated from the roots of Withania somnifera on stress indices in Wistar rats. *J Altern Complement Med* 9: 897–907.

Khare, C.P. 2007. *Indian Medicinal Plants: An Illustrated Dictionary*. Heidelberg: Springer Verlag, pp. 669–671.

Killian, P.H. Kronski, E. Michalik, K.M. et al. 2012. Curcumin inhibits prostate cancer metastasis in vivo by targeting the inflammatory cytokines CXCL1 and -2. *Carcinogenesis* 33(12): 2507–2519.

Lansky, E.P. Harrison, G. Froom, P. Jiang WG. 2005a. Pomegranate (Punica granatum) pure chemicals show possible synergistic inhibition of human PC-3 prostate cancer cell invasion across Matrigel. *Invest New Drugs* 23: 121–122.

Lansky, E.P. Jiang, W. Mo, H. et al. 2005b. Possible synergistic prostate cancer suppression by anatomically discrete pomegranate fractions. *Invest New Drugs* 23: 11–20.

Malik, A. Mukhtar, H. 2006. Prostate cancer prevention through pomegranate fruit. *Cell Cycle* 5: 371–373.

Malik, A. Afaq, F. Sarfaraz, S. et al. 2005. Pomegranate fruit juice for chemoprevention and chemotherapy of prostate cancer. *Proc Natl Acad Sci U S A* 102: 14813–14818.

Matsuda, H. Murakami, T. Kishi, A. et al. 2001. Structures of withanosides I, II, III, IV, V, VI, and VII, new withanolide glycosides, from the roots of Indian Withania somnifera DUNAL and inhibitory activity for tachyphylaxis to clonidine in isolated guinea-pig ileum. *Bio Org Med Chem* 9: 1499–1507.

Meena, H. Pandey, H.K. Arya, M.C. et al. 2010. Shilajit: A panacea for high-altitude problems. *Int J Ayurveda Res* (1): 37–40.

Murthy, K.R.S. *Astanga-Hridaya of Vagbhata. Vol. III. Uttarsthana.* 2005a. Varanasi: Choukhamba Orientalia. p. 277.

Murthy, K.R.S. *Sushruta samhita (700 BC). Vol. II, Chikitsasthan.* 2005b. Varanasi: Choukhamba Orientalia. p. 177–179.

Pantuck, A.J. Zomorodian, N. Belldegrun, A.S. 2006. Phase-II study of pomegranate juice for men with prostate cancer and increasing PSA. *Curr Urol Rep* 7: 7.

Pattanaik, N. Singh, A.V. Pandey, R.S. et al. 2003. Toxicology and free radicals scavenging property of Tamra bhasma. *Indian J Clin Biochem* 8(2): 181–189.

Peña-Méndez, E.M. Havel, J. Patočka, J. 2005. Humic substances – compounds of still unknown structure: applications in agriculture, industry, environment, and biomedicine. *Appl Biomed* 3: 13–24.

Sartippour, M.R. Seeram, N.P. Rao, J.Y. et al. 2008. Ellagitannin-rich pomegranate extract inhibits angiogenesis in prostate cancer in vitro and in vivo. *Int J Oncol* 32: 475–480.

Sastry, J.L.N. *Introduction to oncology, cancer in Ayurveda.* 2001. Varanasi: Chaukhambha Orientalia; p. 1–24.

Seeram, N.P. Adams, L.S. Henning, S.M. et al. 2005. In vitro antiproliferative, apoptotic and antioxidant activities of punicalagin, ellagic acid and a total pomegranate tannin extract are enhanced in combination with other polyphenols as found in pomegranate juice. *J Nutr Biochem* 16: 360–367.

Seeram, N.P. Aronson, W.J. Zhang, Y. et al. 2007. Pomegranate ellagitannin-derived metabolites inhibit prostate cancer growth and localize to the mouse prostate gland. *J Agric Food Chem* 55: 7732–7737.

Sharma, P.V. 2007. *Charaka samhita. Vol. I. Sutrasthan.* Varanasi: Choukhamba Orientalia. p. 129–130.

Singh, R.H. 2002. An assessment of the Ayurvedic concept of cancer and a new paradigm of anticancer treatment in Ayurveda. *J Altern Complement Med* 8: 609–614.

Spelman, K. Burns, J. Nichols, D. et al. 2006. Modulation of cytokine expression by traditional medicines: a review of herbal immunomodulators. *Altern Med Rev* 11(2): 128–150.

Umadevi, P. 1996. Withania somnifera Dunal (Ashwagandha): potential plant source of promising drug for cancer chemotherapy and radiosensitization. *Indian J Exp Biol* 34: 927–932.

Wickenberg, J. Ingemansson, S.L. Hlebowicz, J. 2010. Effects of Curcuma longa (turmeric) on postprandial plasma glucose and insulin in healthy subjects. *Nutr J* 9: 43.

Ziauddin, M. Phansalkar, N. Patki, P. 1996. Studies on the immunomodulatory effects of Ashwagandha. *J Ethnopharmacol* 50: 69–76.

CHAPTER 14

Siddha Medicine for Prostate Cancer

**S. Selvarajan, T. Anandan, A. Rajendra Kumar, S. Syed Hissar,
V. Gayathri Devi, and Muthuirulappan Srinivasan**

CONTENTS

14.1 INDIAN TRADITIONAL MEDICINE SYSTEMS

Traditional medicine systems play an important role in meeting global healthcare needs. Systems of medicine which are considered to be Indian in origin and systems of medicine which have come to India from outside and have been assimilated into Indian culture are known as the Indian Systems of Medicine. India has the unique distinction of having six recognized systems of medicine. They are Siddha, Ayurveda, Unani, Homoeopathy, Sowa-Rigpa (Amchi), Yoga, and Naturopathy. These now function under the Ministry of AYUSH, Government of India. Among these systems, the Siddha system of medicine is the most ancient traditional system.

14.1.1 An Introduction to the Siddha System of Medicine

India is a herbal hub in which the Siddha system, an ancient and important Indian traditional system of medicine, has flourished. The Siddha system of medicine is practiced in some parts of South India, especially in the state of Tamilnadu. This system is closely involved with Tamil culture and civilization. The term *Siddha* comes from *Siddhi*, which means "achievement." Siddhars are those who have achieved supreme knowledge in the field of medicine, yoga, or tapa (meditation). Before the advent of the Aryans in India, a well-developed civilization flourished in South India, especially on the banks of the rivers Cauvery, Vaigai, Tamiraparani, and others. This civilization seems to be the precursor of the present-day Siddha system of medicine. According to tradition, 18 Siddhars contributed to the development of Siddha medicine, yoga, and philosophy. There is a great deal of literature currently available regarding this system of medicine.

14.1.2 Concepts behind the Siddha System of Medicine

According to the Siddha concepts, the universe is made up of five proto-elements. The fundamental concepts of the Siddha system are the three-humor theory and the five proto-elements. Diagnosis in the Siddha system is based on the *envagaithervu* (examination of eight parameters) that encompasses examination of nadi (pulse), kan (eyes), mozhi (voice), sparisam (touch), niram (color), naa (tongue), malam (feces), and neer (urine). These examination procedures are documented in detail in the Siddha textbooks and classical literature.

14.1.3 Principles of Treatment

The principles of Siddha medicine are based on oppurai (synergism), ethirurai (antagonism) and kalappurai (mutualism). In the Siddha system, treatment methods are divided into three categories: deva maruthuvam (divine medicine), asura maruthuvam (surgical treatment), and manida maruthuvam (rational method), and drug administration routes are divided into 64 types: 32 internal and 32 external. The treatment method in the Siddha system focuses on the individual in a personalized manner according to their constitution (temperament).

According to Siddha Materia Medica, the concepts pertaining to drug composition are from plant, mineral, metal, and animal origins. The mineral- and metal-based drugs in the Siddha system are categorized as follows:

1. Uppu (lavanam): drugs that are dissolved in water and become decrepitated when put into fire, giving rise to vapor.
2. Pashanam: drugs that are water insoluble but give off vapor when put into fire.
3. Uparasam: similar to pashanam chemically, but have different actions.
4. Ratnas and uparatnas: drugs based on precious and semiprecious stones.
5. Loham: metals and metal alloys that do not dissolve in water but melt when put into fire and solidify on cooling.
6. Rasam: drugs that are soft, sublime when put into fire, changing into small crystals or amorphous powders.
7. Gandhakam (sulphur): insoluble in water and burns off when put into fire.

Various compound preparations are derived and developed from the above drugs.

Ancient Siddhars in India developed and protected the knowledge of Traditional Siddha Medicine (TSM) by using specific language codes. These security codes are more complex than modern computer encryption/password technology. TSM was designed in such a way with multiple and integrated security systems with the help of customized language codes and specific compilation templates for user community intimacy. It is really great that TSM has a scientific approach from invention to documentation in order to remain as an eternal monument.

14.1.4 Key Issues for Modern Research into Siddha Medicine

In India, there are many well-established indigenous medicine systems like Siddha. The Siddha system of medicine dates back more than 5000 years. Some supreme concepts and state-of-the-art technologies must have been developed by Indian philosophic scientists in all aspects of human well-being. Researchers from various parts of the world are looking to Indian systems of medicine, as they have been used for thousands of years and are effective in managing various chronic ailments. Siddha medicine is often complicated for modern researchers because it has so many different active compounds in different proportions.

Intensive research has been conducted to find herbal products for effective treatment of many diseases including diabetes and cancer, which are prevalent in India. These diseases have already been identified and treated successfully by our ancient traditional practitioners.

14.1.5 Traditional Practices and Regulatory Issues

The current trend of using herbal products is facing some difficulties due to the introduction of modern scientific application in standardizing herbal formulations. TSM is now considered a potential complementary system worldwide. Establishment of toxicity reports by modern scientific methods is needed in order to globalize these formulations. The federal agencies giving approval for these drugs need details on the mechanisms of action and chemical nature of the compounds along with supporting evidence from proper preclinical and clinical trials. In addition, the introduction of good laboratory practice and good manufacturing practice is vital hence manufacturers can follow the appropriate medical codes needed for standardization.

The World Health Organization defines traditional medicine as including diverse health practices, approaches, knowledge, and beliefs incorporating plant, animal, and mineral-based medicines, spiritual therapies, manual techniques, and exercises applied singly or in combination to maintain well-being, as well as to treat, diagnose, or prevent illness (WHO Traditional Medicine Strategy, 2002). There are many botanical products with a long history of medicinal use that have already been reported on the basis of their geographical areas, identification, parts used, preparation process, formulation, dose, mode of administration, indications, remedy for overdose and toxicity, as well as preservation. In India these data are transcribed from the ancient literature, and necessary materials are translated and are being used as authenticated documents for reference purposes (Siddha Formulary of India, Siddha Pharmacopoeia of India, etc.) as the national standards. These are the legal documents of the Government of India. The use of this information may avoid animal experiments in preclinical testing and reduce the number of clinical trials in humans.

A report from the FDA reveals that waiver of toxicology studies for initial clinical trials such as a single-dose toxicity test was considered for an herbal medicine intended to be used as a prescription. Single-dose toxicity studies in animals are required for herbal medicines as being developed under the Investigational New Drug (IND) Application or the New Drug Application (NDA), where there is sufficient evidence available, obtained through TSM practices, most of which are in day-to-day use (Muthuirulappan and Sridhar, 2013).

However, chronic toxicity studies and drug–drug interaction safety studies are areas of concern and are recommended for further development of the traditional system of medicine on scientific grounds.

In view of modern research into TSM regarding using heavy metals, the TSM system has identified many metals and minerals in addition to herbal sources that can be used for severe illness by adopting technology such as nanoparticles, nanotechnology, etc. According to TSM literature there are nine herbal/metal elements (Navapashanam, which are nine herbo-mettallic preparations, purified and converted in to potent medicines by the ancient Siddhars) such as mercury, arsenic etc., that are classified as metallic drugs in the Siddha system of medicine. These nine elements in micro concentration together with various herbs do produce a potent compound, in a process classified as alchemy.

When some of these compounds are subjected to a series of different purification and preparation processes as per the Siddha literature, most of them produce either white or red colored drugs called Parpam and Chendooram, respectively. These drugs have unique features in that they are tasteless, odorless, insoluble in water and alcohol, do not fuse with metals at red hot conditions, they float on water, are in the form of a fine powder, and are stable for many decades, but their therapeutic applications are different. After the discovery of modern analytical instruments, it was found that the unique character and potency of these drugs are due to the presence of nanoparticles.

In the literature of TSM, it is clearly documented that while using raw drugs of metal origin, they have to be purified in the proper manner to detoxify them.

The concepts of modern science and traditional knowledge differ in many ways. Although the traditional system of medicine has been in practice for more than 5000 years, it is still unable to achieve many of the expectations of modern scientific standards. This is due to the complex nature and the logics of the TSM. It is suggested that more emphasis must be laid on TSM literature for further evaluations.

Another justifiable reason is that most of the traditional medicine preparations involve several processes such as adding various herbal juices, some grinding techniques, different heating methods, etc., and hence standardization becomes a challenging task for modern scientists

14.1.6 General Cancer Therapeutic Herbs

Medicinal plants have become the paramount source of drug discovery in research for treating diverse diseases, including cancer. Evidence-based research to explore those medicinal plants with potent anticancer activity is needed. The literature analysis based on traditional systems including modern parameters reveals that several medicinal plants have their own specific effects on specific types of cancer.

Plant-derived phytochemicals possessing anticancer activities have received considerable attention in recent years because of the adverse effects produced by chemotherapy and radiation therapy. Phytochemicals derived from traditional medicinal plants have been found to possess anticancer and chemoprotective effects. They are safer for long-term use in cancer patients. They provide nutrition and reduce the side effects of conventional cancer therapy due to their effective antioxidant activity.

Medicinal herbs play an important role in primary healthcare systems among rural populations, as synthetic anticancer remedies are beyond the reach of many people because of the cost factor. Herbal medicines have a vital role in the prevention and treatment of cancer. They execute their therapeutic effect by inhibiting cancer-activating enzymes and hormones, stimulating DNA repair mechanisms, promoting production of protective enzymes, inducing antioxidant activities, and enhancing immunity. The Siddha system of medicine provides a good base for the scientific exploration of potent anticancer drugs.

Integrative oncology is a field of medicine where the traditional systems of medicine can collaborate with modern allopathic cancer treatment modalities used to manage symptoms, control the untoward effects of conventional modalities, and improve quality of life. The ancient Indian medicinal approach to cancer treatment and management includes a wide array of herbs and practices. There is an increasing demand for traditional and natural medicine for cancer patients. Conventional oncologic surgeons and physicians need to be aware of the role of CAM and provide treatment that focuses on the physical and mental state of wellness in combating cancer (Ramamoorthy et al., 2015).

Much of the current research in cancer therapeutics is aimed at developing drugs or vaccines to target key molecules for combating tumor cell growth, metastasis, proliferation, or changes in the associated stromal microenvironment. Studies of a wide spectrum of plant secondary metabolites extractable as natural products from fruits, vegetables, tea, spices, and traditional medicinal herbs show that these natural plant products can act as potent anti-inflammatory, antioxidant, or anticancer agents (Aravindaram and Yang, 2010).

In the classical Siddha texts, drugs such as *Abrus precatorius*, *Calotropis procera*, *Tinospora cordifolia*, *Oroxylum indicum*, *Aegle marmelos*, *Moringa oleifera*, *Semecarpus anacardium*, *Glycyrrhiza glabra*, *Curcuma longa*, etc. are indicated for cancer treatment. Modern research on these herbs provides scientific proof and substantiates their use in various cancers (Gopal et al., 2013).

An anticancer drug should be (1) cytotoxic, to inhibit the cancer cell's metabolism – particularly synthesis of proteins and nucleic acids – in order to prevent cell growth, differentiation and vascularization of new growth, etc.; (2) mitostatic, to disrupt the process of cell division and prevent an uncontrolled number of cycles of cell division and growth, to retard the proliferation of the cancerous tissue; (3) nontoxic to the rest of the body of the patient, and should not cause any side effects such as renal or hepatic dysfunction, neurotoxicity, etc.; and (4) target-oriented in its action, acting only on the cancerous region without causing damage to other parts of the body. Moreover, the drug should be effective in small doses, should not be expensive, should have longer shelf life and should be freely available in the market. It is hard to find any drug, synthetic or natural, that meets with all these qualifications. Cisplatin and other drugs used in conventional cancer chemotherapy are limited by their side effects of nephrotoxicity, acute cochlear toxicity, and peripheral neuropathy.

The National Cancer Institute (United States) has launched an extensive program for the development of natural products for the treatment of various forms of cancer. Many clinically useful drugs have been discovered from various plants. These include vinblastine and vincristine from *Catharanthis roseus*, taxanes from the bark of *Taxus brevifolia*, *T. canadensis* and *T. baccata*, camptothecines derived from the bark and wood of *Camptotheca acuminate*, etc. Camptothecin and a number of camptothecin analogs are currently being developed as anticancer agents.

Several other plant-derived compounds such as goniodiol, citronellol and geraniol, lignans, flavonoids, curcumin, eugenol and hydroxylchavicol, taxanes, and certain alkaloids appear to possess antitumor properties.

Curcumin (diferuloyl methane), a natural compound from the root of turmeric (*Curcuma longa*), is described as a potent chemopreventive agent. Due to the high prevalence and slow progression of prostate cancer, primary prevention appears to be an attractive strategy for its eradication. In addition to its anticarcinogenic properties, curcumin exhibits anti-inflammatory, antiproliferative, antiangiogenic, and antioxidant properties in various cancer cell models.

Ellagic acid in fruits, nuts, and vegetables inhibits chemically-induced cancer in the lungs, liver, skin, and esophagus of rodents. Many flavonoids act as potent antitumor agents, and they exhibit antimutagenecity. Certain gossypol derivatives have been developed as antitumor agents. Gossypol Schiff's bases with enhanced antitumor activity has been studied and reported. The cytogenetic effects of gossypol and its derivatives have also been reported. Experimental antitumor activity of taurine gossypol and barbital gossypol was also reported. Isoflavones have been investigated in detail for their role in the prevention and therapy of prostate cancer; experiments proved that high dietary isoflavone intake reduced the risk of developing prostate cancer. The reduced incidence of prostate cancer in Asian countries has been attributed to high intake of soy diets. Major soy isoflavones, in particular daidzein and genistein, are thought to be the source of the beneficial and anticancer effects of soy foods. Compared to purified single isoflavones, cooked and digested soy were more effective on induction of prostate cancer cell apoptosis, which indicated synergistic interactions between various bioactive compounds in the whole soy.

Plants play an important role in the prevention and treatment of cancer by their antioxidant, antiproliferative, antiangiogenic, immunomodulatory, and anticancer activities. Plumbum (karuvangam) and stannum (velvangam) play an important role in the treatment of cancer by immunomodulatory, antiproliferative, and anticancer activities.

14.1.6.1 Antioxidant Activity

Dietary antioxidants, such as vitamin E and green tea extracts, have also been used against prostate cancer and exhibit anticancer effects both *in vitro* and *in vivo*. Plant extracts, a mixture of bioactive non-nutrient phytochemicals, have long served as the most significant source of new leads for anticancer drug development. Explored for their unique medicinal properties, the leaves of *Piper betel*, an evergreen perennial vine, are a reservoir of phenolics with antimutagenic, antitumor, and antioxidant activities. Pomegranate (*Punica granatum*) is rich in polyphenols with potent antioxidant activity, inhibits cell proliferation and invasion, and promotes apoptosis in various cancer cells. Turmeric (*Curcuma longa*) has been shown to possess anti-inflammatory, antioxidant, and antitumor properties.

Modern experiments reveal that herbal medicines possess their antioxidant and immunomodulator qualities due to the presence of secondary metabolites and trace elements, which play various therapeutic roles in curing several disorders. Moreover, the synergistic effects of the herbal drugs support quality of life.

The ethanolic extract from neem (*Azadirachta indica*) leaves exhibited free radical scavenging activities and reduced the power of ferric ion (Fe^{3+}) to ferrous ion (Fe^{2+}) in dose responses (Fattahi et al., 2013). The aqueous extract of stinging nettle (*Urtica dioica*) showed antioxidant effects with a correlation coefficient of $r(2)=0.997$. Dose-dependent and antiproliferative effects of the extract were observed only on MCF-7 cells after 72 hrs with an IC50 value of 2 mg/mL (Fattahi et al., 2013).

Reactive oxygen species (ROS) levels were downregulated and catalase activity was upregulated after treatment with Kushecarpin D. Zingiberaceae (ginger) rhizomes are a potential source of natural antioxidants and could serve as basis for the development of future anticancer drugs and food supplements (Alafiatayo et al., 2014). Ginger extract has an antioxidant protective efficacy against PbAc-induced hepatotoxicity (Mohamed et al., 2015).

The ethanolic extract from neem leaves has strong antioxidant activity and an antiproliferative effect on cancer cells (Pangjit et al., 2014). It has been demonstrated that guava leaf extract significantly inhibits lipopolysaccharide-induced production of nitric oxide and prostaglandin E2 in a dose-dependent manner. It suppressed the expression and activity of both inducible nitric oxide synthase and cyclooxygenase-2 (Jang et al., 2014).

14.1.6.2 Revitalizing Activity

Herbs that have been used in Indian traditional medicine to promote physical and mental health, improve the body's defense mechanisms, and enhance longevity are considered revitalizers. The anabolic activity is evaluated by weight gain of the muscle, ventral prostate gland, and seminal vesicles in rats as compared to untreated control. Experiments on induced models and parameters such as antistress activity, leucopenia, and anemia are the evaluating parameters for the revitalizing activities of some herbs and their preparations (Azmathulla et al., 2006). Higher intake of antioxidant-rich foods is clearly associated with better health and functional longevity. The specific agents and mechanisms responsible are not yet clear, but there is convincing evidence that including more plant-based, antioxidant rich foods, herbs, and beverages in the diet is effective in promoting health and lowering the risk of various age-related diseases (Benzie and Choi, 2014).

Luteolin, one of the most common abundant flavonoids in vegetables and herbs, has antitumor effects on various tumors by inducing apoptosis, antioxidant effects, and inhibition of angiogenesis. Data have demonstrated that cigarette smoke extract-induced oxidative damage was inhibited by luteolin. Hence, luteolin may serve as a chemopreventive agent for the prevention and treatment of lung cancer (Tan et al., 2014; Xu et al., 2012). Natural antioxidants such as alpha-tocopherol, caffeic acid, catechin, quercetin, carvacrol, and plant extracts have been incorporated into food packaging. The demand for natural antioxidant active packaging is increasing due to its unquestionable advantages compared with the addition of antioxidants directly to the food. Therefore, the search for antioxidants perceived as natural, namely those that naturally occur in herbs and spices, is a field attracting great interest (Sanches-Silva et al., 2014; Ghasemzadeh and Jaafar, 2013). Eugenol is a major ingredient in herbs such as clove, and experiments suggest that eugenol could be available as an excellent agent for prevention of metastasis related to oxidative stress (Nam and Kim, 2013). Curcumin exerts a hypolipidic effect, which prevents the fatty acid accumulation in the hepatocytes that may result from metabolic imbalances, and which may cause nonalcoholic steatohepatitis.

14.1.6.3 Antiproliferative Activity

Worldwide anticancer drug design has gained considerable attention due to the antiproliferative effects of phytochemicals. Sinigrin is the major compound present in *Brassica nigra*. Cell cycle analysis has indicated that sinigrin caused cell cycle arrest in the G0/G1 phase. Sinigrin induced apoptosis of liver cancer cells through upregulation of p53 and downregulation of Bcl-2 family members and caspases (Jie et al., 2014).

One study demonstrated the effect of *Ficus carica* latex in glioblastoma multiforme cells and observed on let-7d expression, which may be an important underlying mechanism of the antiinvasive effect of this extract (Tezcan et al., 2015).

Azadirachta indica (neem) leaf extract inhibited human promyelocytic leukemic cell line (HL-60 cells) growth in concentration response (0–500 μg/mL) for 24-hour treatment (Pangjit et al., 2014). Antiproliferative activity of *Urtica dioica* leaf was associated with an increase of apoptosis, and there is an increase in the amount of calpain 1, calpastatin, caspase 3, caspase 9, Bax, and Bcl-2 – all proteins involved in the apoptotic pathway (Fattahi et al., 2013).

Coptis chinese Frach and *Evodia rutaecarpa* have significant anticancer activities due to induction of mitochondria-dependent apoptosis pathway (Xu et al., 2014). Methanol extracts of the peels of *Citrus aurantium* L. induced caspase-dependent apoptosis demonstrated on human leukemia cells for anticancer activity revealed significant cancer cell destruction (Han et al., 2012).

Ocimum sanctum Linn, commonly known as "Tulsi" or "Holy Basil," is considered to be the most sacred herb of India. Several anatomical parts of *O. sanctum* are known to have an impressive number of therapeutic properties and accordingly find use in various traditional systems of medicine. Scientific investigations have demonstrated the biochemical and molecular mechanisms involved in the antineoplastic effects of *O. sanctum* (Bhattacharyya and Bishayee, 2013).

14.1.6.4 Antiangiogenic Activity

Nontoxic antiangiogenic phytochemicals are useful in combating cancer by preventing the formation of new blood vessels to support tumor growth. Kushecarpin D showed antiangiogenic activity via inhibitory effects on cell proliferation, cell migration, cell adhesion, and tube formation. Essential oil of *Origa numonites* L. could markedly inhibit cell viability and induce apoptosis of 5RP7 cells and also could block *in vitro* tube formation and migration of adipose tissue endothelial cells, and prevent angiogenesis-related diseases (Bostancioglu et al., 2012).

14.1.6.5 Immunomodulatory Activity

Physicians are increasingly encountering patients who use herbal products. Some of these products are known to modulate the immune system, but their scientific basis is not well established. Because these products can affect the host immune system, they could be beneficial in the treatment of immune related diseases, or alternatively, they could cause inadvertent side effects (Wilasrusmee et al., 2002).

Hundreds of botanicals are used in CAM for therapeutic use as antimicrobials and immune stimulators. While there exists many centuries of anecdotal evidence and few clinical studies on the activity and efficacy of these botanicals, limited scientific evidence exists on the ability of these botanicals to modulate immune and inflammatory responses (Denzler et al., 2010).

Crude polysaccharides were isolated from the fruit pulp of jackfruit. The major monosaccharide residues were rhamnose, glucose, galactose, and arabinose. Jackfruit polysaccharides showed immunomodulatory effects by enhancing the thymus weight index and the phagocytic rate in mice (Tan et al., 2013). Lamiaceae herbs have a potential enhancement in pathogen recognition and antioxidant defense (Vattem et al., 2013).

Astragalus membranaceus, *Sambucus cerulean*, and *Andrographis paniculata* are immune-stimulatory herbs. The presence of potent lipopolysaccharide in these herbs do demonstrate the immune cell activation, migration, and various inflammatory responses pertaining to destruction of cancer cells. (Denzler et al., 2010). The immunomodulatory properties of amla (*Emblica officinalis*) and shankhpushpi (*Evolvulus alsinoides*) were evaluated in adjuvant induced arthritic (AIA) rat model. Observations suggested that both herbal extracts caused immunosuppression in AIA rats, indicating that they may provide an alternative approach to the treatment of arthritis (Ganju et al., 2003).

Curcumin proved to have an immunomodulatory effect involving activation of host macrophages, and natural killer cells (Singh et al., 2013). Curcumin and piperine have been proven to have potent medicinal benefits to treat various diseases, and they are most commonly used in combination with various Indian systems of medicine (Ramaswamy et al., 2014; Purwar et al., 2012).

Amukkara chooranam, a Siddha polyherbal formulation, was examined for its analgesic and antiinflammatory activity at a dose of 500 mg/kg and it showed significant activity (Saraswathy et al., 2009). The effect of *Withania somnifera* on glycosaminoglycan synthesis in the granulation tissue of carrageenin-induced air pouch granuloma was studied. *W. somnifera* was shown to exert a significant inhibitory effect on incorporation of 35S into the granulation tissue. *W. somnifera* also reduced the succinate dehydrogenase enzyme activity in the mitochondria of granulation tissue (Begum and Sadique, 1987).

14.1.6.6 *Anticancer and Cytotoxic Activity*

Menispermaceae is a medium-sized family of flowering plants, with 70 genera totaling 420 extant species, mostly climbing plants. Plants belonging to this family are rich in alkaloids, especially bisbenzylisoquinoline type. A study showed that *Cissampelos hirsutus* and *Cissampelos pareira* have *in vitro* cytotoxic activity against HeLa cell line (Thavamani et al., 2013). *Cissampelos pluricaulis* is an important indigenous medicine. It has a long list of medicinal applications for liver disease, epilepsy, microbial disease, and cytotoxic and viral diseases (Agarwal et al., 2014).

Embelia ribes, more commonly known as vidanga, possesses hydroxybenzoquinone active constituent embelin which acts as an NF-kappa B blocker and potential suppressor of tumorigenesis. It also exhibits potent cytotoxic, antioxidant, and cancer chemopreventive effects (Poojari, 2014). Molecular evidence shows that the Ashwagandha leaves and its active component triethylene glycol have selective cancer cell growth arrest activity and hence may offer natural and economic resources for anticancer medicine (Wadhwa et al., 2013; Vaishnavi et al., 2012).

Gymnema montanum induced apoptosis in human leukemic cancer cells, mediated by collapse of mitochondrial membrane potential, generation of ROS, and depletion of intracellular antioxidant potential (Ramkumar et al., 2013). Piplartine is a biologically active alkaloid/amide from peppers, as from long pepper (*Piper longum* L.). This compound is selectively cytotoxic against cancer cells by induction of oxidative stress, induces genotoxicity, is an alternative strategy to killing tumor cells, has excellent oral bioavailability in mice, and inhibits tumor growth in mice (Bezerra et al., 2013).

All fractions of frankincense essential oil from *Boswellia sacra* are capable of suppressing viability and inducing apoptosis of a panel of human pancreatic cancer cell lines. Gallic acid as a major bioactive cytotoxic constituent appears to have promising anticancer activity (Russell et al., 2011; Sandhya and Mishra, 2006; Kaur et al., 2005). *Boesenbergia rotunda* (Roxb.) Schlecht is a rhizomatous herb that is distributed from northeastern India to southeast Asia. It has been demonstrated that an active compound of this plant, boesenbergin-A, induced apoptosis of CEMss cells through Bcl2/Bax-signaling pathways with the involvement of caspases and G2/M phase cell cycle arrest.

A study was designed to examine the *in vitro* cytotoxic activities of saline extract prepared from ginger extract on HEp-2 cell line. Results show that the extract exerts dose-dependent suppression of cell proliferation; the IC (50) value was found to be 900 μg/mL (Vijaya et al., 2007) (Table 14.1).

Table 14.1 Major Targets in Cancer Therapy

Popular herbs used in cancer treatment	Major Targets in Cancer Therapy								
	NF-κB suppression	AP-1 suppression	Proliferation and apoptosis activation	Growth factor suppression	JAK–STAT pathway suppression	Multi-drug resistance suppression	COX-2	Angiogenesis suppression	Cyclins
Guggulsterone (*Commiphora mukul*)	Y						Y		
Curcumin (*Curcuma longa*)	Y	Y	Y	Y	Y	Y	Y	Y	Y
Resveratrol (*Vitis vinifera*)	Y				Y		Y	Y	Y
Flavopiridol (*Dysoxylum binectariferum*)	Y								Y
Zerumbone (*Zingiber zerumbet* Smith)	Y						Y		
Withanolide (*Withania sominifera*)	Y		Y					Y	
Boswellic acid (*Boswellia serrata*)	Y					Y			
Green tea components									

14.1.6.7 Summary

The herbs most widely used for cancer therapy and treatment are summarized in Table 14.1 opposite. Corresponding observations and findings with regard to those herbs are expanded below:

- NF-κB is an inducible transcription factor for genes involved in cell survival, cell adhesion, inflammation, differentiation, and growth.
- Activated protein-1 (AP-1) is another transcription factor that regulates the expression of several genes involved in cell differentiation and proliferation.
- Downregulation of NF-κB sensitizes the cells to apoptosis. The mechanism through which NF-κB promotes these proliferation and cell survival mechanisms has become increasingly clear.
- The potent cell proliferation signals generated by various growth factor receptors, such as the epidermal growth factor.
- Several genetic or epigenetic mechanisms that contribute to a number of abnormal oncogenic signaling pathways by preventing apoptosis through increased expression of anti-apoptotic proteins.
- Multidrug resistance in human cancer is often associated with overexpression of the mdr-1 gene, which encodes transmembrane protein.
- Cyclooxygenase-2 (COX-2) overexpression is a consequence of the deregulation of transcriptional and post-transcriptional control. Several growth factors, cytokines, oncogenes, and tumor promoters stimulate COX-2 transcription.
- Angiogenesis, the regulated formation of new blood vessels from existing ones.
- Cyclins are enzyme complexes that play a role in checkpoints and disrupt the normal cell cycle control.

14.2 AN INTRODUCTION TO SIDDHA FORMULATIONS

14.2.1 Different Types of Formulations

Siddhars have documented several alchemical procedures and techniques, such as calcination, sublimation, distillation, dissolution, fusion, separation, combination, coagulation, fermentation, extraction, purification, incineration, and so on. The science related to environmental factors such as season, geography, habitat, occupation, race, and pharmacological properties of metals, minerals, plants, and animals are familiar to all Siddhars. Hence, they are able to customize the formulations in any form and at any size for a select individual upon a specific need. Some of the following categories of formulations are often prescribed for general ailments.

- *Chendooram:* A category of medicine that generally has reddish color and is in a powdery form, usually obtained from heat treatment of preprocessed drugs. Strong heat is required for conversion of metals and their salts into a stable, nonreactive form of drug. After cooling, they are ground and sieved by fine mesh. Some modes of preparations are listed below.
  - Araippu Chendooram: Prepared by prolonged grinding
  - Erippu or Varuppu Chendooram: Prepared by red hot heating
  - Puda Chendooram: Prepared by capsule heating under white hot condition
  - Kuppierippu Chendooram: Prepared by sand bath process
  - Laghu puda Chendoorams: Prepared by applying heat in the range close to 100°C
- *Parpam:* Equivalent to calx (ash), which is prepared by a process of calcination. The process is similar to the preparation of Chendooram, but the resultant color is usually white.
- *Chooranam:* These are fine, dry powdered drugs. They are prepared from single or multiple drugs. Usually, unprocessed drug powders are prepared separately and mixed for homogeneity. A mortar and pestle are used for grinding and it is then sieved by fine mesh.

- *Chunnam:* These are the medicaments prepared by heat, just like Chendooram, but the raw materials used for preparation are calcium compounds (limestone, shells, etc.). The end product is alkaline and white in color.
- *Karuppu:* This is prepared by heat, just like Chendooram, but the raw materials used for preparation are usually mercury and sulfur. The end product is black in color.
- *Mezhugu, Kuzhambu, Kalimbu and Mai:* This category of medicine has a waxy or semisolid consistency. The consistency is obtained by the addition of mucilaginous materials such as oils, fats, waxes, butter, etc. This preparation is more complex than Chendooram. It is prepared without strong heating.

14.2.2   Quality Test for Chendooram and Parpam

Chendooram and Parpam are usually practiced by skilled Siddha physicians. Characteristic color for Chendooram is reddish and white for parpam. The following screening tests are performed for safe therapeutic purposes.

- In order to test the proper finishing of the drug, a small quantity of the finished product is pressed between two fingers. Product must be a fine powder that when rubbing between fingers, the fingerprints must be visible on the pressed surface or fine particles must be lodged in the fingerprint grooves when rubbed between fingers, and remain in grooves even after gentle wiping with a cloth.
- When a pinch of sample is laid over a water surface it must float, and this floating capacity must be able to bear a load of at least one rice grain or a material equivalent to food grain having similarity in size, density and weight of about 65 mg.
- It should not have any property similar to that of a metal like luster and taste.
- When fused with metallic silver under red hot heat, the end product should not react or fuse.
- Reverting the metal from a parpam by a metal revert test must be negative. This is performed by mixing a pinch of parpam with cane jaggery, hemp power, ghee, and honey then placed inside a sealed crucible and heated for several hours in a red hot oven. Parpam must be stable and intact. This test ensures that there are no harmful metal ions or traces for toxicity.

14.2.3   Storage and Shelf Life of Different Formulations

Air-tight glass vials and bottles are suitable for all types of preparations. Simple preparations like Chooranam and liquid forms have a shorter shelf-life than heat-treated solids Chendooram and Parpam. The shelf lives of some categories are listed below.

- Chooranam: 3 months
- Kalimbu and Mai: 5 years
- Chendooram: 75 years
- Karuppu: 100 years
- Parpam: 100 years
- Chunnam: 500 years

14.2.4   Doses of Different Formulations

Recommended doses differ for each formulation. Dose also depends on the health status of the patient.

Chendooram:	50–150 mg	1–2 times/day	2–3 days
Chooranam:	1–2 g	2–4 times/day	1–2 weeks
Chunnam:	200–500 mg	2–3 times/day	3–7 days
Karuppu:	50–150 mg	1–2 times/day	2–3 days
Kalimbu and Mai:	50–150 mg	1–2 times/day	2–3 days
Parpam:	50–150 mg	1–2 times / day	2–3 days

In certain chronic cases duration of treatment depends on the health status of the patient.

14.2.5 Units of Volume

Units in Siddha	Equivalent in Siddha Unit	Equivalent in SI Unit
360 Nel	1 Sodu	33.6 mL
5 Sodu	1 Aazhakku	168 mL
2 Aazhakku	1 Uzhakku	336 mL
2 Uzhakku	1 Uri	672 mL
2 Uri	1 Nazhi / Padi	1.34 L
1 Thekkarandi	1 dram	4 mL
1 Kuppi	24 ounce	700 mL
1 Neikkarandi	–	4 mL

14.2.6 Units of Weight

Units in Siddha	Equivalent in Siddha Unit	Equivalent in SI Unit
1 Thilam	–	3 mg
2 Thilam	1 Kakini	6 mg
4 Kakini	1 Virigi	24 mg
1 Ulundu	1 grain	65 mg
4 Yavam	1 Kunri / ~2 grains	130 mg
1 Manjadi	4 grains	260 mg
6 Kunri	1 Masham	780 mg
32 Kunri	1 Varaganedai	4.16 g
10 Varaganedai	1 Palm	41.6 g

14.2.7 Units of Time

Units in Siddha	Equivalent in Siddha Unit	Equivalent in SI Unit
1 Nodi	–	1 sec
60 Nodi	1 Nimidam	1 min
1 Nazhigai	–	24 min
1 Muhurtham	–	90 min
1 Jamam	–	3 h
1 Madham	–	30 days
1 Mandalam	–	45 days

14.2.8 Administration of Siddha Formulations

Siddha medicines should only be consumed under direct supervision of a qualified Siddha physician.

14.3 ANUBANAM (ADJUVANTS) USED WITH DIFFERENT FORMULATIONS

This is a drug delivery vehicle used for the following purposes:

- Solubility and palatability are increased
- Very small doses are distributed effectively
- Adverse reactions and side effects are minimized
- The drug is mitigated and released slowly and steadily, over a longer time
- Helps in absorption, distribution, metabolism, and elimination
- It plays a great role in site directed action and selection among diversified actions; in modern terms they are called site directed or target delivery systems

Examples of formulation Kowsikar kuzhambu, used with the following anubanam for the desired action:

Anubanam	Indication
Hot water	Fever
Milk	Peptic ulcer
Buttermilk	Piles
Black goat urine	Liver diseases
Thiriphalai	Hypoprotenemia
Direct application on skin	Scorpion sting
Direct application into eye	Snakebite

Pathiyam (diet restriction) is to be followed during the treatment. Salt, sour, and spicy diets reduce the therapeutic efficacy and bioavailability and so should be avoided during medication.

14.4 SIDDHA LITERATURE

Some of the original ancient Tamil scripts are explored and followed for formulations, preparations, and the practice of Siddha medicines. These documents deal systematically with various concepts. A well-developed language technology has been used in translation to avoid misunderstanding, manipulation, and misreading.

The coexistence of medical and language technology along with philosophy and dedication are the assets of these authors, who are called Siddhars. The medicine system is known as Siddha system of medicine. Adjacent numbers indicate the collection of verses/set of scripts/pages/notes.

- Agasthiyar Amudha Kalai Gnanam
- Agasthiyar Baala Vaakatam
- Agasthiyar Chendooram – 300
- Agasthiyar Chillarai Kovai
- Agasthiyar Erathina Churukkam
- Agasthiyar Paripooranam – 400
- Agasthiyar Vaidhdhiyam – 600
- Agasthiyar Vaidhya Chillarai Kovai
- Agasthiyar Vaidhya Kaaviyam – 1500
- Baala Vaakatam
- Bogar Vaidhiyam – 700
- Bogar Vaidhyam – 700 and Vallathi – 600
- Brammamuni Karukkadai – 300

- Chimittu Eraththina Churukkam
- Dhanvanthiri Vaidhya Kaviyam – 1000
- Kalnandu Soothiram
- Kowsika Muni Nool
- Patharthaguna Vilakkam of Kannuswami Pillai
- Pulipani Vaidhdhiyam – 500
- Raasa Vaidhya Pothini
- Siddha Vaidhya Thirattu
- Sikichcha Raththina Deepam of Kannuswamy Pillai
- Theraiyar Karisal – 300
- Theraiyar Padal Thirattu
- Theraiyar Padal Thirattu – 1001
- Theraiyar Thaila Varkkam
- Theraiyar Tharu
- Theraiyar Yamakam
- Vaidhya Chinthamani
- Veeramamuni Vaakata Thirattu
- Yugi Chinthamani – 500
- Yugi Karisal– 151

14.5 SIDDHA PRINCIPLES AND CANCER THERAPY

According to the Siddha concepts, the universe is made up of five proto-elements. The fundamental concepts of the Siddha system are the three-humor theory and the five proto-elements.

The three-humor theory is the physiological base of the Siddha system of medicine. The treatment plan is based on this theory. These three basic functions, *vazhi* (wind), *azhal* (fire), and *Iyyam* (water), operate through a constant interplay between the environment and the individual to maintain the integrity of a living system. In benign neoplastic conditions, one or two of the three humors are deranged and may not lead to a harmful state, since the body may be able overcome this condition. Malignant tumors (*Vippuruthi, Putru*) are very harmful because all three major humors fail to exert mutual coordination, causing tissue proliferation that results in a morbid state (Sambasivampillai, 1998). Siddha literature deals with various types of malignant conditions. Saint Yugi used the terms *Vippuruthi* and *Dhunmangism*, which can be correlated with cancer, in his text *Yugi vaidhya chinthamani*. Some other texts such as *Agathiyar rana vaithyam*, *Nagamuni nayana vithi*, and *Agathiyar nayana vithi* deal with cancer as *Putru*. *Naakku putru*, *Sevi putru* and *Vaai putru* are cancer of the tongue, ear, and mouth, respectively (Kuppusamy Mudhaliar and Utthamarayan, 1998).

Several medicinal plants that can be used for cancer are mentioned in Siddha texts. The concept of single-drug administration has been mentioned in Siddha as *Yega mooligai prayogam* (single-drug therapy). The three humors of subtle energy on which Siddha literature is based mutually coordinate to perform the normal functions of the body. *Yugi vaidhya chinthamani*, a book on Siddha pathology, addresses *Vippurudhi roga nidhanam* (diagnosis of cancer) in detail, according to which seven types of cancer are established regarding functional disorders with organ involvement. Based on the functional disorders, they are classified as *Vazhi vippurudhi*, *Azhal vippurudhi*, and *Iyya vippurudhi*. Based on the organs involved, they are classified as *Kuvalai* (lung) *vippurudhi*, *Karpa* (uterus) *vippurudhi*, *Sandu* (bone and joint) *vippurudhi*, and *Oodu* (metastatic) *vippurudhi*. The etiological factors for *vippurudhi* are excessive intake of salty and spicy food, excessive intake of meat, excessive intake of minerals, frequent sexual intercourse, and sexual contact with elderly women. According to another text, *Anubava vaithya dheva raghasiyam*, there are 10 major areas that are prone to *vippurudhi*. They are *Nabi* (umbilicus), *Vasthi* (bladder), *Kalleeral* (liver),

Manneeral (spleen), *Kanaiyam* (pancreas), *Iraipai* (stomach), *Abanam* (anorectal), *Karuppai* (uterus), *Thodaiiduku* (groin), and *Moothirakiranthi* (prostate gland).

14.5.1   Noi Guna Iyal (Pathophysiology)

Azhal, which is responsible for digestion and various metabolic functions, is present in every cell. In cancer, there is a decrease in agni (fire), which is inversely proportional to Iyyam (↓ agni = ↑ iyyam), resulting in excessive tissue growth. *Vazhi* can be related to the anabolic growth phase. *Iyyam* can be related to the catabolic phase of morbidity. In cancer, the metabolic crisis develops with decrease in agni followed by a counter-increase in *vazhi* and *Iyyam* forces, interacting with each other and resulting in proliferation. According to the Siddha system of medicine, the stages of cancer can be categorized based on the type of humor deranged and the choice of traditional medicinal plants and their preparations. An increase in *azhal* is pacified by *kaippu* (bitter), *inippu* (sweet), and *thuvarpu* (astringent) tastes. An increase in *vazhi* is pacified by *inippu* (sweet), *pulippu* (sour), and *uppu* (salt) tastes. The increase in *Iyyam* is pacified by *kaippu* (bitter), *karppu* (pungent), and *thuvarpu* (astringent) tastes (Shanmugavelu, 1987). Many herbs that have been used for cancer in the traditional system of medicine constructed on the Siddha philosophy of three humors have now gained predominant focus in research and are paving the way for new drug discovery

14.5.2   Rasagenthi Lehyam (RL) Therapy – Siddha Medicine Compound May Hold Clues to Prostate Cancer Prevention

In previous studies, it is reported that the herbal preparation Rasagenthi Lehyam (RL), an herbal formulation used in Siddha medicine, is an effective treatment for prostate cancer in an animal model. The most potent compound of RL is psoralidin, which proved to have more potent anti-cancer effects in prostate cancer cells compared to the other isolated compounds identified in RL. The action of psoralidin inhibits cancerous cell growth and tumor survival. Importantly, the researchers found that psoralidin targets cancer cells without causing significant toxicity to normal prostate cells (Srinivasan et al., 2010).

The future focus of the said study is to know that the compound psoralidin functions to inhibit the growth of prostate cancer cells and tumors. The results of the study may lead to the identification of biomarkers for prostate cancer and the development of chemotherapeutic and/or chemopreventive strategies for prostate cancer.

14.5.3   Textual Reference for Different Types of Cancer

Some of the cancers are treated based on the literature given below

Name of Drug	Type of Cancer	Textual Reference
Vanga chendooram	In penis	Yagobu vaidya chindamani
Kantha chendooram	In vulva	Yagobu vaidya chindamani
Rasa chendoram	In penis	Pulippani vaidyam 500
Gandaga parpam	In penis and vulva	Agasthiyar chendooram 300
Parangi pattai rasayanam	In cheek	Bohar 7000
Rasa parpam	In sex organs	Bohar 7000

14.6 PROSTATE CANCER AND SIDDHA TREATMENT

14.6.1 Introduction

Prostate cancer (purasthakola putru noi) is a disease that affects the prostate gland in the male reproductive system. Other terms for prostate cancer in Tamil are purasthakola perukkam, purasthakola veekkam, and purasthakola vanmeegam. Prostate cancer is predominantly seen in males between 65 and 75 years of age, but although prostate cancer seems to be a geriatric health problem, the imbalances that predispose to it begin much earlier in life. Most prostate cancers can be prevented by adopting lifestyle and dietary modifications.

Clinical and experimental observations suggest that hormones, genes, heredity, diet, animal fat, and environmental factors contribute pivotal roles in the occurrence of prostate cancer. According to Siddha concepts, the exact cause for prostate cancer is kanma vinai (consequence of deeds). In addition, the following habits may also be contributing factors.

1. Intake of food items that increase body heat
2. Excessive exposure to sunlight
3. Chronic alcoholism and/or smoking
4. Prolonged neglected spermatorrhoea
5. Excessive sexual urge and sexual intercourse

The above habits increase body heat and pave the way to increase azhal (protective factor). This increased azhal leads to deranging the humors vazhi and iyyam, and the deranged vazhi and iyyam produce the symptoms of the disease.

The main symptoms of prostate cancer are described in ancient Tamil books such as Dhanwandari's Vatha Varthi Kiricharam and Moothira Kiranthi (kiranthi means glandular swelling that denotes prostate gland).

- Difficulty in urination or scanty urination
- Dribbling of urine
- Increased frequency of urination
- Hematuria
- Painful urination; pain in the lower abdomen and urethra
- Edema in the lower limbs
- Red or white color urine and turbid appearance

14.6.2 Prevention of Prostate Cancer

Pini anuka vithiis, a poem from the book *Siddha Maruthuvanga Surukkam*, suggests the following lifestyle for preventing prostate cancer.

- Natural urgency of defecation and micturition should not be controlled
- Excessive sexual intercourse must be avoided
- Food preparation and consumption must follow these procedures:
  - Water must be boiled before drinking (Neer Surukki)
  - Buttermilk must be diluted before consumption (Mor perukki)
  - Ghee must be melted before use (Nei urukki)

14.6.3   Diagnosis of Prostate Cancer

The eight diagnostic tools for presenting symptoms of prostate cancer are:

- Naadi: Pulse
- Sparisam: Physical examination by touch
- Naa: Tongue examination
- Niram: Color
- Mozhi: Voice examination
- Vizhi: Eye examination
- Malam: Stool examination
- Moothiram: Urine examination

Naadi is always iyya-vazhi. Urine is thick with red or white in color.

14.6.4   Principles of Treatment

14.6.4.1   Purgation Therapy

According to Siddha, disease is caused by *vazhi* (Vatha malathu meni kedathu – Theraiyar). Hence, vazhi humor must be normalized by purgation therapy for maintaining equilibrium.

- Agasthiyar kuzhambu: 65 mg
  Anubanam: Plant extract (*Pandanus odoratissimus* – Thazhai vizhuthu)
  Once in early morning on empty stomach
- Magarajanga Ennai: 5 to 10 drops with milk at night, after food, for 3 days
- Lavanagunathi Ennai: 1 to 2 mL at night, after food, for 3 days

14.6.4.2   Restoration Therapy

Any one of the following general tonics may be given for restoration of normal health:

1. Amukkura Lehiyam
2. Thetran Kottai Lehiyam
3. Nellikkai Lehiyam

14.6.4.3   Rejuvenation Therapy

A potential rejuvenator may be given to rebuild the deranged humors with any one of the gold preparations such as Thanka uram, Poorna chandrodayam, etc.

14.6.4.4   Symptomatic Line of Treatment

Urinary outflow can be facilitated by any one of the following medicines: Silasathu parpam, Kungilium parpam, Jalamanjari.

14.6.5 Medications

14.6.5.1 Oral Drugs: Herbal-Based Preparations

- Amukkura choornam   : 1 to 2 g with hot water, twice daily
- Poonaikali vithai choornam : 1 to 2 g with milk, twice daily
- Thriphala choornam   : 1 to 2 g with hot water, thrice daily
- Thriphala karpam   : 1 to 2 tablets with hot water daily for 45 days.
- Seenthil choornam   : 1 to 2 g with milk, twice daily
- Seenthil sarkkarai   : 1 g with milk, twice daily

14.6.5.2 Oral Drugs: Herbo-Mineral–Based Preparations

These categories of medicines are more powerful than the pure herbal-based drugs.

- Thamira kattu chendhooram: 25 mg twice daily with honey, after food
- Narasimma lehiyam: 5 g twice daily with milk, after food

In addition to the above, Plumbum (karuvangam) and stannum (velvangam) preparations may be administered under the direct supervision of a qualified Siddha practioner to obtain the appropriate results.

14.6.5.3 External Applications

To reduce swelling and pain of the prostate gland, the external applications mentioned below can be adopted. This is to be applied on a skin surface where the patient feels pain and has found swelling on his body, usually in the abdomen region, i.e., lower abdomen.

1. Karchunnambu and egg white mixed together and applied externally to reduce swelling.
2. *Abutilon indicum* leaves with turmeric powder, boiled in steam and applied externally to relieve pain.
3. Annabhedi ground with water and applied externally for improving quality of life.

14.7 CONCLUSION

In this document the authors have discussed the history, concept, formulations, and other issues with regard to the Siddha system of medicine on prostate cancer. The details herein have been conceptualized according to the knowledge and experience of the authors. We hope this will pave the way for planning and performing treatment of prostate cancer. Further research is needed to explore the various benefits of the Siddha system of medicine for humankind.

ACKNOWLEDGMENTS

The authors express their sincere gratitude to Prof. Dr. R.S. Ramaswamy, Director General, Central Council for Research in Siddha, Chennai under Ministry of AYUSH, Government of India, New Delhi, for providing the appropriate facilities for completing this work. We also express our sincere thanks to Dr. Shyamala Rajkumar, Research Officer (Siddha), Central Council for Research in Siddha, Chennai, for support during the preparation of this document. We express our sincere gratitude to Smt. Anitha John, Research Officer (Chemistry), SRRI, Thiruvananthapuram, Central Council for Research in Siddha for providing the appropriate support during the preparation of this document. In addition, we thank Dr. G.S. Lekha, Medical Officer (Siddha), SCRI, Chennai, Central Council for Research in Siddha, Chennai, Dr. Annie Jasmine, Swapna Consultant (Siddha), SRRI, Thiruvananthapuram, Central Council for Research in Siddha, and internees Dr. S. Haripriya, Dr. B. Anupama, Dr. C.J. Chithira, Dr. S. Kiran Krishna, and Dr. Renjini Ashok of Santhigiri Siddha Medical College, Pothencode, Thiruvananthapuram for their help in preparing this document.

REFERENCES

Agarwal, P. Sharma, B. Fatima, A. et al. 2014. An update on Ayurvedic herb Convolvulus pluricaulis Choisy. *Asian Pac J Trop Biomed* 4: 245–252.

Alafiatayo, A.A. Syahida, A. Mahmood, M. 2014. Total anti-oxidant capacity, flavonoid, phenolic acid and polyphenol content in ten selected species of Zingiberaceae rhizomes. *Afr J Tradit Complement Altern Med* 11: 7–13.

Aravindaram, K. Yang, N.S. 2010. Anti-inflammatory plant natural products for cancer therapy. *Planta Med* 76: 1103–1117.

Azmathulla, S. Hule, A. Naik, S.R. 2006. Evaluation of adaptogenic activity profile of herbal preparation. *Indian J Exp Biol* 44: 574–579.

Begum, V.H. Sadique, J. 1987. Effect of Withania somnifera on glycosaminoglycan synthesis in carrageenin-induced air pouch granuloma. *Biochem Med Metab Biol* 38: 272–277.

Benzie, I.F. Choi, S.W. 2014. Antioxidants in food: content, measurement, significance, action, cautions, caveats, and research needs. *Adv Food Nutr Res* 71: 1–53.

Bezerra, D.P. Pessoa, C. de Moraes, M.O. et al. 2013. Overview of the therapeutic potential of piplartine (piperlongumine). *Eur J Pharm Sci* 48: 453–463.

Bhattacharyya, P. Bishayee, A. 2013. Ocimum sanctum Linn. (Tulsi): an ethnomedicinal plant for the prevention and treatment of cancer. *Anticancer Drugs* 24: 659–666.

Bostancioglu, R.B. Kurkcuoglu, M. Baser, K.H. et al. 2012. Assessment of anti-angiogenic and anti-tumoral potentials of Origanum onites L. essential oil. *Food Chem Toxicol* 50: 2002–2008.

Denzler, K.L. Waters, R. Jacobs, B.L. et al. 2010. Regulation of inflammatory gene expression in PBMCs by immunostimulatory botanicals. *PLoS.One* 5: e12561.

Fattahi, S. Ardekani, A.M. Zabihi, E. 2013. Antioxidant and apoptotic effects of an aqueous extract of Urtica dioica on the MCF-7 human breast cancer cell line. *Asian Pac J Cancer Prev* 14: 5317–5323.

Ganju, L. Karan, D. Chanda, S. et al. 2003. Immunomodulatory effects of agents of plant origin. *Biomed Pharmacother* 57: 296–300.

Ghasemzadeh, A. Jaafar, H.Z. 2013. Profiling of phenolic compounds and their antioxidant and anticancer activities in pandan (Pandanus amaryllifolius Roxb.) extracts from different locations of Malaysia. *BMC Complement Altern Med* 13: 341.

Gopal, R. Lakshmi, A.V. Kumar, R. 2013. Anticancer herbs in Ayurveda: a review. *Int J Res Ayurveda Pharm* 4(2): 284–287.

Han, M.H. Lee, W.S. Lu, J.N. et al. 2012. Citrus aurantium L. exhibits apoptotic effects on U937 human leukemia cells partly through inhibition of Akt. *Int J Oncol* 40: 2090–2096.

Jang, M. Jeong, S.W. Cho, S.K. et al. 2014. Anti-inflammatory effects of an ethanolic extract of guava (Psidium guajava L.) leaves in vitro and in vivo. *J Med Food* 17: 678–685.

Jie, M. Cheung, W.M. Yu, V. et al. 2014. Anti-proliferative activities of sinigrin on carcinogen-induced hepatotoxicity in rats. *PLoS.One* 9: e110145.

Kaur, S. Michael, H. Arora, S. et al. 2005. The in vitro cytotoxic and apoptotic activity of Triphala – an Indian herbal drug. *J Ethnopharmacol* 97: 15–20.

Kuppusamy M.K.N. Utthamarayan, K.S. 1998. *Siddha Vaithiya Thirattu*, Department of Indian Medicine & Homeopathy, Chennai, India.

Mohamed, O.I. El-Nahas, A.F. El-Sayed, Y.S. et al. 2015. Ginger extract modulates Pb-induced hepatic oxidative stress and expression of antioxidant gene transcripts in rat liver. *Pharm Biol* 16:1–9.

Muthuirulappan, S. Sridhar, R. 2013. Trend on traditional system of medicine and modern Ethnopharmacology-Perspective view. *Int J Res Pharm Sci* 4: 7–11.

Nam, H. Kim, M.M. 2013. Eugenol with antioxidant activity inhibits MMP-9 related to metastasis in human fibrosarcoma cells. *Food Chem Toxicol* 55: 106–112.

Ng, K. B. Bustamam, A. Sukari, M. A. et al. 2013. Induction of selective cytotoxicity and apoptosis in human T4-lymphoblastoid cell line (CEMss) by boesenbergin a isolated from boesenbergia rotunda rhizomes involves mitochondrial pathway, activation of caspase 3 and G2/M phase cell cycle arrest. *BMC Complement Altern Med* 13: 41.

Ni, X. Suhail, M. M. Yang, Q. et al. 2012. Frankincense essential oil prepared from hydrodistillation of Boswellia sacra gum resins induces human pancreatic cancer cell death in cultures and in a xenograft murine model. *BMC Complement Altern Med* 12: 253.

Pangjit, K. Tantiphaipunwong, P. Sajjapong, W. et al. 2014. Iron-chelating, free radical scavenging and antiproliferative activities of Azadirachta indica. *J Med Assoc Thai* 97: Suppl 4, S36–S43.

Poojari, R. 2014. Embelin – a drug of antiquity: shifting the paradigm towards modern medicine. *Expert Opin Investig Drugs* 23: 427–444.

Pu, L. P. Chen, H. P. Cao, M. A. et al. 2013. The antiangiogenic activity of Kushecarpin D, a novel flavonoid isolated from Sophora flavescens Ait. *Life Sci* 93: 791–797.

Purwar, B. Shrivastava, A. Arora, N. et al. 2012. Effects of curcumin on the gastric emptying of albino rats. *Indian J Physiol Pharmacol* 56: 168–173.

Ramamoorthy, A. Janardhanan, S. Jeevakarunyam, S. et al. 2015. Integrative oncology in Indian subcontinent: an overview. *J Clin Diagn Res* 9: XE01–XE03.

Ramaswamy, S. Kuppuswamy, G. Dwarampudi, P. et al. 2014. Development and validation of simultaneous estimation method for curcumin and piperine by RP-UFLC. *Pak J Pharm Sci* 27: 901–906.

Ramkumar, K.M. Manjula, C. Elango, B. et al. 2013. In vitro cytotoxicity of Gymnema montanum in human leukaemia HL-60 cells; induction of apoptosis by mitochondrial membrane potential collapse. *Cell Prolif* 46: 263–271.

Russell, L.H. Jr. Mazzio, E. Badisa, R.B. et al. 2011. Differential cytotoxicity of triphala and its phenolic constituent gallic acid on human prostate cancer LNCap and normal cells. *Anticancer Res* 31: 3739–3745.

Sambasivampillai, T.V. 1998. Dictionary based on Indian medicinal science. Directorate of Indian Medicine and Homeopathy, Chennai, India.

Sanches-Silva, A. Costa, D. Albuquerque, T.G. et al. 2014. Trends in the use of natural antioxidants in active food packaging: a review. *Food Addit Contam Part A Chem Anal Control Expo Risk Assess* 31: 374–395.

Sandhya, T. Mishra, K.P. 2006. Cytotoxic response of breast cancer cell lines, MCF 7 and T 47 D to triphala and its modification by antioxidants. *Cancer Lett* 238: 304–313.

Saraswathy, A. Devi, S.N. Pradeep Chandran, R.V. 2009. Analgesic and antiinflammatory activity of Amukkarac curanam. *Indian J Pharm Sci* 71: 442–445.

Shanmugavelu, M. 1987. *Siddha Maruthuva Noi Nadal Noi Mudal Naadal, Part I*, Tamil Nadu Siddha Medical Board, Chennai.

Singh, V. Pal, M. Gupta, S. et al. 2013. Turmeric – A new treatment option for lichen planus: a pilot study. *Natl J Maxillofac Surg* 4: 198–201.

Srinivasan, S. Kumar, R. Koduru, S. et al. 2010. Inhibiting TNF-mediated signaling: a novel therapeutic paradigm for androgen independent prostate cancer. *Apoptosis* 15(2): 153–161.

Srinivasan, M. Rajendren, S. 2012. Current concepts in herbal medicine research. *Int J Mod Biol Med* 2(1): 46–51.

Tan, X. Jin, P. Feng, L. et al. 2014. Protective effect of luteolin on cigarette smoke extract-induced cellular toxicity and apoptosis in normal human bronchial epithelial cells via the Nrf2 pathway. *Oncol Rep* 31: 1855–1862.

Tan, Y.F. Li, H.L. Lai, W.Y. 2013. Crude dietary polysaccharide fraction isolated from jackfruit enhances immune system activity in mice. *J Med Food* 16: 663–668.

Tezcan, G. Tunca, B. Bekar, A. et al. 2015. Ficus carica latex prevents invasion through induction of let-7d expression in GBM cell lines. *Cell Mol Neurobiol* 35: 175–187.

Thavamani, B.S. Mathew, M. Dhanabal, S.P. 2013. In vitro cytotoxic activity of menispermaceae plants against HeLa cell line. *Anc Sci Life* 33: 81–84.

Vaishnavi, K. Saxena, N. Shah, N. et al. 2012. Differential activities of the two closely related withanolides, Withaferin A and Withanone: bioinformatics and experimental evidences. *PLoS.One* 7: e44419.

Vattem, D.A. Lester, C. Deleon, R. et al.2013. Dietary supplementation with two Lamiaceae herbs (oregano and sage) modulates innate immunity parameters in Lumbricus terrestris. *Pharmacognosy Res* 5: 1–9.

Vijaya, P.V. Arul Diana, C.S. Ramkuma, K.M. 2007. Induction of apoptosis by ginger in HEp-2 cell line is mediated by reactive oxygen species. *Basic Clin Pharmacol Toxicol* 100: 302–307.

Wadhwa, R. Singh, R. Gao, R. et al. 2013. Water extract of Ashwagandha leaves has anticancer activity: identification of an active component and its mechanism of action. *PLoS One* 8: e77189.

WHO Traditional Medicine Strategy. (2002–2005). WHO/EDM/TRM/2002.1 Original: English, Distribution: Geneva, pp. 1–53.

Wilasrusmee, C. Kittur, S. Siddiqui, J. et al. 2002. In vitro immunomodulatory effects of ten commonly used herbs on murine lymphocytes. *J Altern Complement Med* 8: 467–475.

Wu, K. M., Ghantous, H., and Birnkrant, D. B. 2008. Current regulatory toxicology perspectives on the development of herbal medicines to prescription drug products in the United States. *Food Chem Toxicol* 46: 2606–2610.

Xu, L. Qi, Y. Lv, L. et al. 2014. In vitro anti-proliferative effects of Zuojinwan on eight kinds of human cancer cell lines. *Cytotechnology* 66: 37–50.

Xu, T. Li, D. Jiang, D. 2012. Targeting cell signaling and apoptotic pathways by luteolin: cardioprotective role in rat cardiomyocytes following ischemia/reperfusion. *Nutrients* 4: 2008–2019.

CHAPTER 15

Homeopathic Medicine for Prostate Health

Hakima Amri and Christopher Funes

CONTENTS

15.1 INTRODUCTION

Homeopathy has been in practice since its establishment in the late 1800s and patients around the world have used homeopathic remedies since then, primarily in Europe, and a number of countries in southeast Asia (India and Sri Lanka). While homeopathy gained acceptance and recognition in the United States more than a century ago, the American Medical Association's (AMA) opposition to its teachings and practice accelerated its demise. Despite this opposition from allopathic physicians, an increasing trend of its use in the United States has been noted (D'Huyvetter and Cohrssen, 2002; Merrell and Shalts, 2002). Antagonism was consistent and harsh, and claims were made that homeopathy was no more than a pseudoscience, thus forcing homeopaths to either assimilate or to stop practicing medicine and treating patients. Unfortunately, the antagonism is still ongoing. Homeopathic institutions were either forced to join allopathic institutions or simply close down

(Jonas et al., 2003). However, allopaths and homeopaths have adopted practices from one another – homeopaths adopted conventional treatments such as diphtheria antitoxin, while allopaths borrowed homeopathic remedies, such as the use of nitroglycerin in the treatment of cardiovascular pathology. It is estimated that homeopathic physicians use conventional medications in a quarter of the patients they consult (Jonas et al., 2003). Despite scrutiny from physicians and scientists, this medical system has seen an unprecedented growth in the number of patient users globally in recent years.

In the United States alone, 1 in 3 patients have used integrative, complementary, and alternative medicine (ICAM) practices at some time, with 3.4% of those patients using homeopathy (D'Huyvetter and Cohrssen, 2002). A survey by the Centers for Disease Control (CDC) in 2007 found that 4 in 10 adults and 1 in 9 children used at least one ICAM therapy in the past year. Patients who seek homeopathic consultations tend to be more affluent, more frequently white, and be younger than patients seen by conventional physicians (Jonas et al., 2003). Sixty-eight percent of family practice physicians demonstrated interest in learning more about homeopathy, and there is evidence of increasing patient demand for high-quality research and availability of ICAM treatment options (Merrell and Shalts, 2002). Since homeopathic consultations are rarely covered by insurance, all of the expenditure from the consumer is out of pocket, reaching nearly $200 million per year in early 2000 (D'Huyvetter and Cohrssen, 2002). This amount increased to $3.1 billion, as reported by Nahin et al. (2009) and Barnes et al. (2008). The tenets of homeopathy are not well understood, yet patients using homeopathic remedies are increasing in numbers and in demographic range (Merrell and Shalts, 2002).

15.2 BASIC PRINCIPLES AND TENETS

In homeopathic medicine, symptoms of a person do not equate to the disease; rather they are thought of as the adaptation of the body to the stress caused by the disease. The main tenet of homeopathy is therefore to shift the body's energy, or *vital force*, back toward homeostatic balance (D'Huyvetter and Cohrssen, 2002; Merrell and Shalts, 2002). Restoring homeostatic balance is achieved by introducing substances that stimulate auto-regulatory and self-healing processes (Jonas et al., 2003). This vitalistic theory of health and illness is based on the self-healing and self-recovery potential of the individual and emphasizes a close connection between mind and body. Illness therefore is a result of an imbalance in one of the many vital forces within every individual (Merrell and Shalts, 2002). When considering what homeopathic remedy to prescribe, homeopaths take into consideration the "Totality of Symptoms" and "Constitutions" (D'Huyvetter and Cohrssen, 2002; Merrell and Shalts, 2002). Organs and organ systems are not thought to respond individually to disease; the manifestation of symptoms is viewed in terms of the whole organism. A person is thought of as a constellation of symptoms that represent the best way the individual's integrative system can deal with a particular event at a particular time (Merrell and Shalts, 2002). A person's "constitution" includes moral and intellectual character, habits, relationships, likes and dislikes, what makes that person feel better or worse, and even the time of day and side of the body that the symptoms first appeared (D'Huyvetter and Cohrssen, 2002). In essence, all the biological, psychological, and social determinants of health are taken into consideration when matching the individual's symptoms to a homeopathic remedy.

The first principle of homeopathy is *similia similibus curentur*, the Law of Similars. According to this principle, a substance that produces symptoms of a disease in a healthy person will cure the same symptoms in an ailing person (D'Huyvetter and Cohrssen, 2002). In 1796, Samuel Hahnemann formulated this concept when he self-administered *Cinchona* bark (the source of quinine) and found that he developed symptoms characteristic of malaria. The astringent taste of *Cinchona* bark was reported in the *Materia Medica* as the reason to treat malaria. This argument was far from convincing to Hahnemann, since other astringent and bitter plants do not treat malaria. So, he experimented on himself and took *Cinchona* bark, which triggered similar symptoms to malaria except for the fever; the symptoms disappeared when he stopped and reappeared as soon as he started taking it again. From this, he postulated that *Cinchona* could therefore be used to treat malaria (Merrell and Shalts, 2002).

The second principle of homeopathy, the Law of Infinitesimal Doses (ultra-high dilution and potentization), postulates that potentization allows for the energy of a substance to remain in a solution even when no molecule of the original substance is present (Merrell and Shalts, 2002). The process of potentization consists of a series of dilutions and succussions, and it is believed that the process extracts the "vital" or "spirit-like" nature of the substance so that even highly diluted substances can retain biological and therapeutic activity (Merrell and Shalts, 2002; Jonas et al., 2003). With the new developments in the fields of quantum physics, digital biology, and bioenergy, the mechanism(s) of homeopathy could be illustrated using new concepts of physics (Schulte and Endler, 2015; Smith, 2015; Thomas, 2015).

The homeopathic *Materia Medica* is the original collection of medical works by Samuel Hahnemann and currently holds within it the detailed recordings of over 2000 substances and the reactions that these substances produce in healthy volunteers. It serves as a system of remedy selections that homeopaths use as a guide to prescribe (D'Huyvetter and Cohrssen, 2002; Merrell and Shalts, 2002; Dantas et al., 2007). Provings, or homeopathic pathogenic trials (HPTs), involve the administration of a nontoxic dose of a substance to a healthy volunteer so that the homeopath or prover can meticulously record the effects that the substance produces. When the correct remedy is found, it can potentially cause worsening of symptoms if the remedy is not strong enough to provoke aggravation of the symptoms, or too weak to bring about a cure (D'Huyvetter and Cohrssen, 2002; Merrell and Shalts, 2002; Dantas et al., 2007).

Once the correct remedy has been found for the ailing individual, the remedy must be prepared. Remedies can be prescribed as an acute treatment of a single symptom or condition that is short acting, or as a constitutional treatment in which the patient is treated as a whole and includes mental, emotional, and physical manifestations of the condition (D'Huyvetter and Cohrssen, 2002). Typical homeopathic remedies are prepared from plants, animals, and minerals and come in various forms, including but not limited to herbal assortments, tinctures, ointments, and capsules. The substance or its extracts are placed in a solvent, typically water or ethanol, resulting in a mother tincture that then undergoes potentization. Dilutions are generally prepared in C (centesimal, or 1:100) or X (decimal, or 1:10) potencies following a series of dilutions and succussions (potentization); the substance is typically diluted below Avogadro's number of particles. It is therefore unlikely that any particle of the original substance exists in the final preparation (D'Huyvetter and Cohrssen, 2002).

One single homeopathic remedy may have different effects on different individuals. Unlike conventional medicine, homeopathic remedies are tailored to the individual; two patients with the same clinical condition may receive two different remedies based on the unique characterization of symptoms and the mental and environmental states of the particular individual (D'Huyvetter and Cohrssen, 2002; Merrell and Shalts, 2002). In a recent study, 44 out of 48 homeopaths recommended different remedies for the same clinical case. Very little data has examined the consistency of homeopaths when making clinical decisions, and no studies have yet explored the role of intuition in the actual process of making remedy decisions in homeopathy (Brien et al., 2004).

Homeopathy has been used historically in the treatment of numerous ailments, the top ten being asthma, depression, otitis media, allergic rhinitis, headache/migraine, neurotic disorders, allergy, dermatitis, arthritis, and hypertension (Jonas et al., 2003). For some conditions, such as allergies, evidence is positive and supports the clinical efficacy of homeopathic remedies. One study found that the homeopathy treatment group had a trend toward greater reduction in bronchial reactivity with an increase in histamine resistance, as well as an overall improvement in nasal airflow (Taylor et al., 2000). Moreover, it was found that a homeopathic gel is as effective and well tolerated as the conventional nonsteroidal anti-inflammatory drug-based gel used as a topical treatment of osteoarthritis, with slightly more benefits found in the homeopathy group compared to placebo (Taylor et al., 2000; Haselen and Fisher, 2000). On the other hand, research on ailments such as headaches and migraines, while positive, has largely been attributed to bias and likely due to no more than a placebo effect (Straumsheim et al., 2000).

15.3   SAFETY AND EFFICACY OF HOMEOPATHIC MEDICINE

In controlled clinical trials, the adverse effects associated with homeopathic remedies occur more frequently when compared to the adverse effects in a placebo group, suggesting some degree of pharmacological activity of the homeopathic remedy. However, the effects tended to be minor and transient, and ultimately resulted in best treatment outcomes compared to the placebo group (D'Huyvetter and Cohrssen, 2002; Paterson, 2002). It is unlikely for homeopathic remedies to provoke severe adverse reactions when prescribed by a trained homeopath. Surprisingly, although high dilutions are equated to placebo, direct adverse effects have been reported (Posadzki et al., 2012). The most common side effects observed were headaches, tiredness, skin eruptions, dizziness, bowel dysfunctions, and symptom aggravation (D'Huyvetter and Cohrssen, 2002). Homeopathic remedies cause far less and fewer adverse effects than conventional drugs, largely due to the ultra-low concentration of the active ingredient, yet such a comparison may be misleading. The absolute risk of the intervention itself may not be great, but it is the risk-benefit balance that should determine the risk of any medical treatment. The most prominent risk currently is the use of homeopathic remedies in place of conventional treatments, which could prolong treatment or aggravate the ailment (Posadzki et al., 2012). Recently, the Food and Drug Administration (FDA) has been looking into revisiting the regulatory framework of homeopathy in the United States. Since homeopathic remedies generally use ultra-diluted doses, almost all authorities assume that homeopathy is safe and should have no interactions with conventional drugs (Jonas et al., 2003). Regulation of homeopathic substances has existed since the creation of the FDA. It has since then labeled homeopathic remedies as drugs, based on the official Homeopathic Pharmacopoeia of the United States (Merrell and Shalts, 2002).

Despite being regarded as generally safe and nontoxic, the efficacy of homeopathic remedies is still under question and debate. Since the mechanism by which homeopathic remedies show effect seems impossible in the current zeitgeist, many leading authorities and scientists have assumed it is a nonspecific placebo effect (Shang et al., 2005). The first meta-analyses to suggest that the clinical effects of homeopathy are not completely due to placebo stated that there was insufficient evidence from the existing studies to suggest it is efficacious for any single condition, but that the effects of homeopathic remedies are superior to that of the placebo effect (Linda et al., 1997). However, a more recent analysis of large trials of higher quality resulted in no convincing evidence that homeopathy was superior to the placebo, whereas in conventional medicine the significant effect remained over the placebo. Therefore, the clinical effects of homeopathy, but not those of conventional medicine, were found to be unspecific placebo or context effects (Shang et al., 2005). This last study in particular generated a long debate in the scientific community that pointed to the bias in the study design that favored conventional medicine.

15.4   PROPOSED MECHANISM OF ACTION OF HOMEOPATHIC REMEDIES

At present, there is no convincing explanation of the mechanism by which homeopathic drugs affect biological systems (Merrell and Shalts, 2002). However, there are numerous proposed mechanisms that attempt to explain homeopathy and its major principles, the most prominent being the "Water Memory Effect" theory. When the homeopathic substance is in a solution, it forms clathrates, which are bonds between water molecules and surrounding molecules that behave like a crystal compound. The formation and subsequent growth of these clathrate compounds is achieved by succussion in the potentization process, which mimics the oscillatory nature of crystal growth. Physicochemical properties of water can be modified by a solute and remain that way for a certain period of time, even in the absence of the solute itself (D'Huyvetter and Cohrssen, 2002; Vallance, 1998).

Current evidence suggests that apoptotic genes (bax, blc-2, bcl-x, capsase-1, caspase-2, and caspase-3) are not modulated by homeopathic medicines in cancer cell lines. In a different separate study, lymphocytes treated with homeopathic remedies did not have a significant increase in chromosomal aberrations amongst other genotoxic effects (Seligmann et al., 2003; Thangapazham et al., 2006). These findings suggest that homeopathic remedies are unlikely to affect cancer by alterations in gene expression.

On several occasions, homeopaths have paralleled numerous homeopathic principles to allopathic observations. Drugs and other substances, for example, may induce the symptoms they are trying to relieve, but they can also have the opposite effect than expected. Some proponents of homeopathy also suggest that the pre-exposure to low reagent concentrations may modulate the response to subsequent exposures. A significant number of animal model studies were conducted in the 1970s and 1980s and confirmed the latter observation (Bildet et al., 1978; Cambar et al., 1983). Still, allopaths do not regard these examples as convincing or accurate (Merrell and Shalts, 2002).

Overall, the methodological quality of most research papers is inadequate. Evidence is positive to a large extent, but higher quality studies are needed to increase the strength of findings (D'Huyvetter and Cohrssen, 2002). Although some evidence suggests homeopathic treatments are more effective than placebo, the level of this evidence is low because of low methodological quality. It was found that trials of low methodological quality are a major source of bias (Shang et al., 2005). Moreover, it was found that more rigorous trials are associated with smaller effect sizes, which, in turn, render the overall effect less significant. The more rigorous trials tend to yield less optimistic results than trials with fewer precautions against bias. Confirmatory and independent replications are lacking (Shang et al., 2005; Linde et al., 1999; Linde and Melchart, 1998).

Despite the seemingly implausible mechanism of action remaining unclear, evidence exists that supports the use of diluted homeopathic remedies. These findings contradict the current laws of physics and chemistry since a tincture diluted beyond Avogadro's number most likely does not contain a single molecule of active substance. Despite contemporary physics and chemistry, it was found that ultra-high dilutions of mercuric chloride had significant inhibitory and stimulatory effects of the activity of diastase, an enzyme important in the digestion of starch (Vallance, 1998). Further, a different study found increases in coronary flow could be achieved by the infusion of ultra-high dilution of ovalbumin, the findings of which have been reproduced successfully (Vallance, 1998). Moreover, several ultra-high dilution studies found that *Arsenicum album* and *Kali iodide* inhibited spore germination of *Alternaria alternaria*, whereas other remedies were ineffective (Vallance, 1998). It is important to note that studies involving plants and animals could offer plausible insights into the association of homeopathy with placebo. Despite the shortcomings in the quality of these research studies, the trials provide a large number of positive results (Vallance, 1998).

15.5 CHALLENGES TO RESEARCH IN HOMEOPATHY

One of the central tenets of homeopathy is the use of individualized remedies in the treatment of clinical conditions. Patients with the same diagnosis are each treated with different homeopathic remedies based on their characteristic symptoms (Jonas et al., 2003). Thus, it is difficult to study the effects of homeopathic remedies since only one remedy is used for the symptoms of diagnostic criteria in current research models, yet it does not hold true to the actual nature of homeopathic practice and treatment approach. Clinical trials use a standardized homeopathic treatment in all patients, which is not ideal since it is not true to the practice of homeopathy (Merrell and Shalts, 2002). Clinical research is complicated when the experimental sample is selected according to conventional criteria but the therapy is based on homeopathic criteria (Jonas et al., 2003). Another complication arises through numerous methodological problems, including lack of objective or validated outcome measures, sample size, and bias (Merrell and Shalts, 2002). Even in placebo-controlled trials, bias is found in the conducting and reporting of trials, which can possibly explain the positive findings (Shang et al., 2005). Even the best systematic reviews cannot distinguish between components of bias that may exist, but they cannot rule out the true effects since they may be obscured by the heterogeneous nature of the population sample. In essence, it is nearly impossible to draw definitive conclusions (Jonas et al., 2003).

15.6 HOMEOPATHY IN CANCER CARE

During the last 20 years, an increase in use of CAM for neoplastic diseases, mainly cancer, has been observed. Nearly 1 in 3 cancer patients use a CAM practice in conjunction with their conventional treatment (Montfort, 2000). In most of Europe, homeopathic remedies are given with, if not before, conventional treatment options. In fact, 30% of all referrals made to the Homeopathic Hospitals in the United Kingdom are directly from oncologists (Thompson and Kassab, 2000). However, to this day, no published evidence exists for the use of homeopathy as a complementary treatment to conventional therapies for potentially curable cancers. As a palliative or supportive treatment, homeopathy is used mainly to strengthen the body in its fight against cancer, to improve general well-being, and to alleviate pain resulting from disease or the side effects of conventional treatments (Milazzo et al., 2006). Evidence suggests that certain homeopathic remedies may contain anticancer properties and may be beneficial in the treatment of cancer symptoms and treatment-related side effects, yet there is no support that homeopathy can cure any type of cancer (Paterson, 2002).

15.7 HOMEOPATHIC REMEDIES FOR PROSTATE HEALTH AND PATHOLOGY

15.7.1 Saw Palmetto

PC-SPES, an herbal combination used in traditional Chinese medicine, contains extracts from eight different herbs and has been available commercially since 1996, but was later removed from the market following controversies over the quality of the herbal mixture preparation (Taille et al., 2000; Ikezoe et al., 2001). Although it is not typically prescribed as a homeopathic remedy, some of the herbal components have been studied as homeopathic dilutions. The top homeopathic remedies used in research of prostate health and pathology are *Conium maculatum*, saw palmetto, *Thuja occidentalis*, and curcumin (Jonas et al., 2006). Saw palmetto, also known as *Serenoa repens* or *Sabal serrulata*, is most commonly used for prostate health and benign pathologies. In numerous trials this phyotherapeutic agent has been demonstrated to be beneficial in the treatment of prostate cancer, and moreover it has a specificity to prostate cancer, a characteristic lacking in conventional cancer therapies such as chemotherapy and radiation therapy (MacLaughlin et al., 2006).

Research on the effects of saw palmetto on prostate cancer cell lines at different doses demonstrated a reduced proliferation in a temporal and dose-dependent manner. It should be noted that not all of these studies focused on the use of ultra-low concentrations typical of homeopathic dilutions. The inhibitory action on cell proliferation was exclusive to the three prostate cancer cell lines observed (LNCaP, PC-3, and DU 145), with no effect observed on breast cancer cell lines, suggesting a specificity of saw palmetto for prostate cancer cell lines, *in vitro* (MacLaughlin et al., 2006; Kubota et al., 2000; Yang et al., 2007). Further, saw palmetto increased the percentage of cells in the G0-G1 phase of the cell cycle in PC-3 and LNCaP cell lines, and increased the percentage of cells in the G2-M phase in the DU 145 cell lines (Kubota et al., 2000). Throughout all cancer cell line cultures used, the percentage of cells in the S phase decreased in a statistically significant manner. Histological analysis of the tumors grown *in vivo* in mice models revealed that the tumors treated with saw palmetto had significant necrosis and fibrosis as well as cytological changes associated with apoptotic events (Kubota et al., 2000). Saw palmetto appears be effective in part via the regulation of the cell cycle. When compared to the control group, a two-fold increase in level of p53, a protein important in cell cycle checkpoints, was observed. Other important proteins, such as p21, were also increased significantly, while levels of p27 were not modulated (Yang et al., 2007). Saw palmetto was also observed to downregulate the level of prostate-specific antigen (PSA), a biomarker commonly used in the diagnosis of prostate health. Further, androgen receptor (AR) was downregulated by 80%. AR is important in prostate cancer because it binds to 5alpha-dihydrotestosterone (DHT), a hormone associated with prostate functioning (Yang et al., 2007). Saw palmetto appears to block DHT. In LNCaP prostate cancer cells, DHT-induced elevated PSA levels decreased by 70% after treatment with the herbal extract. Furthermore, it was found that saw palmetto blocks IL-6 induced levels of PSA by 88%, and does so by blocking the phosphorylation of STAT-3 (Yang et al., 2007). The growth and weight of prostate cancer tumors, as well as the volume of tumors, were significantly decreased in the treatment group of mice compared to the control group (Figures 15.1 and 15.2). MacLaughlin et al. (2006) reported that the volume and weight of prostate tumors were reduced in mice treated with saw palmetto while no significant change was

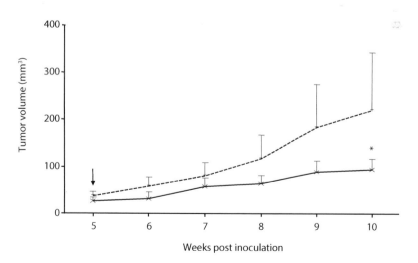

Figure 15.1 Inhibitory effect of homeopathic dilution (200C) of saw palmetto (*Sabal serrulata*) on the tumor growth in nude mice inoculated with human prostate cancer cells (PC-3). Mice were treated for five weeks and followed for five additional weeks. The arrow marks the administration of the last treatment. At ten weeks, the tumor size was significantly reduced in the treated mice (solid line) in comparison to the untreated animals (dashed line) (ANOVA, p<0.05). Graph adapted from MacLaughlin et al. 2006.

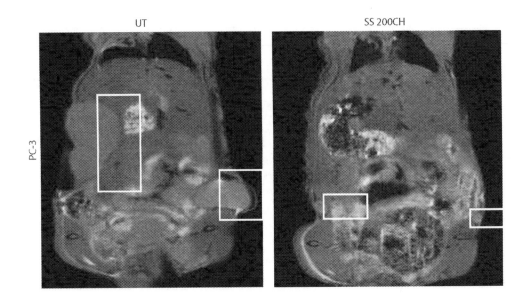

Figure 15.2   Representative MRI imaging of mice treated with homeopathic dilution (200C) of saw palmetto (*Sabal serrulata*) on the tumor growth in nude mice inoculated with human prostate cancer cells (PC-3), as described in Figure 15.1. UT: untreated; SS 200CH: *Sabal serrulata* 200CH following the Hahnemannian dilution process; the white rectangle delineates the tumor in the abdominal area of the mouse.

noted on breast cancer tumors, as shown by manual measurements and MRI. There were significant marked fibrosis and inflammatory cells in the tumors of mice receiving saw palmetto. Interestingly, the organs from mice treated with saw palmetto did not show any changes compared with the controls, again suggesting the affinity of saw palmetto for prostate cells (Yang et al., 2007).

Saw palmetto is also the most commonly used herbal compound in the treatment of men with voiding symptoms secondary to benign prostatic hyperplasia (BPH) (Gerber et al., 1998). This study found no significant improvements in mean peak urinary flow rate, post-void residual urine volume, or bladder pressure for 6 months following treatment with saw palmetto. However, there were significant improvements in lower urinary tract symptoms, an overall of 50% in 6 months following the treatment (Gerber et al., 1998). A separate study found that the changes in prostate size, residual volume after voiding, the BPH impact index, serum PSA, creatinine, and testosterone levels did not differ significantly between treatment groups and control groups, and the conclusion was made that saw palmetto is not superior to the placebo for improving urinary symptoms and objective measures of BPH. More recent research suggested that there was no evidence for the effects of saw palmetto over the placebo in the improvement of patients with BPH (Bent et al., 2006). Although research exists on *Thuja occidentalis* and *Conium macalutum*, evidence is scarce and inconsistent. When tested *in vitro* and in the mouse model, these homeopathic remedies did not show any effects on prostate cancer cell lines' proliferation or tumor growth (MacLaughlin et al., 2006).

15.7.2   The Canova Method

The Canova Method, a complex homeopathic remedy produced mostly in Brazil, acts mainly by increasing the immune response through the activation of macrophages and is at times indicated in the treatment of cancer, as well as other diseases that suppress the immune system such as AIDS

(Seligmann et al., 2003). This homeopathic remedy is produced as drops, inhalants, and intravenous forms. The final product contains an intricate mixture of *Aconitum napellus*, *Bryonia alba*, *Thuja occidentalis*, *Arsenicum album*, and *Lachesis muta* in 1% ethanol and distilled water (Sato et al., 2005). One study in sarcoma 180–bearing mice found significant tumor regression in the treatment group compared to the control group, indicative of the remedy's anticancer properties. The proposed mechanism of action postulates that Canova acts as an immune modulator. The argument as to whether or not a homeopathic remedy can influence immune cells has long been debated. Davenas and colleagues found that the degranulation of human basophils could be achieved when the basophils are exposed to a very dilute anti-IgE antibody serum and are marked with the release of histamine (Davenas et al., 1988). These findings were scrutinized when subsequent studies were unsuccessful in replication of the findings (Hirst et al., 1993). However, more recent investigations have found that basophil degranulation is indeed modulated by homeopathic histamine administration (Lorenz et al., 2003). A delay was observed in the development of tumors as well as a reduction in size. Secondary to the effects on the cancer cells, there was increased infiltration of lymphoid cells, an increase in granulation tissue formation, and fibrosis in the area around the tumor (Sato et al., 2005).

15.7.3 Traumeel S

Traumeel S is a homeopathic preparation containing arnica, calendula, millefolium, chamomilla, symphytum, belladonna, aconitum, *Bellis perennis*, hypericum, *Echinacea angustifolia*, *Echinacea purpurea*, hamamelis, Mercurius solubilis, and Hepar sulfuris (Milazzo et al., 2006). One study investigated the effects of Traumeel S on the development of stomatitis, a general inflammatory damage of mucous membranes in patients receiving chemotherapy; 33% of patients in the Traumeel S treatment group did not develop stomatitis compared to only 7% in the control group. Moreover, of those that did develop stomatitis in either group, only 47% of the patients in the Traumeel S treatment group experienced worsened stomatitis compared to 93% of the placebo group (Oberbaum et al., 2001). The symptoms were more severe in the placebo group compared to the Traumeel S treatment group. Reaction index for radiotherapy-related side effects was lower in both intervention groups compared to placebo, although no significant differences were observed in tumor reduction (Milazzo et al., 2006). In another study, a non-significant trend favoring belladonna treatment during radiotherapy was found, while a significant benefit in recovery period for those receiving homeopathic treatment was observed. However, the study was weakened by the use of non-validated scales of measures for radio-dermatitis, such as skin color, warmth, swelling, and pigmentation (Paterson, 2002).

15.7.4 Carcinogens

A more controversial use of homeopathic remedies is based upon the homeopathic principle, the Law of Similars. According to this principle, an introduction of carcinogenic/mutagenic compounds in low doses should be therapeutically beneficial in the treatment of cancer. In essence, a carcinogen is introduced in the body with the intention of treating cancer (Montfort, 2000). A three-patient clinical case study provided evidence that suggests the property of carcinogenic compounds could increase p53 protein levels, which are capable of stopping replication of damaged DNA in cancer cells. Further, in small doses, the carcinogenic compounds are capable of inducing incomplete differentiation, apoptosis, and degradation of oncogenic proteins. One example is the modulation of hepatic alkyltransferase that was achieved in animals by a hepatic carcinogen, suggesting that its homeopathic doses promote DNA repair (Montfort, 2000). However, the use of carcinogens to treat cancer is anecdotal evidence and requires further investigation.

15.8   CASE REPORTS

While visiting Sri Lanka, the author (HA) had the opportunity to discuss several case reports dealing with a variety of prostate problems at a homeopathic clinic in Colombo. The late physician in charge, D.V.K., MD, DTH, MB, DCH, MFH, had pursued studies in conventional medicine and theoretical homeopathy in the United States as well as clinical homeopathy and homeopathic pharmacy in England and Germany, respectively. The case reports ranged from early-stage BPH to malignant cancer, and had been successfully treated. We are well aware of the lack of statistical data regarding the incidence of the disease, the treatment's success rate, as well as follow-up information addressing the duration of remission and the incidence of relapse. The lack of financial support in this field is one of the main reasons for these limitations in epidemiological and clinical studies.

15.8.1   Case Report 1: Prostate Hypertrophy

Mr. J, 60 years of age, complained of urinary retention, frequency, urgency, and severe stress incontinence. He also reported dimness of vision when reading and redness of eyes with occasional tearing. Iritis is an associated symptom of prostate enlargement. The patient was given saw palmetto 12C once a day until complete recovery.

15.8.2   Case Report 2: Prostate Hypertrophy with a Benign Mass

Mr. K, 50 years of age, complained of despondency, irritability, severe tenesmus, pain at the bladder neck, persistent urinary incontinence, constipation, and coldness of external genitals extending to the abdomen. Rectal examination revealed a mass of 4.5 cm in diameter. Saw palmetto 6X was prescribed three times a day for 6 weeks, leading to a decrease in urinary frequency as well as resolution of pain and urinary incontinence. The patient was also given Hepar sulphuricum 30C, one dose at bedtime, to prevent urinary sepsis. Saw palmetto 30C was continued, once a day, until complete resolution of all symptoms.

15.8.3   Case Report 3: Prostate Hypertrophy with a Malignant Tumor

Mr. M, 45 years old, suffered from gradually worsening micturition, tenesmus, and hematuria for 2½ years. Hematuria was accompanied by intense burning and pain located over the perianal area, with the patient being unable to sit in the same position for any length of time. The patient's abdomen was distended and he experienced low-grade temperatures as well as bilateral lower extremity edema in the evenings. The patient also reported lack of appetite and appeared anemic. Rectal examination revealed the presence of a hard mass. CT scan and further work-up confirmed the presence of a malignant tumor. Due to the seriousness of the condition, saw palmetto was started at 3X and administered every 4 hours in conjunction with Thuja 200C, every 6 hours times 3 days every 6 days. Thuja was prescribed to alleviate symptoms other than prostate-related problems. By the time he completed the course of Thuja, the patient had experienced rapid improvement of these symptoms. His temperature had normalized and he denied any abdominal distension or lower extremity edema. He reported good appetite and normal bowel movements. Urinary frequency was reduced but continued. Saw palmetto was changed to 30C twice a day for 6 weeks, at which point the urinary frequency had completely resolved and the patient reported normal flow and denied any pain. Saw palmetto 30C was reduced to one dose a day. Rectal examination at this point revealed no palpable masses and follow-up CT scan was negative. The patient was advised to continue saw palmetto 30C every other day for 3 more months in the absence of symptoms.

These case reports clearly indicate a potential role for Saw palmetto in prostate cancer therapy.

REFERENCES

Barnes, P.M. Bloom, B. Nahin, R.L. 2008. Complementary and alternative medicine use among adults and children: United States, 2007. *Natl Health Stat Report* 12: 1–23.

Bent, S. Kane, C. Shinohara, K. et al. 2006. Saw palmetto for benign prostatic hyperplasia. *N Engl J Med* 354(6): 557–566.

Bildet, J. Saurel, M. Aubin, M. et al. 1978. Etude de l'action de divers complexes sure l'hepatite experimentale au tetrachlorure de carbone. *Ann Homeo Fr* 4: 277–286.

Brien, S. Prescott, P. Owen, D. et al. 2004. How do homeopaths make decisions? An exploratory study of inter-rater reliability and intuition in the decision making process. *Homeopathy* 93: 125–131.

Cambar, J. Demouliere, A. Cal, J.C. et al. 1983. Mise en evidence de l'effet protecteur de dilutions homeopathiques de mercurius corrosivus vis-a-vis de la mortalite au chlorure mercurique chez la souris. *Ann Homeo Fr* 5: 6–12.

Dantas, F. Fisher, P. Walach, H. et al. 2007. A systematic review of the quality of homeopathic pathogenetic trials published from 1945 to 1955. *Homeopathy* 96: 4–16.

Davenas, E. Beauvais, F. Amara, J. et al. 1988. Human basophil degranulation triggered by dilute antiserum against IgE. *Nature* 333: 816–818.

D'Huyvetter, K. Cohrssen, A. 2002. Homeopathy. *Primary Care* 29: 407–418.

Gerber, G. Zagaja, G. Bales, G. et al. 1998. Saw palmetto (serenoa repens) in men with lower urinary tract symptoms: effects of urodynamic parameters and voiding symptoms. *Urology* 51(6): 1003–1007.

Haselen, R. Fisher, P. 2000. A randomized controlled trial comparing topical piroxicam gel with a homeopathic gel in osteoarthritis of the knee. *Rheumatology* 39(7): 714–719.

Hirst, S. Hayes, N. Burridge, J. Pearce, F. Foreman, J. 1993. Human basophil degranulation is not triggered by very dilute antiserum against human IgE. *Nature* 366: 525–527.

Ikezoe, T. Chen, S. Heber, D. et al. 2001. Baicalin is a major component of pc-spes which inhibits the proliferation of human cancer cells via apoptosis and cell cycle arrest. *Prostate* 49: 285–292.

Jonas, W. Kaptchuk, T. Linda, K. 2003. A critical overview of homeopathy. *Ann Intern Med* 138: 393–399.

Jonas, W. Gaddipati, J. Rajeshkumar, N. et al. 2006. Can homeopathic treatment slow prostate cancer growth? *Integr Cancer Ther* 5: 343–349.

Kubota, T. Hisatake, J. Hisatake, Y. et al. 2000. Pc-spes: a unique inhibitor of proliferation of prostate cancer cells in vitro and in vivo. *Prostate* 42: 163–171.

Linda, K. Clausius, N. Ramirez, G. et al. 1997. Are the clinical effects of homeopathy placebo effects? A meta-analysis of placebo-controlled trials. *Lancet* 350: 834–843.

Linde, K. Scholz, M. Ramirez, G. et al. 1999. Impact of study quality on outcome in placebo-controlled trials of homeopathy. *J Clin Epidemiol* 52(7): 631–636.

Linde, K. Melchart, D. 1998. Randomized controlled trials of individualized homeopathy: a state-of-the-art review. *J Altern Complement Med* 4(4) 371–388.

Lorenz, I. Schneider, E. Stolz, P. et al. 2003. Sensitive flow cytometric method to test basophil activation influences by homeopathic histamine dilutions. *Forsch Komplementarmed Klass Naturheilkd* 10(6): 316–324.

MacLaughlin, B. Gutsmuths, B. Pretner, E. et al. 2006. Effects of homeopathic preparations on human prostate cancer growth in cellular and animal models. *Integr Cancer Ther* 5(4): 362–372.

Merrell, W. Shalts, E. 2002. Homeopathy. *Med Clin North Am* 86(1): 47–62.

Milazzo, S. Russell, N. Ernst, E. 2006. Efficacy of homeopathic therapy in cancer treatment. *Eur. J Cancer* 42: 282–289.

Montfort, H. 2000. A new homeopathic approach to neoplastic diseases: from cell destruction to carcinogen-induced apoptosis. *Br Homeopath J* 89: 78–83.

Nahin, RL. Barnes, PM. Stussman, BJ. et al. 2009. Costs of complementary and alternative medicine (CAM) and frequency of visits to CAM practitioners: United States, 2007. *Natl. Health Stat Report* 18: 1–14.

Oberbaum, M. Yaniv, I. Ben-Gal, Y. et al. 2001. A randomized, controlled clinical trial of the homeopathic medication TRAUMEEL S in the treatment of chemotherapy-induced stomatitis in children undergoing stem cell transplantation. *Cancer* 92(3): 684–690.

Paterson, I. 2002. Homeopathy: what is it and is it of value in the care of patients with cancer. *Clini Oncol* 14: 250–253.

Posadzki, P. Alotaibi, A. Ernst, E. 2012. Adverse effects of homeopathy: a systematic review of published case reports and case series. *Int J Clin Pract* 66(12): 1178–1188.

Sato, D. Wal, R. Oliveira, C. et al. 2005. Histopathological and immunophenotyping studies on normal and sarcoma 180-bearing mice treated with a complex homeopathic medication. *Homeopathy* 94: 26–32.

Schulte, J. and Endler, PC. 2015. Update on preliminary elements of a theory of ultra high dilutions. *Homeopathy* 104 (4): 337–342.

Seligmann, I. Lima, P. Cardoso, P. et al. 2003. The anticancer homeopathic composite "canova method" is not genotoxic for human lymphocytes in vitro. *Genet Mol Res* 2(2): 223–228.

Shang, A. Huwiler-Muntener, K. Nartey, L. et al. 2005. Are the clinical effects of homeopathy placebo effects? Comparative study of placebo-controlled trials of homeopathy and allopathy. *Lancet* 366: 726–732.

Smith, CW. 2015. Electromagnetic and magnetic vector potential bio-information and water. *Homeopathy* 104 (4): 301–304.

Straumsheim, P. Borchgrevink, C. Mowinckel, P. et al. 2000. Homeopathic treatment of migraine: A double blind, placebo controlled trial of 68 patients. *Br Homeopath J* 89(1): 4–7.

Taille, A. Buttyan, R. Hayek, O. et al. 2000. Herbal therapy pc-spes: in vitro effects and evaluation of its efficacy in 69 patients with prostate cancer. *J Urol* 164: 1229–1234.

Taylor, M. Reilly, D. Llewellyn-Jones, R. et al. 2000. Randomized controlled trial of homeopathy versus pacebo in perennial allergic rhinitis with overview of four trial series. *BMJ* 321(7259): 471–476.

Thangapazham, R. Rajeshkumar, N. Sharma, A. et al. 2006. Effect of homeopathic treatment on gene expression in copenhagen rat tumor tissues. *Integr Cancer Ther* 5: 350–355.

Thomas, Y. 2015. From high dilutions to digital biology: the physical nature of the biological signal. *Homeopathy* 104(4): 295–300.

Thompson, E. Kassab, S. 2000. Homeopathy in cancer care. *Br Homeopath J* 89: 61–62.

Vallance, A. 1998. Can biological activity be maintained at ultra-high dilution? An overview of homeopathy, evidence, and Bayesian philosophy. *J Altern Complement Med* 1: 49–76.

Yang, Y. Ikezoe, T. Zheng, Z. et al. 2007. Saw palmetto induces growth arrest and apoptosis of androgen-dependent prostate cancer LNCaP cells via inactivation of STAT 3 and androgen receptor signaling. *Int J Oncol* 31: 593–600.

CHAPTER 16

Yoga, Naturopathy, Acupuncture, and Prostate Cancer Therapy

Athira Thampy

CONTENTS

16.1 ACUPRESSURE AND ACUPUNCTURE IN PROSTATE CANCER TREATMENT

Prostate cancer is becoming the most common cancer among men; studies predict an alarming 230,000 new prostate cancer diagnosis in United States alone (Torre et al., 2015).

16.1.1 What Is Acupressure and Acupuncture?

Acupressure and acupuncture are medical procedures that help to reduce pain and restore health. They can be used for positive promotion of health. In acupressure, the thumb and palms are used to deliver treatment. In acupuncture, the same points will be stimulated by the application of needles. Prostate cancer chemotherapy can damage the nervous system. Rather than choosing to have a new set of painkillers, a qualified medical practitioner in the field of acupressure and acupuncture can help to reduce pain.

Acupressure and acupuncture are parts of the traditional Chinese system of healing. They have a significant place in alternative medicine. References about acupuncture have been written in Chinese history. Acupuncture can be traced back 2000 years, at the time when metals had not been invented, and pointed stones were used for performing acupuncture. With the invention of metals, gold and silver were introduced as acupuncture needles. Later, stainless steel needles were invented. *The Yellow Emperors Classic of Internal Medicine* is the oldest acupuncture book available. Color therapy, magneto therapy, massage therapy, acupressure, hydrotherapy, acupuncture, and yoga together make up naturopathy medicine.

16.1.2   The Concept of Acupuncture

The human body has various channels that conduct bioelectricity. These channels are called meridians. The meridians have many pressure points, or acupuncture points. Needles are applied to these pressure points. The size, thickness, and method of application of needles vary from individual to individual. The length of the needle can vary from 0.5 tsun to 8 tsun.

Acupuncture is the therapeutic method in medical science that utilizes needle stimulation. Every act of the universe is said to be brought about by *Qi*, or life force, which functions by bipolarity. In Indian philosophy it is known as prana. It is the invisible force responsible for all the movements of life.

During needling, the subjective effects are felt by the patient alone and they cannot be scientifically explained. Some of the needling points recommended are

UB-23:   This is the point in deficiency conditions; it also alarms the kidney points such that this point helps to regularize the body system

UB-28:   This is an alarm point for urinary bladder and is commonly used for urinary complications

CV-3,4: These points are very useful for genitourinary disorders

ST-28:   This point is essential in removing toxins from the body

All these points can improve or get rid of the above ailments, and they can also help to rejuvenate the body by bringing the universal energy flow into balance. When the apt acupressure point is pricked, the patient feels a numb or cold sensation.

The needles can be applied to the points for 20 to 25 minutes. Acupuncture can be done daily or on alternate days. Single-course duration can vary from 7 to 10 days. There should be a gap of 15 minutes between each course.

Acupuncture points are applied along channels or meridians. There are 14 channels, 12 of which are pairs.

1. Lung meridian
2. Large intestine meridian
3. Stomach meridian
4. Spleen meridian
5. Heart meridian
6. Small intestine meridian
7. Urinary bladder meridian
8. Kidney meridian
9. Pericardium meridian
10. Triple warmer meridian
11. Gallbladder meridian
12. Liver meridian

The above 12 meridians are bilateral. The conception vessel meridian and the governing vessel meridian are the other two non-paired meridians. The conception vessel meridian or ren channel is to be used for urinary tract and genital organ diseases.

16.1.3 Comparison of Acupressure and Acupuncture

Acupressure has almost the same effect as that of acupuncture, and fear of needles can be avoided. In reality, needles used in acupuncture do not cause much pain, but if a person is worried or anxious about using needles, then acupressure will be the best choice. The only difficulty a medical practitioner can face here is to apply pressure only on exact points. Because needles are very thin, only the special points along the meridian get stimulated. Fingernails should never be used for acupressure; only the thumb and palms should be used, with appropriate pressure.

Acupuncture is also used for treatment of hot flashes, which is a common adverse effect of hormonal therapy for prostate cancer. In one study, 25 patients were recruited with hot flash score (HFS) >4 in the study. A qualified professional provided the service, twice each week for the first 4 weeks and once per week for an additional 6 weeks. Twelve of the patients had over 55% reduction in HFS, thus providing a significant effect of acupuncture. Another study involving 17 patients with hot flashes and androgen ablation therapy showed 80.3% improvement after 8 months (where mean of HFS was decreased from 37.409 to 7.385) (Beer et al., 2010; Ashamalla et al., 2011).

16.2   CHROMOTHERAPY

Chromotherapy is the only treatment that is focused on the color therapies. Color therapy is dependent on the relationship between humans and the universe. Each color of the universe has its own meaning, and is a marvelous gift to humans.

Color therapy has the ability to control the human mind and body. Color can influence the appetite. If you want to reduce your weight, try to have your food in a purple colored plate. Color therapy discovers and treats the deficiencies in the human body. How can one find out which color is needed? In general, we can point out colors according to the disease condition, but an expert naturopath can take a patient through color meditation and find appropriate colors for that individual.

In general, yellow is the color that is mostly suggested for prostate diseases. This powerful and awesome color helps to stimulate the nerves and also helps to remove morbid matters from the body by its action. While the major color suggested for a prostate disease patient is yellow, other colors can be added according to a patient's needs. If the patient is suffering from insomnia, then a blue light can be used in his bedroom if blue-colored walls and curtains might not be possible. Then we can put a blue-colored shawl or towel on a chair and have him try to look at it for some time. If the patient suffers from pain and headache, then relaxing in a garden and looking at trees (green color) will give a lot of relief.

This chromotherapy helps us to be healthy and also helps with the deficiencies of the body. This brings us towards healthy life by regaining all the positive energies.

16.3   PROSTATE DISEASES AND NATUROPATHIC INTERVENTION

16.3.1 Hydrotherapy (Water) Treatments

Water treatments are well known for their healing effects. They are miraculous healers for hormonal issues, constipation, gastric issues, insomnia, and aches and pains. The desired results are brought about by using different water treatments. The temperature used for each treatment varies. Naturopathy and hydrotherapy work well when customized. A generalized plan might give minimal results, but when a physician creates a better healing environment for the patient by analyzing the patient's progress and healing signs, the results will be far better. Hydrotherapy when combined with other naturopathy treatments can root out diseases.

16.3.2 Hydrotherapy Treatments for Prostate Disease

1. Sitz bath: A sitz bath is a warm bath that cleanses the perineum, which is the space between the rectum and the scrotum. You can take the bath in your bathtub or using a plastic kit that fits over your toilet. If you are taking it in your bathtub, then fill the tub with 3½ to 4 inches of warm water. The temperature should be comfortable; it should not cause burns or discomfort.

   The kit is simply a round, shallow basin that often comes with a plastic bag. The bag has long tubes on the end and the bag can be filled through these tubes. The basin is larger than a standard toilet bowl, allowing it to be easily and securely placed underneath the toilet seat. This makes you feel comfortably seated while taking the sitz bath. The kit is available in pharmacies.

   A sitz bath is a soothing treatment for pain and/or itching in the genital area.
   * A doctor's prescription is not needed
   * It is very easy to do
   * Relieves itching, irritation
   * Soothes pain
   * Increases blood flow to the external genital areas, promoting better and faster healing
   * No side effects; the only problems that could occur are if the plastic bags or tubs are not properly cleaned

   Note: Do not do these baths if you have acute bacterial prostatitis.

2. Hip bath: A contrast hip bath is an effective remedy for enlarged prostate.
   * Hot baths will help to reduce swelling and promote healing. In addition, it relaxes the pelvic muscles.
   * Cool baths help to reduce pain.

   Fill one tub with warm water and three tablespoons of Epsom salts. Fill another tub with cold water and 3 drops of lavender essential oil. First, sit in the hot tub for 5 minutes, and next sit in cold tub for 2 minutes. Repeat this two to three or more times.

3. Hot foot immersion bath: Fill a tub with warm water and immerse your feet in it. The water should be about 2½ inches above the ankle joints. This will help with sleep, is beneficial for stress management, and enhances the healing phase of disease.

4. T wet pack: T packs come under the general category of hydrotherapy, water therapy. Naturopathy evolved as a system of medicine through hydrotherapy. Wet packs are given to patients by folding cloths in desired measurements; as the name denotes, they are immersed in water then wrung out so excess water is removed. We can make the packs cold, hot or lukewarm, all according to the temperature of water we use. This T pack is more like the Indian langotti. Folding a lengthy piece of cloth horizontally, it can be fashioned in such a way that it can be worn like a belt. As a belt, you can tie it around your waist and take another piece of cloth and wear it like a langot (loincloth); that is, tuck in one end at the front of the belt and take it towards your back and tuck in the other end at the back of the belt. At naturopathy clinics, you can get these cloths dipped in medicated water and sun dried, and those cloths can be used for tying T wet packs.

   And medicated water is used in the same way as untreated water in these baths.

16.4   PROSTATE DISEASES AND YOGIC MANAGEMENT

Yoga is not an ancient myth buried in oblivion. It is the most valuable inheritance of the present. It is the essential need of today and the culture of tomorrow.

Swami Satyananda Saraswati

Yoga is the ancient science of healing that cuts across age, caste, religion, and sex. It is a powerful tool in managing chronic prostatitis and chronic pelvic pain syndrome.

How yoga acts in your body:

1. Increases blood flow
2. Increases immunity
3. Lowers stress
4. Helps to build strength
5. Enhances flexibility
6. Improves sleep
7. Helps with pain management (the most important part of yoga's effect)

Recently, a Canadian study reported the possible benefits of yoga in prostate cancer patients. The study duration was 14 weeks (7-week class-based yoga program [adherence phase], followed by 7 weeks of self-selected physical activity [maintenance phase]). Results indicated that yoga is one of the feasible physical activity options for cancer patients. No adverse effects were found. Yoga was also found to decrease stress and fatigue (Ross Zahavich et al., 2013).

The beneficial effects of yoga in prostate cancer patients while they are undergoing external beam radiation therapy were also studied. Yoga practice twice weekly was helpful in reducing cancer-related fatigue. The international prostate symptom score sheet (IPSS) was used to determine the severity of urinary symptoms and it was found that IPSS scores were increased during yoga treatment (Ben-Josef et al. 2015).

Yoga was developed by ancient sages and seers; the healing art has its roots in Indian culture. Now this healing tool is not limited to sages, and it had been modified to meet the needs of today.

REFERENCES

Ashamalla, H. Jiang, M.L. Guirguis, A. et al. 2011. Acupuncture for the alleviation of hot flashes in men treated with androgen ablation therapy. *Int J Radiat Oncol Biol Phys* 79(5): 1358–1363.

Beer, T.M. Benavides, M. Emmons, S.L. et al. 2010. Acupuncture for hot flashes in patients with prostate cancer. *Urology* 76(5): 1182–1188.

Ben-Josef, A.M. Wileyto, E.P. Chen, J. et al. 2015. Yoga intervention for patients with prostate cancer undergoing external beam radiation therapy: a pilot feasibility study. *Integr Cancer Ther* 2015 Nov 20. [Epub ahead of print]

Ross Zahavich, A.N. Robinson, J.A. Paskevich, D. et al. 2013. Examining a therapeutic yoga program for prostate cancer survivors. *Integr Cancer Ther* 12(2): 113–125.

Torre, L.A. Bray, F. Siegel, R.L. et al. 2015. Global cancer statistics, 2012. *CA: Cancer J Clin* 65 (2): 87–108.

Index

Printed in the United States
by Baker & Taylor Publisher Services